THE IMPACT OF TELEMEDICINE ON HEALTH CARE MANAGEMENT

Studies in Health Technology and Informatics

Editors

Volume 64

Earlier published in this series

Vol. 31. The SEISMED Consortium, Data Security for Health Care I, Management Guidelines
Vol. 32. The SEISMED Consortium, Data Security for Health Care II, Technical Guidelines
Vol. 33. The SEISMED Consortium, Data Security for Health Care III, User Guidelines
Vol. 34. J. Brender, J.P. Christensen, J.-R. Scherrer and P. McNair (Eds.), Medical Informatics Europe '96
Vol. 35. M. Di Rienzo, G. Mancia, G. Parati, A. Pedotti and A. Zanchetti (Eds.), Frontiers of Blood Pressure and Heart Rate Analysis
Vol. 36. M. Sosa-ludicissa, N. Oliveri, C.A. Gamboa and J. Roberts (Eds.), Internet, Telematics and Health
Vol. 37. J.A. Sevastik and K.M. Diab (Eds.), Research into Spinal Deformities 1
Vol. 38. R.A. Mortensen (Ed.), ICNP in Europe: TELENURSE
Vol. 39. K.S. Morgan, H.M. Hoffman, D. Stredney and S.J. Weghorst (Eds.), Medicine Meets Virtual Reality
Vol. 40. G. Lowet, P. Rüegsegger, H. Weinans and A. Meunier (Eds.), Bone Research in Biomechanics
Vol. 41. J. Mantas (Ed.), Health Telematics Education
Vol. 42. J. Brender, Methodology for Assessment of Medical IT-Based Systems
Vol. 43. C. Pappas, N. Maglaveras and J.-R. Scherrer (Eds.), Medical Informatics Europe '97
Vol. 44. G. Riva (Ed.), Virtual Reality in Neuro-Psycho-Physiology
Vol. 45. J. Dudeck, B. Blobel, W. Lordieck and T. Bürkle (Eds.), New Technologies in Hospital Information Systems
Vol. 46. U. Gerdin, M. Tallberg and P. Wainwright (Eds.), Nursing Informatics
Vol. 47. W. Ceusters, P. Spyns, G. De Moor and W. Martin (Eds.), Syntactic-Semantic Tagging of Medical Texts: The Multi-TALE Project
Vol. 48. J. Graafmans, V. Taipale and N. Charness (Eds.), Gerontechnology
Vol. 49. L. van den Broek and A.J. Sikkel (Eds.), Health Cards '97
Vol. 50. J.D. Westwood, H.M. Hoffman, D. Stredney and S.J. Weghorst (Eds.), Medicine Meets Virtual Reality
Vol. 51. J. Mantas (Ed.), Advances in Health Telematics Education
Vol. 52. B. Cesnik, A.T. McCray and J.-R. Scherrer (Eds.), MedInfo '98
Vol. 53. M.C. Sievert, D.E. Moxley, N.J. Ogg and T.B. Patrick, Thesaurus of Health Informatics
Vol. 54. O. Ferrer-Roca and M. Sosa-Iudicissa (Eds.), Handbook of Telemedicine
Vol. 55. H.M.J. Goldschmidt, M.J.T. Cox, R.J.E. Grouls, W.A.J.H. van de Laar and G.G. van Merode, Reference Information Model for Clinical Laboratories
Vol. 56. I. Iakovidis, S. Maglavera and A. Trakatellis (Eds.), User Acceptance of Health Telematics Applications
Vol. 57. In production
Vol. 58. G. Riva, B.K. Wiederhold and E. Molinari (Eds.), Virtual Environments in Clinical Psychology and Neuroscience
Vol. 59. I.A.F. Stokes (Ed.), Research into Spinal Deformities 2
Vol. 60. In production
Vol. 61. R.A. Mortensen (Ed.), ICNP® and Telematic Applications for Nurses in Europe
Vol. 62. J.D. Westwood, H.M. Hoffman, R.A. Robb and D. Stredney (Eds.), Medicine Meets Virtual Reality
Vol. 63. R. Rogers and J. Reardon, Recommendations for International Action

ISSN: 0926-9630

The Impact of Telemedicine on Health Care Management

Edited by

M. Nerlich
Department of Trauma Surgery, University of Regensburg Medical Centre, Regensburg, Germany

and

R. Kretschmer
Centre for Health Care Quality, University of Missouri – Columbia, Columbia, MO, USA

IOS Press
OHM Ohmsha

Amsterdam • Berlin • Oxford • Tokyo • Washington, DC

ISBN 90 5199 484 2 (IOS Press)
ISBN 4 274 90292 7 C3047 (Ohmsha)

Publisher
IOS Press
Van Diemenstraat 94
1013 CN Amsterdam
Netherlands
fax: +31 20 620 3419
e-mail: order@iospress.nl

Distributor in the UK and Ireland
IOS Press/Lavis Marketing
73 Lime Walk
Headington
Oxford OX3 7AD
England
fax: +44 1865 75 0079

Distributor in the USA and Canada
IOS Press, Inc.
5795-G Burke Centre Parkway
Burke, VA 22015
USA
fax: +1 703 323 3668
e-mail: iosbooks@iospress.com

Distributor in Germany
IOS Press
Spandauer Strasse 2
D-10178 Berlin
Germany
fax: +49 30 242 3113

Distributor in Japan
Ohmsha, Ltd.
3-1 Kanda Nishiki-cho
Chiyoda-ku, Tokyo 101
Japan
fax: +81 3 3233 2426

PRINTED IN THE NETHERLANDS

Contents

Oncology

Cardiology

Endocrinology

Ophthalmology

Dermatology

Pathology

Radiology

Family Practice and Home Care/Home Monitoring

Psychiatry

Introduction

Editorial

It has been a great honor and pleasure to host the world's telemedicine trendsetters in the course of the GHAP SP4 meeting, "The Impact of Telemedicine on Health Care Management", held November 21-23, 1998 in Regensburg, Germany. In numerous impressive presentations covering almost the entire spectrum of medical specialties, it was clearly demonstrated that telemedicine has the potential to significantly alter structures, procedures, and eventually outcomes in health care systems worldwide.

Today the field of telemedicine is still dominated by very committed efforts of research and development. However, there are a growing number of concepts and applications which have been implemented in clinical routine or are ready to be used in it. Health care providers, patients, third party payers, and not least policymakers should be informed about these rapidly emerging applications, which could have a considerable impact on the delivery of health care.

To offer a comprehensive source of information not only for the experts but also for the target groups mentioned above, we decided to develop a summary of the Regensburg meeting.

Contents of the proceedings therefore are:

- an outline of the Global Health Care Applications Project (GHAP) and its subprojects which represent the research and development framework of the G7/8 countries and other nations;
- background information on legal aspects, issues concerning further development, and evaluation of telemedical applications;
- presentations of numerous projects covering the clinical fields of emergency medicine, surgery, oncology, cardiology, endocrinology, ophthalmology, dermatology, radiology, pathology, psychiatry and other clinical specialties;

and, recognizing the Internet as a major source of information on issues related to telemedicine and information technology in general,

- a "Webliography" providing links to a selection of the most relevant Web sites on the Internet.

The Editors

Prof. Michael Nerlich

Dr. Rainer Kretschmer

Acknowledgements

We have enjoyed the opportunity to work closely with numerous recognized experts who contributed actively to the Regensburg meeting and to the compilation of these proceedings. Thank you!

We would like to thank all members of the Regensburg Program Committee for their exemplary commitment in the preparations of the Regensburg meeting. Special thanks to our local team members, who helped tremendously in organizing the conference.

The conference and these proceedings would not have been possible without the generous support of some organizations, especially:

- the German Federal Ministry of Health,
- the DLR "Deutsches Zentrum für Luft- und Raumfahrt e.V", Köln and
- Roche Diagnostics.

Special thanks for their splendid help in compiling these proceedings to:

- Patrick Asbach, Trauma Surgery, University of Regensburg, for carefully revising the layout of the manuscripts;
- Melanie Johnson-Moxley and David Moxley, Health Management & Informatics, University of Missouri – Columbia, USA, for compiling the Webliography and the trouble they took with the linguistic and grammatical check of the non-native English-speakers' manuscripts; and
- Dr. Ekkehard Hundt and Mr. Ron Jansen at IOS Press for their exemplary cooperation in the realization of this book.

The Editors

The Impact of Telemedicine on Health Care Management

Opening remarks by the German Federal Minister for Health, Andrea Fischer

at the G 8 Global Health Care Applications Project (GHAP) Conference in Regensburg on 21st November 1998

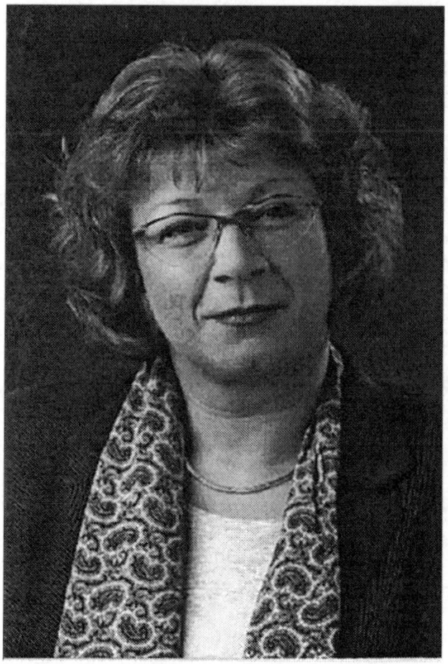

Visions describe an objective, strategies the route to attaining it. What was nothing more than a vision just twenty years ago has, in the meantime, become a matter of course. In the interval, millions of people have come to utilise the possibilities afforded by modern information technologies. In the health care system, too, the use of telecommunication and information technologies is increasingly becoming everyday routine.

Against this background, allow me to make an appeal to the developers of telematic applications: I am aware of the fact that, for them, the overriding criterium in identifying the solution to a problem is technological feasibility. However, I ask you to keep in mind that the solutions you suggest can only be actually applied in the day-to-day provision of care, if they are also workable in medical practice and conducive to public health purposes.

Since it is our aim to have patients derive tangible benefits from the application of health telematics, we may not limit ourselves to island solutions. This goes for both the national and the international level and it is also the reason why I attach great importance to the G8 Health Project.

The possibilities and developments inherent in telematics raise a number of questions we have to address. These include: the details of making the infrastructure and framework conditions available, data protection considerations, organisational and legal issues and others relating to the national economy and financing. This congress provides an excellent forum for discussing possible solutions on the basis of international experience. As a consequence, I am particularly pleased that it is being hosted by Germany and would like to extend a cordial welcome to all of the participants from the 19 countries represented here.

International cooperation can serve to further the development process in the individual Member States. The G 8 Sub-project 6, which deals with harmonising the use of data cards in the health care system, is a fine example of this. In Germany, health care providers will be meeting, in a joint action forum on telematics in health care, to prepare a telematics platform designed to effectively combine island solutions. The Federal Ministry for Health will support these efforts as far as possible. In order to ensure coordination with the Federal Laender, cooperation between the Federal and Laender governments has already been initiated.

I am happy to see that you have also chosen an approach based on international and interdisciplinary cooperation for the benefit of patients and their care in the future. These efforts must continue to be encouraged and supported, monitored and observed and, following the completion of your pilot projects in the course of the coming year, the resulting solutions will need to be examined to determine their transferability. At this point, I would like to thank all of those participating in the project for the great input they have made so far under difficult conditions and wish them every success in their future work.

Andrea Fischer

Federal Minister for Health, Germany

The G8-Global Health Care Applications Project (GHAP) and its Role for the Development of National Telemedicine Activities

Gottfried T.W. DIETZEL
G 8 - Health Project Co-ordinator for Germany, Federal Ministry for Health, Bonn (Project-Group for Health Telematics)

At the summit in Naples in July 1994, G7 leaders emphasized the necessity of encouraging the development of a world-wide information society. Ministers responsible for promoting the development of the information society met in Brussels in February 1995 and identified 11 pilot projects where international co-operation could be an asset. Results will be reported in the upcoming G8-summit in Cologne in June 1999:

- Global Inventory Project (led by the European Commission and Japan)
- Global Interoperability of Broadband Networks (Canada and Japan)
- Trans-cultural Education and training (Tel*Lingua) (France and Germany)
- Electronic Libraries (Bibliotheca Universalis) (France and Japan)
- Multimedia Access to World Cultural Heritage (Italy and France)
- Environment and Natural Resources Management (USA)
- Global Emergency Management (Gemini) (Canada)
- Global Healthcare Applications (GHAP - European Commission)
- Government On-Line (UK)
- Global Marketplace for SMEs (European Commission, Japan, USA)
- Maritime Information Society (MARIS) (European Commission, Canada)

The key objectives for these **G7 Global Information Society Pilot Projects** were to

- create an opportunity for information exchange leading towards the further development of the information society,
- identify and select projects of an exemplary nature having tangible and clearly understandable social, economic and cultural benefits which will demonstrate to the public the potential of the information society,
- identify obstacles to the implementation of practical applications serving the creation of a global information society,
- establish the basis for productive forms of co-operation among G7 partners.

The pilot projects should avoid creating new bureaucracies or institutions, and should be financed by existing programmes.

The **Global Healthcare Applications Project** aims at improving quality and cost efficiency of healthcare delivery through telematic tools. It comprises 10 sub-projects:

1. Towards a global public health network (completed)

This sub-project focussed on the design of an international data exchange on vital statistics and Communicable Disease surveillance. WHO will take this initiative forward, in co-operation with the EU's European Antimicrobial Resistance Surveillance System and the US-EU Task Force on communicable diseases.

2. Improving prevention, early detection, diagnosis and treatment of cancer

International co-operation is promoted through an international network of reference cancer centres, accessible through telematic networks. Implementation of a pilot network of centres is underway. Standards have been agreed by major user groups. Demonstrators have been developed for: remote consultation of pathologists and remote-controlled microscopy for diagnosis on frozen sections in real time during surgery; Internet use for continuing medical education; second opinion over distance, and planning of treatment in radiotherapy.

3. Improving prevention, diagnosis and treatment of major cardiovascular diseases

This sub-project concentrates on the development of common standard clinical databases for improving the cost/benefit ratio by integrating patient care data and health economics analysis in to a „shared stratified system of care". Work includes integration of Intranet databases with health cards. The project has produced a multimedia working model demonstrator for such a system of care. Validation has started in Italy.

4. International concerted action on collaboration in telemedicine

This sub-project encourages information exchange on the use of telemedicine. Links have been established to the EU Teleplans project. The International Multipoint Project of Advanced Communications in Telehealth is a limited-scale pilot-project. As a key project of importance for horizontal questions the project under Canadian guidance has found special attention and is organising widely recognised Forum-conferences concentrating on specific issues of telemedicine today, such as standards or cost/benefit relationships.

5. Enabling mechanisms for a global healthcare network including Internet connectivity

A web site and closed discussion group are being set up, with information and expert views on barriers to achieving a global information society in the health field. The final report (early 1999) will focus on legal, security and codification issues. For Internet connectivity, results include information about routing, the number of connecting points, and the variation of time needed to reach the destination.

6. International harmonisation of the use of data cards in healthcare

Architecture and software have been developed according to general specifications, allowing interoperability between technical platforms used world-wide. A pilot-project has been prepared and interoperability between EC data cards and Japanese health cards has been demonstrated. Coherent implementation of health networks, patient data cards and health professional cards will be attempted.

7. Evidence and effectiveness

This sub-project is developing: a register of randomised controlled trials; criteria for costs, risks and benefits of data capture for research and management; on-line access to best medical knowledge accessible to clinicians and the public: and a virtual institute of evidence of effectiveness. Work on a protocol for stroke management involves 24 hospitals and five countries.

8. Multilingual anatomical digital database

This sub-project is producing multi-lingual anatomical labels for the US National Library of Medicine's Unified Medical Language System project and the future Visible Human Data Base.

9. Medical image reference centre

The objectives are to support clinical activities, contribute to medical education and training and facilitate medical research. The reference centre includes clinical and pathological images (still and moving) for cancer and cardiovascular diseases (including typical, rare and difficult to diagnose cases), and access to image databases via Internet. Data collection mechanisms, on-line publishing, organisation (including regional co-ordination centres) etc. have been proposed. A technical group will ensure interoperability with other image databases.

10. Special Interactive TV & MultiMedia Programmes for Professionals and Public in Dentistry and International On-line Academy for Dentistry and Oral Medicine

This new sub-project **SIPP/IOA** - using telematic tools to support education and training in dentistry by creating an International On-line Academy - started 1998 and aims - together with major telecommunication providers and institutions responsible for education in dentistry - at developing a complete system of computer assisted and on-line available education material.

What are the special features of these international co-operation efforts in comparison to the many events of exchange of experiences via international conferences which are organised these days dealing with the global information society in healthcare and with the key words of Health-Telematics and Telemedicine? What are the differences if you only share and discuss the results of your research in a conference or if you are already co-operating

internationally in the process of retrieving new knowledge? Is it possible to overcome national barriers and international competition and to develop new ideas in a joint co-operation effort without the fear of plagiarism?
The G 7 Health Project started with 6 sub-projects focussed around key medical questions of our time. The member states are now including Russia and the recently added tenth project SIPP/IOA already has had a link to Russia from the very beginning. The key questions of the G 7 Ministers to be answered suggested that an early exchange of ideas and information can speed up and contribute to the development of a common information society.

- The projects should serve as an example and should demonstrate a real social and health benefit.
- Nevertheless obstacles related to the implementation of practical applications should be identified.
- Common knowledge should be broadened.

Were these goals achieved? Beyond the contents of the individual sub-projects I will try to condense the experiences of the past years. Success does not just come from a stimulated international co-operation. There are individual success-stories. Success depended on

- the existence of a powerful presenter who would serve as a successful co-operator
- already existing international co-operative networks (especially the cardio-people were used to international co-operation before the G 7 projects started, public health representatives to a minor degree).
- The more mere feasibility considerations are put into practice the more decisive the cultural context and the already existing familiarity with the use of computers proved to be.
- And broad implementation is only possible if the resources needed are available.

Especially the G 7 project is not only a story of success. There was not always a convincing presenter available, and especially the sub-projects 4 and 5 are describing and defining the institutional obstacles in the way to the information society in healthcare.

There are obvious common areas where the sub-projects were hit by these obstacles

- unsolved legal issues of responsible tele-advice and patient data protection
- needed classifications and coding standards
- availability of computer-trained personnel.

The more a sub-project dealt with implementation and with everyday routine the more decisive the national environment turned out to be. Technology is international but its implementation - this was especially shown by the 'evidence-based medicine' sub-project 7 - cannot be separated from the specific financial, organisational and legal national framework. In this way the G 8 projects have not only contributed to the search for internationally valid solutions to nationally urgent questions, but have - especially while pursuing the same goals - also drawn the attention to the need for an individual national implementation strategy. Our key questions - as found out by sub-project 4 and 5 - are very similar. But they have apparently been tackled by an implementation policy which takes into account the specific organisation of health care which is different from country to country. Through the experiences of the G 8 project we are able to anticipate which questions can be solved by international agreement (as achieved in sub-project 6 dealing with the standardisation of health professional cards) and which questions are in need to be decided by accompanying national institutions which are familiar with the specific implementation conditions of their countries.

Technology is global, and we have joint problems, and especially the following applications require stronger attention in the future, benefiting at the same time from internationally shared experiences and exchange of knowledge:

- The integrated electronic patient record
- Standardisation to assure interoperability between nationally organised applications
- Electronic prescription
- Use of cards for patients and health professionals.

It would be a waste of efforts if we were to discuss these applications only from a national perspective. Thus, for example, sub-project 3 combined Italian clinical approaches in the field of cardiovascular diseases with health promotion efforts in Canada.

What is also happening suddenly in all our countries through the joint commitment to the G 8 sub-projects: we are experiencing convergence in the development of telematic and telemedicine implementation strategies in our Member States. We are attracting the attention of our Health Ministers to the important contribution which comes from the use of modern communication technology.

This discussion of implementation strategies is not only challenging the governments but is also a social action involving health authorities, physicians' associations, leading also to private actions of healthcare providers, finally changing the medical culture of our countries. Therefore I do not only appreciate the official establishment of an "Action-Forum for Telematics in Healthcare" for Germany which will create an internationally interoperable platform for health-telematics but I also appreciate the user-oriented activities organising the demands of our customers as expressed in the "Initiative Health-Telematics in Germany" (Initiative Gesundheitstelematik in Deutschland), which had its inauguration in 1998.

All these activities will be successful only if they do not only lead to the use of more technology but to intelligent and user-friendly applications which allow a better and more comprehensive treatment of our patients. Information society technologies are only successful and will only be financed if the underlying vision of the information society is citizen- and patient-oriented, and therefore accepted by this constituency of our healthcare delivery systems.

Address for correspondence

Gottfried T.W. Dietzel
G 8 - Health Project Co-ordinator for Germany
(Project-Group for Health Telematics)
Federal Ministry for Health
Am Propsthof 78
D-53121 Bonn, Germany
Tel.+49 228 941-1850, Fax +49 228 941-4913
E-mail: dietzel@bmg.bund400.de

M. Nerlich and R. Kretschmer (Eds.)
IOS Press, 1999

International Concerted Action on Collaboration in Telemedicine: G8 sub-project 4

André LACROIX
Canadian representative and chair, G8 SP-4
Professor of Medicine, Telemedicine Unit, Research Centre, Centre Hospitalier de l'Université de Montréal (CHUM)
Montréal, Québec, Canada

Abstract: The main objective of G-7/8 Global Healthcare Applications sub-project 4 is to enable an international concerted action on collaboration in telemedicine. To promote and facilitate the implementation of telemedicine or health telematics networks around the world, it was felt necessary to solve certain key issues. Five thematic solution-seeking FORUMS are each addressing a specific item. The first FORUM held in Montréal, Canada on May 28-30 1998 focussed on Interoperability of telemedicine and telehealth systems. Other FORUMS address other themes such as: Impacts of Telemedicine on health care management (Regensburg, Germany, November 21-23 1998); Evaluation and Cost Effectiveness of Telemedicine (Melbourne, Australia, February 19-20 1999); Clinical and technical quality and standards (Washington, USA, April 29-30 1999); Medico-legal aspects of national and international applications (Oxford, UK, fall 1999).

The main objective of these *FORUMS* is to arrive at best practices through consultation amongst experts who seek together the best solutions to facilitate global international telemedicine networks.

Towards this goal, G-8 sub-project-4 will also conduct the IMPACT (International Multipoint Project of Advanced Communication in Telemedicine) feasibility study which will aim at conducting multipoint exchanges between telemedicine units in the academic centers of the participating G-8 and other countries. More detailed information on this project and summaries of the initial FORUMS are found on our Web site at www.g7sp4.org.

1. Introduction

The ministers responsible for the promotion of the development of a global information society in G7 countries met in Brussels in February 1995 and selected eleven pilot projects of international collaboration. Amongst those, the one on Global Healthcare Applications Projects (GHAP) set the objective to improve quality and cost-efficiency of healthcare delivery through the use of telematics tools. Within GHAP, six sub-projects were approved initially and have now been extended to a total of ten sub-projects. The GHAP sub-project 4 (SP-4) was focussed initially on the use of telemedicine tools in the area of emergency medicine.

2. Initial phase of GHAP SP-4

The Global Emergency Telemedicine Service (GETS) was originally one of the projects of the European Union's Fourth Framework Program and was led by Professor Louis Lareng from the European Institute of Telemedicine in Toulouse, France. The objective was to establish a trans-national and multilingual emergency system to improve the promptness and effectiveness of interventions and services through telemedicine connections. An expanded form of this project became one of the 6 initial GHAP sub-projects with the objective of a "24-hour multilingual and multidisciplinary Telemedicine surveillance and Emergency service around the world". A feasibility study launched in December 1995 was conducted mainly as a French-Italian collaboration with participation of other G-7 countries; the conclusions were presented at the world conference on emergency telemedicine in Rome on December 16th 1996. It was concluded that, from a technological viewpoint, the telemedicine world-wide network was feasible and could be implemented gradually and stepwise.

The various GHAP projects were reviewed during a G-7 National coordinators meeting held in Bethesda, USA on January 27-28 1997; despite the technical feasibility of SP-4, it was felt that there was not a sufficient demand to justify the investment from G-7 governments for the setting-up of the service at this point in time. On the other hand, it was agreed that the growing number of regional and national initiatives in the area of telemedicine required a reinforced co-operation between G-7 countries. New orientations should be defined to extend the scope to telemedicine in general and not to emergency telemedicine only; co-operative work on horizontal aspects of Telemedicine should address subjects such as inter-operability, cost-efficiency of applications, legal aspects and health care management. Canada was designated to lead this action; this was accepted by Dr Jo Hauser, the Canadian National co-ordinator and by Dr André Lacroix, the Canadian representative on G7 GHAP sub-project 4. New projects based on these recommendations were to be discussed and selected before the end of 1997 in order to reorient the efforts of G7 international collaboration in telemedicine.

3. Reorientation of G7 GHAP SP-4

Following the recommendations of the G7 GHAP national coordinators, a new orientation of sub-project 4 was planned during a business meeting of its new national representatives held during the 3rd International Conference on the Medical Aspects of Telemedicine in Kobe, Japan, on June 1, 1997. The national representatives to each sub-project were nominated by their respective national GHAP co-ordinator; the list of the national representatives for GHAP SP-4 is presented in Table 1. Please note that, following the addition of Russia to the group of initial countries in 1998, the project became G8 GHAP SP-4. Australia had indicated its interest to participate in G7 GHAP projects from its initiation and thus also has representatives in this working group. This project was very fortunate to be able to count on a group of experts which have accumulated a vast experience in conducting collaborative health telematics and telemedicine activities in their own countries as well as within several international projects.

Country	Representatives
Canada	André Lacroix (chair)
France	Louis Lareng/Guy Rossignol
Germany	Dittmar Padeken
Italy	Marcello Bracale
Japan	Yoich Ogushi/Yoshikazu Okada
Russia	Oleg I. Orlov
United Kingdom	Richard Wootton/James McGee
United States of America	Jay H. Sanders
Australia	Ian McDonald/ Sandra Prerost

Table 1: G8-GHAP SP-4 national representatives

In addition to the national representatives of the G8 countries, GHAP SP-4 has largely benefited from the advises and efforts from other experts from the G8 and non G8 countries in the planning and implementation of its activities.

It was felt that Global telecommunications networks could contribute significantly towards the achievement of a healthier world. However, in order to promote and facilitate the implementation of telehealth networks around the world, it was felt necessary to solve certain key issues. The G8 SP-8 representatives decided that one of our two major objectives should be to hold a series of international workshops to examine these key issues and to propose solutions.

4. Planning of G-8 Sub-project 4 FORUMS on Telemedicine

The objectives of these thematic FORUMS is to bring together national healthcare authorities, key decision makers and users of telemedicine and health telematics applications, to share their views and experiences on requirements, necessary information and planning for the establishment of international collaboration in telemedicine and health telematics networks. The G8 FORUMS will review the various national positions on telemedicine and health telematics in G8 countries (e.g. CA, DE, FR, IT, JN, RU, UK, and USA) but also in other interested countries such as Australia and other countries.

Five meetings of 2-3 days duration were planned to be held between the end of 1997 and the end of 1999; each meeting will focus on one of the following themes which were felt of primary importance:

- Interoperability in Telemedicine and Telehealth;
- The Impact of Telemedicine on Health Care Management;
- Evaluation and Cost Effectiveness of Telemedicine;
- Clinical and Technical Quality and Standards of Telemedicine;
- Medico-legal aspects of national and international Telemedicine.

Each FORUM is organized and chaired by the National representative of the host country with the help of the steering Committee composed of the representatives of each G-8 country and of Australia. There is no central source of funding for the GHAP sub-projects. For the G8 SP-4 FORUMS, the organisers in the host countries have taken the responsibility to obtain the financial support from local public or private sources in order to provide the facilities for the FORUM. Each national representative is responsible to designate the national delegates who are invited to participate in each FORUM. The objective is to recruit 8-10 experts from each G8 country and Australia to participate at each FORUM; some experts from other non G8 countries can also be invited to participate by the organizing committee. There are no registration fees for the G8 SP-4 national delegates to participate to these meetings; however the travel and lodging expenses of the delegates have to be provided from their own sources or through funding support from their country.

Each FORUM includes plenary presentations by the participants from each country to review their past experiences and lessons learned on the topic under discussion. Working group sessions are also conducted with the objective to agree on the main conclusions and to propose recommendations to further the international collaboration in telemedicine and telehealth. A report summarizing the main issues discussed and the working group recommendations will be prepared for each FORUM.

5. Progress on G8 SP-4 FORUMS

The locations, dates and hosts for the five FORUMS are presented in Table 2.

FORUM	Theme	Date	Location	Program Chair
First	Interoperability in Telemedicine and Telehealth	May 28-30 1998	Montréal, Canada	André Lacroix
Second	The Impact of Telemedicine on Health Care Management	November 21-23 1998	Regensburg, Germany	Michael Nerlich
Third	Evaluation and Cost Effectiveness of Telemedicine	February 19-20 1999	Melbourne, Australia	Ian Heath
Fourth	Clinical and Technical Quality and Standards of Telemedicine	April 29-30 1999	Washington, USA	Jay Sanders
Fifth	Medico-legal aspects of national and international Telemedicine	Fall 1999	Oxford, UK	James McGee

Table 2: Program for G8 GHAP SP-4 FORUMS

The first FORUM was held jointly with a Canadian FORUM on the theme of Table 2: Program for G8 GHAP SP-4 FORUMS: "Interoperability in Telemedicine and Telehealth". The meeting was hosted by the Centre

Hospitalier de l'Université de Montréal (CHUM), thanks to the important contributions from the governments of Canada (Industry Canada, Health Canada) and of Québec; major sponsors included Stentor Alliances-Bell Canada, CANARIE inc, National Research Council of Canada, Teleglobe, Videotron, Andromed and Conceptis Technologies Inc. The meeting was held at the Delta Hôtel in Montréal; this was an invitational meeting and it assembled 91 Canadian and 33 international experts from 10 countries. The FORUM discussed interoperability from the technical, organizational and human points of view. There were 37 plenary session presentations and two working group sessions on each aspect of interoperability. A summary report and the conclusions of this FORUM will be published in 1999 under the sponsorship of CANARIE who has prepared reports of several other Canadian Telehealth workshops in the past. This report, as several of the presentations from this FORUM, will also be accessible on our G8 SP4 Website.

The second FORUM focused on the theme of the Impact of Telemedicine on Health Care Management. It was hosted very efficiently by Professor Nerlich and his collaborators from the Department of Trauma Surgery at the University of Regensburg in Germany, where the meeting was held. The meeting was supported by the City of Regensburg, the Bavarian government and the German Federal Ministry of Health; several industrial sponsors and exhibitors facilitated this very hospitable meeting. This FORUM provided an opportunity to hold joint sessions with members of the GHAP SP-5 on "Enabling Mechanisms for Global Healthcare Networks". There were approximately 280 participants; this included 69 international participants from 16 countries (USA:16, Canada:13, UK: 11, Russia: 9; others from France, Spain, Italy, Japan, Switzerland, Australia, Check Republic, Slovak Republic, Norway, Sweden, Denmark, Ireland) and a large representation from Germany. There were more than 83 oral presentations in plenary or specialized sessions and more than 20 in poster sessions. A joint G8 SP-4 and SP-5 working group session was held. The summary of this meeting is presented in this publication and will also be available in our G8 SP-4 Website.

The third FORUM will be hosted by Dr Ian Heath of the Australian Department of Health and Aged Care and be held at Saint Vincent Hospital in Melbourne, Australia on February 19 and 20 1999. This FORUM will be held in association with the European Union's TELEPLANS Project. The theme will be Evaluation and Cost Effectiveness of Telemedicine. The participants will then be able to attend the GHAP national coordinators meeting in Sydney on February 22-24 where the current applications of Telemedicine in Australia will be presented prior to the review of all G8 GHAP sub-projects.

The fourth G-8 SP-4 FORUM will be held at the Renaissance Washington DC Hotel in Washington on April 29-30 1999. The theme will be "Clinical and technical quality and Standards of Telemedicine". The meeting is organized by Drs. Jay Sanders and Michael Ackerman and is hosted by the U.S. National Library of Medicine. The FORUM will follow the Emerging Health Information Infrastructure (HII 99) meeting also hosted by the NLM at the same location on April 26-29th. Further details on the program of these joint meetings can be found on www.fnlm.org.

The fifth FORUM will be hosted by Prof. James McGee in Oxford, UK in the fall of 1999 to examine the important theme of Medico-legal aspects of national and international Telemedicine. The final date and preliminary program of this FORUM is currently in preparation.

6. International Multipoint Project of Advanced Communication in Telemedecine (IMPACT)

The national representatives to G8 SP-4 felt that it was necessary to utilize the recommendations of the FORUMS to develop effective multipoint telemedicine networks between the telemedicine units in academic centers in G-8 countries and Australia. Using, as a laboratory, the various expert centers in the G8 SP-4 centers, it would be very advantageous to share technical and organizational expertise to develop cost-effective advanced communications networks. The objectives of the G8 SP-4 IMPACT pilot study would be :

- Facilitate interconnectivity between Telemedicine units in G-8 countries and Australia ;
- Develop the best technical protocols and agreements between academic and industrial partners ;
- Test the feasability of multipoint meetings using diversified health telematics equipments ;
- Initiate the project with limited sites in each country ;
- The eventual goal is to link the national networks within an international backbone.

The IMPACT network would allow to conduct the following type of exchanges between the partners :

- ♦ Joint multidisciplinary and multimodality staff meetings of groups of experts in diversified fields of clinical medicine and healthcare ;

- ♦ Simultaneous interactive retransmission of prestigious state of the art lectures or formal teaching ;
- ♦ Availability of teleconsultation in complex cases or during emergency large scale public health crisis ;
- ♦ Facilitate International collaborative research studies in various biomedical fields.

A limited number of pilot sites will be selected in each G8 country and Australia. The pilot sites are selected by the national coordinators and health care authorities ; the sites should fulfill the following criteria:

- Academic University Teaching Centers with broad diversified expertise;
- Technical capacity to conduct multipoint activities;
- Research activities in telemedicine and health telematics;
- Eventual anchor site for a national network.

The meetings will be conducted using videoconferencing and transmission of multiple modalities of medical imaging, voice, etc. An important component of evaluation of technical quality and cost-effectiveness would be conducted during this project. Stepwise implementation will be utilized :

- ➢ Select protocols based on the conclusions of the G-8 SP-4 FORUM on interoperability ;
- ➢ Initiate point-to-point sessions: USA-Canada, Japan-Australia, UK-Germany, France-Italy ;
- ➢ Multipoint sessions: Canada-USA-Japan-Australia; France-Italy-Germany-UK ;
- ➢ Larger multipoint sessions ;
- ➢ Multipoint international sessions linking national networks.

As there is no central source of funding for the G8 GHAP SP-4, each participating center is responsible for securing the financial resources necessary to conduct this pilot project.

7. Progress on G8 SP-4 IMPACT activities

The objectives of the working group is to conduct initial IMPACT activities between selected centers during the period of 1999 ; this would allow us to report on the technical feasibility before the end of 1999. Some pilot sites have been selected (partial non exclusive list) in the following countries :

- Canada : Centre Hospitalier de l'Université de Montréal (CHUM) and Memorial University Saint-John's Newfoundland ;
- France : European Institute of Telemedicine, CHU Toulouse and European Institute of Telesurgery, CHU Strasbourg ;
- Germany : DLR, Cologne and Regensburg University;
- Japan : Tokai University, Tokyo;
- U.K. : Oxford University and Queen's Univ., Belfast;
- USA : Yale University, New Haven, CT.

Some of the initial IMPACT activities include :

1) **A program of telemedical education between Tokai University in Japan and Université de Montréal (CHUM) and Memorial University in St-John's, Newfoundland in Canada.**
   This program is made possible by funding to Tokai University from the Ministry of Health of Japan; the multipoint sessions will allow to transfer either formal lectures to medical students, joint staff meetings, and exchanges on the medial education and health care programs between the three centers. Initially, the activities are conducted using H320 standard videoconferencing with ISDN lines (384 kbps), with capacity of sharing data of T120 compatibility between centers. After a pilot phase, it will be possible to expand the network to include other G8 SP-4 centers. The technical aspects were tested in November 1998 and three joint meetings will be performed before March 1999. This pilot project is expected to be continued until March 2001.

2) **Multicenter exchanges between Yale University, Université de Montréal (CHUM), CHU de Strasbourg (EITS) and University of Regensburg.**
   This group plans to conduct joint multipoint and multidisciplinary staff meetings in the following areas : a) endocrine and digestive pathologies/surgery ; b) breast cancer ; c) orthopedics and traumatology. Videoconfe-rencing will utilize H320 (384 kbps) technology initially ; eventually, the objective is to prepare live audio Internet based sessions, which will also remain available on a G8 SP-4 Website. Initial phase of activities is planned for February 1999.

3) During the second FORUM held in Regensburg, several other G8 SP-4 participants have initiated discussions to plan activities in the context of the IMPACT project. These are still in the preliminary stage.

8. Conclusions

Why should we promote international collaboration in Telemedicine and health telematics ? The economic and social benefits of telemedicine and health telematics in health care delivery are certainly more of regional and national importance. However, the rapid sharing of knowledge and expertise in areas of sciences and human needs now bypass geographical and political barriers. The most industrialized nations bare the responsibility to develop and test new technologies which have a potential to improve the quality of life and of healthcare in less industrialized countries.

Healthcare workers in highly specialized academic centers offer telemedicine services to regional and local colleagues ; they would like to be able to discuss their difficult cases or share knowledge and experiences with other world experts. These exchanges will constitute an extraordinary enrichment for the students in healthcare training programs. Traditional international conferences are of great importance for sharing information, but are far-apart and expensive. Patients acquire rapidly healthcare information via Internet and require more and more high-standard quality care. High levels of travel and population migrations require local healthcare providers to be more knowledgeable of diseases from specific geographical distributions.

The G8 GHAP have provided excellent opportunities to experts in various areas of healthcare to examine how the new information technologies will be able to contribute to a healthier global world. Based on our current evaluation, telemedicine and health telematics promises to contribute significantly to this objective.

Further information on the progress and conclusions from the G8 SP-4 are available on its Website at www.g7sp4.org.

Acknowledgments

The author wishes to thank Dr Jean Larivière, the Canadian National GHAP coordinator, Health Canada and Industry Canada for their support. The dedicated efforts of all national representatives to G8 SP-4 is also greatly appreciated.

Address for correspondence

André Lacroix
Canadian representative and chair, G8 SP-4
Telemedicine Unit, Research Centre
Centre Hospitalier de l'Université de Montréal (CHUM)
3840 rue Saint-Urbain
Montréal, Québec, Canada, H2W 1T8
Tel: +1-514- 843-2735; Fax: +1-514-843-2715
E-mail: lacroixa@ERE.UMontreal.CA

Background Information

The Impact of Telemedicine on Health Care Management
M. Nerlich and R. Kretschmer (Eds.)
IOS Press, 1999

Towards a Methodology for Developing and Implementing Best Practices in Telehealth and Telemedicine

Jocelyne PICOT[1]
Conseillère en télémédecine, Centre Hospitalier de l'Université de Montréal
Infotelmed Communications, Verdun (Quebec) Canada

Abstract: One objective of the growing telehealth and telemedicine literature base is to inform potential adopters and raise their awareness through pilot projects. However, pilot studies often fail to create sustainable solutions because certain conditions are needed for long term success:

(1) *matching needs to appropriate solutions*: while needs assessment can identify needs, adopters must view, test, and experience potential solutions under a number of circumstances;

(2) *change and new technology*: technological implementation brings both foreseen and unforeseen changes, difficult to forecast, and pilot projects can create artificial expectations;

(3) a*wareness of context*: there has been a pervasive tendency to treat telemedicine or telehealth as separate from the context of health care delivery, but telemedicine is only a communication and information tool, and should not be considered as separate from other health care delivery activities; (4) *availability of long term funding:* while loans, government grants and private sector partnering can bridge gaps temporarily, sustainable solutions require that savings from existing systems can be applied to pay for telehealth and telemedicine installations. This paper makes a case for adopting best practices by proposing that a data base of case studies documenting best practices and success factors be developed and made widely available.

1. Introduction

It has often been stated that there is a need for more widespread adoption of health telematics or telehealth and telemedicine applications, and that such widespread implementation would have a positive impact on different aspects of the health care system. A recent Canadian study of the telehealth industry listed 15 key areas where such implementations could contribute positively to health care reform [3]. There appears to be a clear case for adoption of telehealth and telemedicine but many barriers continue to stand in the way. Researchers have recommended a variety of solutions to these barriers, including infrastructure development, standardization, more stable sources of funding, remuneration for practitioners, training, and the adoption of policies which would provide solutions to medico-legal problems. Pilot studies are often introduced or recommended as the preferred method for demonstrating successes and as a solution for overcoming these barriers. This paper suggests that telemedicine and telehealth or health

---

1 Special thanks to Valerie Gideon, PhD candidate, McGill University Graduate Program in Communications, for her help in preparing this paper.

telematic pilot studies do not necessarily lead to viable, long-term and cost-effective solutions. Rather, what is recommended in this paper is that telemedicine and telehealth best practices be documented and made easily accessible to potential adopters and decision makers. These best practices could provide relevant, usable examples, based on approved and tested criteria.

2. Definitions

Telehealth, also referred to as health telematics has been defined simply as the use of communications and information technology to deliver health and health care services and information over large and small distances [3]. Several reports have provided similar definitions. For example, in a report of an expert consultation held in 1996, the Pan American Health Organization (PAHO) defines telemedicine and telehealth as applications related to the practice of health or medical care using interactive audio, visual and data communications. This includes medical care delivery, consultation, diagnosis and treatment, as well as health promotion, education and the transfer of medical data.

For purposes of this paper, "best practices" represent the ideal or optimum cost-effective solution or set of practices, based on evidence that pre-established quality criteria have been satisfactorily met. Simply stated, best practices are good practices that have worked well elsewhere. They are proven and have produced successful results. In medicine best practice describes a process or technique whose employment results in improved patient and/or organizational outcomes.

3. The Literature

In 1994, 152 references were found using the key word *telemedicine* and even fewer references using the word *telehealth*. One year later the same search located 400 references [5]. In 1996 the National Library of Medicine published a telemedicine bibliography containing 1634 citations [7]. A researcher at the University of Queensland in Australia documenting a literature review on telemedicine found over 4,400 references [2].

This growing literature base includes documented collections of telemedicine projects or pilot studies, such as the Health Telematics (AIM) program of the European community [4]. Another collection of telemedicine and telehealth projects was carefully documented by David Wright for the International Telecommunications Union (ITU) [9]. Responses to a questionnaire about telemedicine activities were received from 59 countries. About half the respondents reported they have telemedicine and the others are planning or are interested in implementing telemedicine applications. Focussed on developing countries, the report concludes, in part, that "the first requirement of developing countries is for more information about telemedicine." One solution frequently mentioned, and endorsed at a World Telemedicine Symposium organized by the ITU held in Portugal in July 1997, is that developing countries need telemedicine demonstration or pilot projects.

A *Medline* search yielded 652 references linking best practices to current medical practice, but only 2 instances of telemedicine best practices were found on the Internet, which includes a study-in- progress at the University of Queensland in Australia.

Wojner [8] wrote about the interdisciplinary search for best practices in outcomes management. An article by Fernandez et al [1] reviews best practice technology assessment procedures. The authors propose an ideal model based on evidence-based technology assessment processes, consisting of a reiterative loop for technology assessment involving five processes:

awareness, strategic appropriateness, analysis versus need, acquisition and implementation, and reassessment. The authors also suggest a protocol for technology adoption decisions in which serviceability, acceptance testing, warranty, and cost comparison play parts. This analytical framework which encourages critical thinking could be applied to decisions about telemedicine and telehealth technology.

4. Best Practices Vs Pilot Projects

In telemedicine, the case for demonstrating "how it's done" is often made through pilot projects. Pilot projects are often the preferred vehicle for introducing innovation in traditional organizations. Because of their limited life span, these projects are easier to fund and implement than long-term projects, which require substantive organizational change and the creation of new budget priorities.

However, there is some evidence to suggest that pilot projects do not survive to become permanent solutions [2]. There are a number of reasons for this. First, pilot projects are not always implemented in response to identified needs. Even if needs have been identified and documented, matching needs to appropriate technological solutions present important challenges. Local infrastructure may be inadequate to support the innovation.

Secondly, potential adopters have difficulty imagining themselves in a technological future: they need to both *understand and experience* potential solutions under a number of circumstances.

Thirdly, technological implementation brings both foreseen and unforeseen changes which may be difficult to forecast without prior experience. When looking at the topics which most often surfaced in a review of 200 articles, more than half of the topics which surfaced were about organizational issues [2]. Pilot projects can fail because they are too short-lived to take into account organizational change. They can also create artificial expectations, as the adopters do not envision the unexpected changes brought about by their implementation. As well, pilot studies often demonstrate only one method, one technology, or one system. Alternatives are rarely experienced because comparative testing is simply not feasible.

Fourthly, there has been a pervasive tendency to treat telemedicine or telehealth as separate from the context of health care delivery. Telemedicine is a communication and information tool, and should not be considered as separate from other health care delivery activities. Though it sometimes takes on a life of its own, it is not more important than training, health information, diagnosis, research or therapy.

Sustainable telemedicine development requires the adoption of strategies which lead to long term financing. While loans, government grants and private sector partnering can bridge gaps temporarily, sustainable solutions require that savings from existing systems can be applied to pay for telehealth and telemedicine installations [6].

In light of the above, it would seem that pilot studies do not furnish the best route to acquiring sustainable and successful telehealth or telemedicine programs. They can indeed limit the experience of the adopter to the technologies and applications used in the pilot, and cut off other potentially more useful strategies for meeting health care needs. More importantly, they are designed to have a finite lifespan and unless sustainability is pre-planned and built in, even successful pilot projects can end without being renewed due to lack of operational funding.

5. Making a Case for Best Practices

A number of organizations and fields are promoting the notion of "best practices". The idea of adopting the "best of breed", or aiming for the *best way* to carry out procedures and projects, and obtain results, is very appealing. Best practices have recently been documented in a number of fields.

Several studies such as the ones quoted in this paper conclude that more and better quality information is needed to allow potential adopters of new technology to make sound decisions. The US General Services Administration, for example, has established an Office of Information Technology (IT) Best Practices Program. Some of their principles could be adapted to the health care situation, such as the creation of benchmarking results which are repeatable and comprehensive but not overly complicated.

In seeking to identify best practices in technology assessment, Fernandez found that "the past is not always relevant for making predictions about the future." In some countries technology assessments are not undertaken but in others, there were repeated assessments studies because of "inadequate diffusion and inefficient dissemination of technology assessment to prime users of these analyses." [1] Thus the role of dissemination is as important as the role of identification of best practices.

6. Arriving at Best Practices in Telehealth and Telemedicine

Identifying Telemedicine and Telehealth Best Practices

One of the principal challenges involved in developing best practices is that of developing suitable criteria for their selection. One solution would be to select a panel of experts who would select criteria for best practices, in each of the categories and main components of telemedicine and telehealth, covering such vital aspects as ergonomics, efficacy, safety, suitability, flexibility, robustness, reliability, durability, training, adaptability, and usability. An initial round of consultations with experts might reveal wide variations which could then be narrowed down through literature reviews emphasizing valid studies of comparative testing, evaluation, assessment and experimentation in various milieu.

Best practices in telehealth would include "best of breed" systems and applications. They would need to meet pre-established benchmarks and standards, meet user needs, be interoperable, have proven track records for safety and efficiency, be sustainable, be cost-effective, user-friendly, and environment-friendly and come from suppliers and manufacturers who employ quality practices and provide after-sales guarantees. But the most important aspect of identifying best practices would be dissemination and diffusion of the information.

The Case Study Vs the Pilot Study

The pilot study has been used for introducing innovations such as telehealth applications. Pilot studies suffer from a number of limitations. First they illustrate one solution and (usually) one technology. They have a limited exposure to potential users and uses. They are financed through project funds, a fixed amount for a finite time-span, with no provision made for sustaining the project even if it proves to be a success. Pilot studies are not necessarily transferable, and are detached from the context, because they are 'trials' or 'tests' and not real life changes brought about by consensus.

Case studies have long been used as the unit of illustration for teaching business management practice. In another context, case studies are powerful tools to illustrate and narrate qualitative research results [10]. Case studies can be used to describe projects imbedded in the fabric of the community and the health care system. They are rich in context and description and can be used to illustrate best practices. They can also provide transferable information. They can include quantitative and qualitative in depth information leading to analysis that would assist decision-makers and potential adopters by exposing all the facts. Different cases can illustrate different applications in different contexts. Case studies could easily become the preferred vehicle for providing examples of best practices. They could be updated regularly, made accessible in a searchable database and, using the Internet, be widely disseminated to all who intend to implement telehealth or telemedicine systems.

7. In Conclusion

The impact of telemedicine and telehealth technologies and applications on the health care system as a whole is undeniable. There is a growing database of publications, and an increasing wide range of systems and technologies being developed and tested. In almost every continent the world over, there is a telemedicine or telehealth-related meeting, seminar or conference every few weeks. Clearly there is a need for more practical information about the impacts of telemedicine and telehealth on the health care system. Potential adopters and practitioners alike are thirsty for practical advice about this rapidly expanding and changing field. Many conferences and consultations report on pilot studies. Others recommend them as a means to provide and illustrate telemedicine and telehealth solutions. In this article we make a plea for abandoning the pilot study in favour of the case study, which could be used to document critical success factors, and contribute to adopting best practices rather than implementing another pilot study which might not lead to a long-term solution.

References

[1] Fernandez, Annette M., John J. Schrogie, Wendy W Wilson, and David B Nash, A Review and Description of a "Best Practice:" Technology Assessment Process. Best Practices and Benchmarking in Healthcare November/December 1997 pp 240-253.

[2] Ferrers, Richard, Telemedicine Best Practice Literature Review: Work in Progress, unpublished. University of Queensland, Australia (http://student.uq.edu.au/~s054945/litreview.htm)

[3] Government of Canada - Industry Canada, Telehealth Industry: Part 1: Overview and Prospects, *Sector Competitive Frameworks*. March 1998.

[4] Health Telematics (AIM) Final Report, February 1, 1997 available at http://www.ehto.be/aim/

[5] Johnson, Ellen, Telemedicine: An annotated bibliography: Part I. *Telemedicine Journal* 1 (2, summer 1995).

[6] Lobley, D, The economics of telemedicine, *The Journal of Telemedicine and Telecare* 1997, 3:3, pp 117-125

[7] Scannell, Kristine, *Telemedicine: Past, Present, Future, January 1966 through March 1995 – 1634 Citations*. National Library of Medicine, U.S. Department of Health and Human Services, Bethesda, Maryland, 1995

[8] Wojner, Anne W. Outcomes management: An Interdisciplinary search for Best Practice. *AACN Clinical Issues*, 7:1 1996, pp 133-145

[9] Wright, David, Telemedicine and Developing Countries, A report of Study Group 2 of the ITU Development Sector, *Journal of Telemedicine and Telecare*, vol 4 suppl 1, 1998

[10] Yin, Robert K., *Case Study Research: Design and Methods*. Sage Publications 1984

Address for correspondence

Jocelyne Picot
Conseillère en télémédecine
Centre Hospitalier de l'Université de Montréal
Infotelmed Communications
38-10 Place du Commerce
Verdun (Quebec) Canada H3E 1T8
Tel: +1-514-262-5568; Fax +1-767-9933
E-mail: jpicot@istar.ca
Internet: http://infotelmed.ca

Theory of Use behind Telehealth Applications

Pascale LEHOUX[1], Claude SICOTTE[1], André LACROIX[2]
[1]*Dept. of Health Administration, University of Montreal, Montreal Quebec, Canada*
[2]*Head, Telemedicine Unit, Research Centre Hotel-Dieu campus, Montreal University Teaching Hospital (CHUM)*

Abstract: A variety of telehealth applications have been implemented throughout the industrialized world. Given that telehealth has yet to become routine in the practices of physicians, the impact of such applications on health care management remains difficult to identify. Only by becoming integrated into the 'normal practice' of clinicians can telehealth facilitate smooth communications in health care delivery processes.

In this paper we demonstrate the importance of developing a 'theory of use', describing how clinicians are expected to use teleconsultation in their daily activities. By employing Giddens' Structuration Theory, we can develop a clear vision of the utilization of telehealth, and a better framework with which to assess its added value for health care delivery. We illustrate this claim by referring to our research on the Quebec Inter-Regional Telemedicine Network. In this study we compare the 'theory of use' behind the telemedicine network with the perceptions of physicians regarding their needs in terms of communications and access to expert advice. The breach between the theory and the perceptions of physicians may help to explain how the utilization of telehealth could be enhanced, and how new and sustainable routines for its integration into the health care system might be created

Introduction: Why discuss theory of use behind telehealth?

Bashshur commented on the two "horns of a technological dilemma" [1]. On the one hand, he emphasized the lag between technological advances and our ability to capitalize on them to increase the productivity and effectiveness of health care systems. On the other hand, he stressed that "it is far better to start with the clinical and health care problems we wish to address and search for alternative solutions, technological and not, than to start with the technology and then search for ways to use it effectively in medicine and health care" [1:114]. This technological dilemma has not been addressed extensively in the literature. Nor have researchers offered empirical approaches to indicate ways to reduce the lag between technological advances and clinical needs. In this paper, we argue that a critical assessment of telehealth informed by a theory of technology utilization is extremely desirable.

Some observers in the field of telehealth contend that its usefulness is so obvious that there is absolutely no need to evaluate it. The phone is often the favourite example. For these observers, the need for the telephone was somewhat obvious and its utilization has increased steadily without any formal assessments. We would rather stress that the phone has changed drastically since its introduction at the beginning of the century. Perhaps no formal assessment has been done, but many criticisms, trials, analyses, and modifications were certainly achieved. Additionally, the example of the phone is flawed because the context in which technological R&D occurs has radically changed since the 1920s. In our modern age, and more peculiarly in the context of the budget cuts seen in most health care systems, sub-optimal solutions do not compete seriously: they just vanish! Thus, telehealth can gain from formal assessments — if done properly — and stands to lose if it eschews critical examination.

From this perspective, this paper is largely, though not exclusively, concerned with theory and conceptual tools that can help researchers contribute to the development of telehealth.

Ways of bridging the gap between research on telehealth and its practice are urgently needed. We insist on the importance of developing a 'theory of use,' describing how clinicians might be expected to use telehealth in their daily activities. It is our assertion that to be effective and efficient, telehealth should become routine in users' practices. Accordingly, one means to understanding how telehealth can be integrated into those daily practices is to compare the 'theory of use' of telehealth — the logic behind its use — with what physicians or other users actually do and with their communications needs. In other words, the breach between the theory of use and the practices of health care providers' may help to explain how the utilization of telehealth could be enhanced, and how new and sustainable routines for its future integration into the health care system might be created.

To develop this argument, we focus on teleconsultation. This paper is comprised of five parts: first, the rationale behind a theoretical examination of communications technologies is briefly exposed; second, we argue that a relevant theoretical approach to the study of teleconsultation should articulate notions of technology, communications, and social practices; third, we suggest that such concepts — particularly the notion of 'routinization'— can be found in Giddens' Structuration Theory [2]; fourth, we describe how those concepts are operationalized in our on-going research on the Quebec Inter-Regional Telemedicine Network; and fifth, we clarify the links that can be drawn between a theory of use of telehealth and physicians' perceptions and practices.

1. Technology, communications, and social practices

The first author recently completed a report [3] for the *Quebec Health Technology Assessment Council* based on a literature review, on evaluations that were prepared around three important telemedicine networks in Quebec [4-5], and on a conceptual analysis at the level of the health care system. This report endeavoured to maintain a global perspective over a variety of telehealth applications. One general observation was striking: even though a variety of telehealth applications have been implemented and used throughout the industrialized world, teleconsultation has yet to become *routine* in physicians' practices.

As a consequence of the *ad hoc* patterns of utilization observed across pilot projects, the impact of teleconsultation on clinical practice and on health care management remains difficult to define and document [6]. It is, therefore, rather complicated to formulate convincing arguments for policymakers, managers and health care providers about the value of a wider dissemination of teleconsultation. This lack of knowledge will not be improved upon by conducting more technical efficacy studies: something more fundamental is at stake. At this moment, high expectations have been raised around the resurgence of telehealth and, paradoxically, in most programs, low levels of utilization have been observed. This situation is unstable: if ways of enhancing its use are not identified, teleconsultation might lose legitimacy in the eyes of providers, managers and decision-makers.

Insufficient attention has been paid to the manner in which teleconsultation should be used. Of course, it is meant to support the provision of health care services — that is, to support communications between providers, and between providers and patients. But to reach that goal one must first understand what the communications are, and which related clinical tasks are actually involved in health care delivery processes. In other words, only by becoming integrated into the 'normal practice' of managers and clinicians will telehealth facilitate smooth communications in health care delivery processes. *Normal* practice is stressed here since teleconsultation should not be designed and implemented according to an idealized concept of clinical practice. Therefore, a theoretical investigation is worthwhile in order to examine in more detail how teleconsultation and clinical practices are supposed to work together. This kind of analysis would also strengthen our knowledge about the impact of telehealth on clinical practices.

Theoretical investigations on telehealth have been scarcely promoted. For instance, Pelletier-Fleury and colleagues [7] suggested that the "transaction costs economics" framework offers an appropriate analytical approach to examining the transforming role of communications technologies in health care.

> [...] the principal problems faced by the diffusion of telemedicine may be considered as costs which are not linked to the technology itself, but which stem from the way such technology restructures health-care supply. The use of telemedicine affects the relationships between different producers, especially by modifying their respective hierarchical positions. By doing this, telemedicine alters the decision-making processes, and in particular it makes the respective performance of the producers more visible [7: 2].

The non-financial costs related to the restructuring effect of teleconsultation are in fact important barriers to its wider utilization, at least from the users' point of view. These barriers can be studied empirically in their context with other theoretical frameworks as well. Of the different approaches to the study of technology, the more interesting ones have been developed by sociologists applying ethnographic methods [8-9]. They usually spend a prolonged period observing how individuals and collectives make use of technology in their real life settings, what kinds of changes are wrought by the introduction of a new technology, and which aspects of conventional social interactions are transformed through this process. These scholars argue that technology has to fit, or *integrate into human practices* and, in turn, that human practices *are transformed through the utilization* of technology. Their findings are often formulated in narrative forms, or "thick description", depicting in detail what kinds of problems are encountered with the utilization of technology, and what kinds of strategies are put forward to circumscribe those barriers. Thus ethnographic studies contain a wealth of information for those interested in enhancing both technology and its use. For teleconsultation such an approach means that only through an interactive process will telehealth evolve, change, and become more efficient if users, at the same time, adapt, modify and create new work routines around its use.

In addition, teleconsultation possesses the distinctive features of *information technology* [10]. It is multipurpose, multimedia, interactive and "networkable" [3]. Unlike other tools and equipment used by clinicians, teleconsultation does not perform new clinical interventions, nor does it visibly offer practical and unequivocal usefulness for clinical work. Basically, it *supports* clinical communications, e.g. the transmission of data, information and knowledge related to clinical cases. Which means that for teleconsultation to be integrated into clinical practices it has to be tightly linked to the communications practices of clinicians. These communications routines vary from one medical speciality to the other. The actual communication networks of clinicians are also highly diversified. Telehealth researchers should then aim for a more detailed understanding of the specific communications needs in each medical speciality.

Even though it seems obvious, we rarely recognize that communications in health care relies on *social practices*. Interacting with peers, asking for expert advice, educating patients, training residents, or consulting unknown colleagues — all these social activities involve communications skills as well as the integration of tacit rules. In the course of their daily activities, clinicians behave in a manner, which is largely known and/or shared by their peers, and by the other health care providers with whom they interact. They know how to ask for certain information, when to interrupt or not, when to doubt of the validity of information, when to emphasize a point, and when to resume an exchange. Then, telehealth research should document which aspects of social practices in diverse medical specialities have an impact on the effectiveness of their communications routines.

In summary, the kind of approach relevant to the study of teleconsultation would pay attention to: 1) human factors, 2) organizational dimensions, 3) communication flow and 4) professional dynamics that are a part of normal clinical practices. We suggest that Giddens' Structuration Theory offers such an approach.

2. Giddens' Structuration Theory

Anthony Giddens is a prolific British sociologist; he has published over 200 articles, and has participated in the publication of twenty-nine books. He is presently the Head of the London School of Economics. A search on the Web using his name as a key word would reveal more than 2000 web sites. Twelve books have been written on his work by other authors. In this paper, we primarily draw on his book "The constitution of society. Outline of the theory of structuration"[2], which represents a synthesis of earlier work published in 1976, 79 and 82. Giddens adopts a somewhat eclectic approach; he delves into considerable detail to articulate his own theory, and borrows selectively from findings and concepts developed in other disciplines (such as psychoanalysis, cognitive theory, phenomenology, and anthropology). What makes Giddens' theory different than structuralist and functionalist accounts, is that he insists on the *knowledgeability* of actors (or agents). As he puts it, knowledgeability is: "Everything which actors know (believe) about the circumstances of their action and that of others, drawn upon in the production of that action, including tacit as well as discursively available knowledge" [2:375].

Three assumptions define his general intellectual position and his contribution to social theory. First, he argues that actors are *reflexive*: they observe, monitor and reflect upon their own conduct and those of others, and more importantly, they continually bring changes into social practices. A reflexive monitoring of action is a chronic characteristic of daily living. According to Giddens, it refers to "The purposive, or intentional, character of human behaviour, considered within the flow of activity of the agent; action is not a string of discrete acts, involving an aggregate of intentions, but a continuous process" [2:377]. Second, he insists on the fact that *language* and *cognitive skills* are fundamental in social practices. This assumption has a direct implication for research on telehealth. And, finally, he rejects the idea that social sciences should mimic the *natural sciences*, e.g. they should not strive to establish explanatory laws. Because actors are reflexive, any kind of knowledge produced by sociologists is subject to being appropriated by them and thus, capable of modifying their behaviours. Therefore, the idea that laws explaining social practices could be established is useless, or flawed at best.

We propose, more specifically, to borrow three concepts from Giddens' theory which offer interesting analytical tools to the study of teleconsultation. We introduce briefly: 1) the (re)production of social structures by actors; 2) the double effect of structures; and 3) the role of anxiety and self-esteem in the establishment of routines. From those concepts we also derive three research implications for studying teleconsultation.

First, one famous *leitmotiv* of Giddens is *that actors, through social structures, produce and reproduce social structures*. By structures he refers to the features that take different forms across societies, such as governmental bureaucracy, systems of education, or technological systems. For the purposes of our study, we conceive of technologies as structures, and of actors as users. What is original in his claim? Such an approach posits that technologies do not operate "behind the backs" of users; rather, they are embedded in, and they are extended by the behaviour and knowledge of users. Thus the (re)production process always entails the germs of change. According to Hagendijk [11], this conceptualization avoids an extreme voluntarism: a position following which users are not, by almost any practical means, submitted to material constraints. Giddens' conceptualization also avoids an extreme determinism: a position according to which users' behaviours are directly determined by technologies that operate mainly as constraints. Because of this view which unifies the "two horns of the technological dilemma", Giddens' theory allows for the study of what we would call *change in continuity*. How do users gradually modify the existing technologies? Why do they retain some of these technologies? What are the consequences of such a partial and gradual sociotechnical transformation, e.g. partly social and partly technical?

We contend that the introduction of a new technology, such as teleconsultation into clinical practices, is a phenomenon of 'change in continuity.' The utilization of teleconsultation should be conceived of as a process of sociotechnical change.

Second, the *duality of structures* — their double effect — is a central theme for Giddens. A structuration process occurs because users mobilize rules and resources, including technologies, in the course of their daily lives. Rules are either normative, such as a set of obligations and rights, or interpretative, such as the background discussion that leads to the definition of what, at a certain period in a society, can become an object of rights and obligations. Resources can be authoritative (linked to political and decisional powers) or economic (associated with financial and material resources). Rules and resources are not distributed evenly among users who generally hold unequal social positions. A structuration process is *at the same time* enabling and constraining. Technologies may empower individuals and collectives, and facilitate their actions. But they can equally impose barriers and limits to social interactions. In this process, social relations are gradually transformed as a function of the opportunities and constraints faced by users.

With this concept, teleconsultation should be seen and studied as both enabling and constraining for providers, managers and patients. Those enabling and constraining properties should be central in the analysis of teleconsultation utilization.

Third, the last concept refers to why people do what they do. For Giddens, users' actions are meant to *reduce their anxiety and raise their self-esteem*. Actors generally fulfil their actions within a rational and largely conscious frame of mind. They also draw upon individual and collective memory to orient their actions. However, even though Giddens recognizes that actors are largely knowledgeable about their actions, it is clear to him that they are not entirely conscious of what their intentions are, neither can they offer justifications for everything they do. There are *degrees* to which they are able to express in their motivations, or levels of consciousness. More specifically, he distinguishes three levels of consciousness: discursive consciousness (which can be verbally explained), practical consciousness (on which action is based but that does not need to be formulated discursively), and existential security (to which actors do not have access –it is an unconscious motivation). Filtered through these levels of consciousness, users' anxiety and self-esteem motivate their daily activities. This creates a tension that varies across individuals and groups, and explains the extent to which some users will (or will not) experiment with new activities. Routines are thus a powerful means for giving security to individuals and collectives. Routines in our daily lives are important, since they make our world predictable. We assume that the same process is embodied in clinical practices.

A final implication is that research which emphasizes human factors, including organizational and professional dynamics, and which analyses how teleconsultation could become routinized into clinical practices would facilitate, and improve the utilization of teleconsultation.

We now describe how these three concepts are applied in our empirical research.

3. Methods: Quebec Inter-Regional Telemedicine Network Study

The Quebec Inter-Regional Telemedicine Network, chaired by one of the authors [A.L.], is a pilot project which was initiated in 1996 with 4 hospitals, including the Hôtel-Dieu campus of the Montreal University Teaching Hospital (CHUM). One hospital (Rouyn-Noranda) is located more than 600 kms north of Montreal and has a narrow scope of medical specialists; the other two (*Centre hospitalier régional de Lanaudière* in Joliette, Ste-Marie Hospital in Trois-Rivières) are located less than 200 kms from Montreal and have a fair number and diversity of medical specialists. A first phase of 18 months involved tele-education while the second, partly overlapping, phase of 12 months involved teleconsultation in any medical specialities.

A comprehensive evaluative research by two of the authors [C.S., A.L.] was recently completed [5]. We refer in this paper to another on-going research funded by the Medical Research Council of Canada in order to conduct an in-depth study of the physicians' point of view [12]. To our knowledge, a similar qualitative study has not been published yet. The main objective of this study is to identify, from the physicians' point of view, the conditions in which telemedicine would be superior to their current means of communications.

Regarding the methods, we are conducting semi-directed interviews with consultants and referring physicians who are users (n=12) and non-users (n=35) of teleconsultation. The consultants belong to 5 disciplines: cardiology, dermatology, neurology, pulmonary diseases, and radiology. The referring physicians are internists who work in remote regions. Our interview questionnaires are comprised of three parts (see Table 1). In the first part, the questions are meant to obtain a detailed picture of the actual practice of physicians. We document communications that are not formal consultations, as well as rather informal brief discussions about cases. In the second part, questions seek to obtain information about teleconsultation. If they have used the system, we ask how they adapted and, if they have not, how they would adapt to the utilization of teleconsultation. In the third part of the interview, questions relate to a more abstract level, such as the expected impact on hospitals, and dissemination issues (Tab. 1).

An analysis of the videotaped consultations (n=13), pertaining to cases in the five chosen specialities, is also generated. With the analysis of the videotaped consultations we aim to assess the overall quality of the communication flow, and to document the means of information transfer used in each case. For each patient case that was discussed, we note whether accompanying material was prepared and sent before the teleconsultation took place. For instance, in some cases, video images of skin lesions were requested, or EKGs sent by fax. Quality of communication is assessed by intersubjective indicators such as the characteristics of the audio quality, if physicians ask their interlocutors to repeat, or (re)adjust the volume a number of times. We also note the quality of the image. Was the text easily readable or not? Was the focus precise enough for the different documents presented, etc? Finally, we sum up the verbal interactions that took place by transcribing the phrases that ask for something, or respond to a query, or repeat or confirm a prior statement, or expose what information was gathered what hypotheses were formulated and what concluding terms were chosen. This analysis complements the interviews in an important way: we will have a picture of the communication flow that is more detailed, concrete, and which better depicts "real life" situations –in other words, we will be able to perceive nuances by comparing "what they say they do, with what they do."

<u>First part</u> Consultants:	 Referring physicians:	<u>Second part</u>	<u>Third part</u>
For which cases is their expertise being sought?	For which cases do they usually request an expert's advice?	What are the main advantages and disadvantages that they perceive?	What is the perceived impact of teleconsultation on their hospital?
Who requests the consultation? From which hospitals and regions?	In which hospitals do they reach those experts?	What kind of changes would it bring to their practices?	What impact could it have on the establishment of a peer network? On patient recruitment of physicians starting their practice?
What proportion of their patients do the requests coming from another hospital represent?	For what proportion of their cases do they need such external expertise?	In which conditions would it be superior to their actual routines?	In which hospitals, in which regions, should it be implemented?
What information must be exchanged?	What information must be exchanged?	Why do physicians not use it more widely?	Who should decide? What legal aspects should be considered?
What means are generally used (fax, phone)?	What means are generally used (fax, phone)?		What level of trust would they put in a teleconsultation?
How much time does it take?	How much time does it take?		

Table 1: A sample of questions asked in interviews

4. Discussion: Links between theory of use and physicians' perceptions

As regards the analyses, we will apply Giddens' concepts to examine the breach between the actual practice of users with the theory of use of teleconsultation. More precisely, we aim to clarify empirically why and how, in the specialities chosen, physicians communicate, formally and informally. What kind of access to data, patients, and expert advice do they have? What is their usual communication network? In the interviews, we insist on documenting the constraints and opportunities associated with the actual practice of informants: they have to refer to their clinical routine, not just to an idealized vision of what it should be. The enabling and constraining properties of their usual flow of communication will be contrasted to those of teleconsultation.

We are documenting the needs and expectations of physicians regarding teleconsultation, drawing the relevant distinctions between consultants and referring physicians, and between users and non-users. Anyone would assume that before knowing what one can do with a new technology, one must first try it. However, the performance of technological systems of communication is rapidly evolving. The technology of two years ago is not what it is today, or will be tomorrow. It is therefore crucial to push the analysis beyond a simple identification of the technical features, which annoy users and non-users. Thus, our goal is to identify the *process* by which users would experiment and adapt to the use of the new means of communication embodied by teleconsultation. Our central analytical concern is the process of the gradual sociotechnical transformation, which should take place for teleconsultation to fit into clinical work. Finally, other issues — such as the impact of thrust and prior exchanges with a consultant/referring physician, and his/her training and reputation in the use of teleconsultation— are also explored. What criteria do physicians use to appraise a clinical communication? How do they reduce clinical uncertainty? When are they confident with their actions and judgements?

Preliminary impressions and hypotheses that will be investigated in more detail are associated with the three research implications derived from Giddens' theory.

Change in continuity, or are the actual means of communication satisfactory?

Teleconsultation's fiercest rival is found in the means of communication used everyday (phone, fax, face-to-face exchanges, forms). In a medical specialist's daily practice, hundreds of verbal or written communications occur. Which of these are effective? Which are burdensome? Because of the differences in the kinds of clinical information that are used from one medical discipline to the other, we do not believe that teleconsultation will be appropriated by physicians at an even pace. Furthermore, it is likely that teleconsultation will not entirely replace the usual means of communication. The transformation of the organization of clinical communications due to the utilization of teleconsultation may be less difficult and/or more profitable in certain medical areas. Thus, studying the more rapid "adopters" would shed light on the process of change and the manner in which teleconsultation could effectively complement the conventional means of communication. Social and technical dimensions should be dealt with at the same time since technical modifications will affect social adaptation, and vice versa.

Enabling and constraining properties of teleconsultation

Certain specialities might not gain as much as others from teleconsultation. Some of the information needed by physicians might not be appropriately transmitted by teleconsultation. For example, neurologists often prefer to see and talk with the patient directly before formulating their advice for a complex situation. Others might see their work totally transformed by teleconsultation. Some radiologists or pathologists who barely see any patients have an expertise domain which is so specialized, and a work schedule that is so routinized, that they could end up providing their consultations *only* via electronic means. In these instances, teleconsultation will not be used with the same intensity, nor with the same consequences.

For neurologists, teleconsultation could be an additional option, very slightly transforming the kind of work routines they have already established. For radiologists or pathologists, teleconsultation could entirely supplant the conventional means of diagnosis and communication.

Human, organizational, and professional issues in clinical routines

Clinical communications are more complex than they appear. It takes time and a huge number of interactions before physicians establish their peer network, e.g. a network upon which they rely either when they need advice or when they agree to informally offer their medical opinion. Confidence must be established both ways, and the most reliable criteria to assess who and when to trust has been the experience of repeated face-to-face interactions. Why? Face-to-face interactions are information-rich; one knows quickly enough with whom one is dealing. In addition, teleconsultation at the professional level supposes an asymmetry of expertise [5], which renders any communication via an electronic mode even more sensitive. To request advice is to accept that the interlocutor is more competent in the clinical area being discussed. Thus, human communication bears a wealth of information from which one might feel deprived if communicating through a video-conferencing system, unless one knows the other person(s) well.

Medical specialists become experts on very specific problems in their field. Their clinical work, including communications, even though it can grow in complexity for certain cases, is quite predictable. At the organizational level, it suggests that teleconsultation could be integrated, if a routine suited to the speciality's specific features was established, and if a teleconsultation system is designed in such a way that smoothes out the practical irritants associated with its use. We expect that the situation of internists and general practitioners, who are responsible for solving an array of different medical problems, will differ. Their needs for teleconsultation are often more salient, especially when practising in a region lacking specialists [5]. However, they might have to communicate with an array of consultants. Then their utilization of teleconsultation is dependent on the establishment of routines in all the specialities concerned. That is, for teleconsultation to become routine in internists' practices, it should first be routinized into those of medical specialists. Otherwise, internists will have to maintain different modes of consultation, depending on the type of consultant's advice they require.

These hypotheses, among others, will be explored thoroughly during the analyses. The value of such a qualitative in-depth study is to precisely structure the perceptions and views of physicians on teleconsultation with respect to their clinical practices through a informed theoretical framework and by identifying differences and similarities across informants. We expect our findings to be "speciality" and "organization" specific; the patients they see, the region in which they practice, and the clinical isolation they face [6, 7, and 13] influence the communication patterns of physicians. By employing Giddens' theory, our research will yield a clearer vision of the kind of changes involved in the introduction of teleconsultation in hospitals similar to the ones participating in the Quebec Inter-Regional Telemedicine Network. With similar studies on different medical specialities, in different hospitals, our findings will help explain how the utilization of teleconsultation could be enhanced, and how new and sustainable routines for its future integration into the health care system might be created.

5. Conclusion

High expectations are attached to telehealth and low levels of utilization are still observed in most programs. In this paper we argued that insufficient attention has been paid to the manner in which teleconsultation is supposed to be used. A theoretical approach, focused on utilization processes, can help explain the current situation and suggest ways of moving forward. In particular, research inspired by ethnographic technology studies in this area would provide insightful knowledge on human, organizational and professional dimensions that are seriously lacking [13]. Pursuing such a goal, we exposed three research implications that were derived from Giddens' Structuration Theory: 1) teleconsultation represents a "change in continuity" for clinical practices; 2) teleconsultation should be seen as both enabling and constraining for providers, managers and patients; and 3) research which emphasizes human factors and routinization of teleconsultation into clinical practices should improve its utilization.

For these reasons, evaluative research should recognize that routines are fundamental to communications in health care. The utilization of teleconsultation should be viewed as a process of sociotechnical change, which requires both technical and social adaptation. Research should attempt to build a better understanding of the logic behind the use of teleconsultation is specific to a variety of medical specialities and to the geographical position of hospitals within a teleconsultation network. The kind of research we discussed indicates ways in which both technology and human practice could be modified. The idea is to close the gap between theory of use and telehealth practice.

Acknowledgements

We would like to acknowledge the contribution of our colleagues Jean-Louis Denis, Marc Berg and François Champagne for their collaboration on the research project and Marie-Pierre Moreault, our research assistant. This paper is based on a research funded by the Medical Research Council of Canada (#9709P-38006 HSR).

References

[1] R.L. Bashshur, Critical issues in telemedicine. Telemedicine Journal 3(2) (1997) 113-126.

[2] A. Giddens, The constitution of society. Outline of the theory of structuration. Cambrige, Polity Press, 1984.

[3] P. Lehoux, Télémédecine et télésanté au Québec. État de la question. Report prepared for the Quebec Health Technology Assessment Council, CETS, Montreal, 1998 (english version forthcoming).

[4] J.-P. Fortin and C. Banville, Rapport d'évaluation des projets pilotes en télécardiologie et en téléradiologie. Centre de santé publique de Québec, Université Laval and CEFRIO, Quebec, 1998.

[5] C. Sicotte, F. Champagne, L. Farand, A. Lacroix, L. Rousseau, M. Ayé, and D. Reinharz, Analyse de l'expérimentation d'un réseau inter-hospitalier de télémédecine, Research report, GRIS, University of Montreal, 1998.

[6] IOM Institute of Medicine, Committee on Evaluating Clinical Applications of Telemedicine, Telemedicine: A guide to assessing telecommunications in health care. M.J. Field (Ed). Washington, DC National Academy Press, 1996.

[7] N. Pelletier-Fleury, V. Fargeon, J.L. Lanoé, and M. Falardeau, Transaction costs economics as a conceptual framework for the analysis of barriers to the diffusion of telemedicine, Health Policy 42 (1997) 1-14.

[8] B. Latour, La science en action. Paris, Éditions La Découverte, 1989.

[9] N. Dodier, Les hommes et les machines. La conscience collective dans les sociétés technicisées. Paris, Éditions Métailié, 1995.

[10] R. Coombs, D. Knights, H.C. Willmott, Culture, control and competition: Towards a conceptual framework for the study of information technology in organizations, Organization Studies 13(1) (1992) 51-72.

[11] R. Hagendijk, Structuration theory, constructivism, and scientific change, In Theories of science, S. Cozzens, and T. Gieryn (ed.), Bloomington, Indiana University Press, 1991.

[12] P. Lehoux, C. Sicotte, A. Lacroix, J.-L. Denis, F. Champagne, and M. Berg, Réseau inter-hospitalier de télémédecine. Usage en contexte réel par les médecins, Research proposal, Funded by the Medical Research Council of Canada (MRC) #9709P-38006 HSR, Montreal, 1997.

[13] tanding Comittee on Family and Community Affairs (SCFCA) Health on line. Report into health information management and telemedicine. Report to the Parliament of the Commonwealth of Australia, Canberra, Australian Government Publishing Service, 1997.

Address for correspondence

Pascale Lehoux
Assistant Researcher
Dept. of Health Administration
University of Montreal
Box 6128, Branch Centre-ville
Montreal Quebec H3C 3J7 Canada
Tel.: (514) 343-6111 #1370
Fax: (514) 343-2448
pascale.lehoux@umontreal.ca

The Value of an Evaluation Framework for Telehealth Initiatives

Richard E. SCOTT, Ken COATES, G. Frank McCARTHY
Institute for Health Research, Saint John Regional Hospital,
Saint John, New Brunswick, Canada

Abstract: Healthcare managers and policy makers will, in the immediate and near future, make major decisions about the allocation of scarce healthcare resources for telehealth 'solutions'. In our haste to capitalize on what technology can do we may be obscuring discussion and research about what technology should do. For example, currently much attention is being paid to standardization for technological aspects of telehealth. In contrast few efforts have been made to seek standardization in regards to a broad evaluation framework for telehealth. A body of opinion believes that missing in our rush into the on-line world is a systematic approach to research into the human, social, cultural, economic, and political factors associated with healthcare. As a result we lack the tools and experience necessary to assess the true value and implications of telehealth 'solutions'. Developing general guidelines for an evaluation framework, from needs assessment through integrated research to post-study assessment, would greatly enhance the quality of decision making by healthcare managers and policy makers. We propose a model - the Telehealth Integrated Research Model (TIRM) - as the first step in encouraging discussion and development of an internationally accepted standardized telehealth evaluation framework.

1. Telehealth: Introduction and Definition

Telehealth involves the use of communication and information technologies as a mechanism of providing health care and health care services when distance separates the participants. The majority of telehealth initiatives can be broadly classified into two categories: remote diagnosis and consultation (usually between a specialist and a primary care physician), and distance learning for continuing health education. Although the primary rationale for the development of telehealth is to serve those populations that, for one reason or another, have limited access to health care, telehealth today must also be viewed as a mechanism of centralizing health care specialists. In this regard telehealth has the potential to dramatically reshape the 'face to face' medical model of health care delivery that has existed since its inception.

2. Telehealth Growth

Since its origins 25 or so years ago to 1996, the growth of telemedicine in Canada and the United States has been very slow. The industry, for the most part, has been supported by government subsidies and R&D grants to researchers to promote pilot projects in telemedicine, where telemedicine embodied „all forms of remote medicine". Recently, with the merging of traditional telemedicine with telehealth, „reflecting the changing nature of the twin fields of telemedicine and health and medical information" remote medicine initiatives now account for only 30% of Canada's telehealth network projects [1].

In the past few years, growth in rural telemedicine and telehealth network development has been rapid. For example, the Association of Telemedicine Service Providers (ATSP) data on 96 active telemedicine sites in over 40 U.S. States indicates that the number of telemedicine consults in 1996 (21,000) tripled that of 1995, and in the first quarter of 1997, over 11,000 consults in over 40 medical specialties have been registered [2]. A study of telehealth centers commissioned by the Office of Rural Health Policy in the United States, determined that 29% of the rural health hospitals interviewed (2,472) already use or plan to implement a telehealth network. The Telemedicine Information Exchange lists 142 North American telehealth projects of which 6 are Canadian. Globally, 168 telemedicine projects in 35 countries were registered in 1996; a year later this number had grown to 183 [1].

In Canada, 300 companies are currently active in the telehealth sector. Large companies function as computer manufacturers and telecommunication providers, and a host of smaller companies provide services in software development, consulting, service, and R & D. The combined annual revenue of these companies in 1997 was $330 million and is expected to reach $1 billion per annum by the year 2000. Current telehealth projects in Canada are valued at an estimated $500 million. Homecare, the most important growth component of telehealth in Canada, has grown 15% annually over the past 5 years. In this capacity, the Canadian provincial governments have spent $1.5 billion on homecare in 1996 out of the $72.5 billion health care budget [1].

3. Telehealth Challenges

With the merging of traditional telemedicine with telehealth, this once largely fragmented industry must now respond to two major challenges: rapid technological advances, and increasing demand for its services.

At first glance, one would think that telehealth would only derive support from the technological progress. For example, advances in computer hardware and communications bandwidth are now available at affordable costs, improved high capacity and high speed interoperating technologies support telehealth integration, and the backing of the private sector to facilitate technology transfer and commercialization should serve to encourage a wide variety of telemedicine initiatives. Yet this very technological progress seems fragmented as well, with over 80% of the telehealth industry members in Canada maintaining that the „lack of common technological standards hampered the development of telehealth networks" [1]. Moreover, it is a growing concern that many telehealth developments are overly biased towards the technological aspects of their programs. In 1995, the G7 Ministers of Industry and Telecommunications met to discuss these very concerns and pushed for a global development and implementation strategy for a common telecommunications network [3].

Increasing demands for telehealth were in direct response to its potential to provide telehealth 'solutions'; solutions to better serve an aging population through home telecare, to reduce the costs associated with duplication in health care, to decrease the number of prescriptions (and, therefore, adverse drug interactions in the patient population), to reduce both patient and professional travel, and to provide for health and wellness information through better information management systems. Telehealth, therefore, was to provide not only better access to health care but to increase the quality of health care and to provide it at a reduced cost. The fact remains, however, that of the many pilot projects drawn up to test these very hypotheses, few have survived beyond the funding period.

4. Need for a Telehealth Evaluation Strategy

Today, given the rapid advancements in telecommunication infrastructure and in computer and compression technologies offered at lower costs, coupled with the relentless financial pressures on national health care systems, societal concerns surrounding access to quality health care have provided new incentives for increased and concerted research efforts in telehealth. While considerable attention has recently been paid to standardization for technological aspects of telehealth, few concerted efforts have been made to seek standardization with regards to an evaluation framework.

Given the dramatic growth in telehealth, the National Library of Medicine (NLM) recognized that telehealth is hardly unique among health care services in lacking evidence of its effectiveness. In direct response, the Institute of Medicine (IOM) developed a broad framework for evaluating telehealth. They stated all telehealth evaluations should be : 1) „treated as an integral part of program design, implementation, and redesign; 2) viewed as a cumulative and forward-looking process for building useful knowledge for decision makers rather than an isolated research exercise; 3) designed to compare the benefits and costs of telehealth with those of current practice; and 4) focussed on identifying practical and economical ways to achieve desired results rather than investigating the most exciting or advanced telehealth options." This working paper, although broad in scope, failed to address application-specific measures and criteria, and instead proposed broadly relevant evaluation questions concerning the issues of quality, accessibility, cost and acceptability of telehealth initiatives. Moreover, they did not attempt to address other important issues such as clinical objectives [4].

A common theme emerging at the 1993 Mayo Telemedicine symposium was the lack of published research and evaluation data on the use of telehealth. This data was identified as being „crucial to success", according to Dr. Max House of Memorial University, Newfoundland. He adds, „the evaluation should be built in from the beginning; even if your evaluation may only concern cost effectiveness or technology, it must provide useful information that can be acted upon to improve the service and help to assure its success" [5].

Similarly, Field (1996) proposed a number of relevant telemedicine evaluation questions in order to evaluate: „1) quality of care and health outcomes; 2) access to care; 3) health care costs and cost-effectiveness; 4) patient perceptions; and 5) clinical perceptions. Field echoed many of the views proposed by the IOM in that „evaluation should be viewed as an integral part of program design, implementation, and redesign; it should be understood as a cumulative and forward-looking process for building useful knowledge and as a guidance for program or policy improvement rather than an isolated exercise in project assessment; the benefits and costs of specific telemedicine applications should be compared with those of current practice; the potential benefits and costs of telemedicine should be broadly construed to promote the identification and measurement of unexpected and possibly unwanted effects and to encourage an assessment of overall effects on all significant parties; the accent should be on ways of achieving the least costly and most practical ways of achieving desired results rather than investigating the most exciting or advanced telemedicine options; focus on the clinical, financial, institutional, and social objectives and needs of those who may benefit or suffer from telemedicine" [6].

Douglas Perednia of the Advanced Telemedicine Research Group at Oklahoma State University Telemedicine Center (OHSU) proposed a collaborative model for multi-centered research in telehealth. In it he identifies a number of key questions about the use and performance of telehealth systems. Essentially, the basic form of „technology evaluation“ must relate to the safety and efficacy of the technology „to transmit medically important data so that correct diagnoses can be made and appropriate treatments can be instituted.“ The clinical „gold standard“ for diagnoses, therefore, requires that all safety and efficacy issues be tested in controlled laboratory settings. A second question refers to the clinical utility of the system, i.e., what effect does the new technology have on medical care delivery. These questions must be addressed in the context of the actual telehealth project and determinations should be made on how equivalent cases are handled in the absence of telehealth. Measures of medical effectiveness; accuracy in terms of a diagnostic test and therapeutic effects in the case of a treatment were also identified as being critically important and requiring long term clinical follow-up in the field. Questions of cost effectiveness with respect to the raw technology and the effects of technology on clinical outcomes were also described [7].

Unfortunately, evaluation attempts have been hampered by the fact that rural areas are, by their very nature, sparsely populated, and telehealth projects rarely generate sample sizes large enough to warrant robust statistical analysis. In response to this, Perednia proposed the Clinical Telemedicine Cooperative Group (CTCG), modeled after the successful research consortia the SouthWest Oncology Group (SWOG). In this evaluation model data is pooled from multiple programs by using common data collection instruments and protocols such that quantitative evaluations can be carried out [7]. At this time no such common tools exist.

In this excellent working paper, Perednia concludes by delivering a very sobering thought concerning the status of telehealth evaluations in the United States. He states, „thus, there is probably not a single telemedicine project in the United States that is, by itself, currently capable of providing meaningful data on medical efficacy, clinical utility or cost effectiveness“ [7].

John Mitchell & Associates (JMA) in Australia argued that „telemedicine in Australia is at risk of being derailed by inappropriate evaluation approaches and by confusion about how to measure telemedicine outcomes.“ In 1998, they proposed the JMA 8-Point Workshop Model for Evaluating Telemedicine and Measuring Outcomes. This development further underscores the need for telehealth evaluation initiatives [8].

Dr. Paul Dick, of the Hospital for Sick Children in Toronto, also emphasized the need for strong evaluations in telehealth services relative to design objectives and unintended consequences, and reflected the views of Perednia in that the results of pilot studies should be pooled to yield statistically meaningful results [9].

Not only are evaluation strategies important, but questions as to the timing of evaluations of new and fast-evolving health technologies must be addressed. Regular reporting of outcomes and side effects should be carried out after the initial assessment, and reassessment should rapidly follow the evolving technology. Initial reports by research pioneers, media, and business often support rapid application of the technology before adequate evaluation programs have been carried out. More often than not, the timing of such technological change biases the evaluation solely towards the technological aspects of the application [10].

In 1997, the National Forum on Health in Canada released its final report in which it recommended adoption of an evidence based health system, in which „the systematic application of the best available evidence to the evaluation of options and to decision making in clinical, management and policy settings“ [11]. In the same year, Dr. André Lacroix, Canadian representative at the international telehealth conference in Kobe, Japan, stated „the most industrialized nations bear the responsibility to develop and test new technologies, which have a potential to improve the quality of life in less industrialized countries“ [1].

5. Telehealth Integrated Research Model (TIRM)

At the TExpo '98 meeting (Fredericton, NB, Canada), 7 speakers discussed current telehealth initiatives within New Brunswick alone, including the Virtual Interactive Telehealth Assistance Links (VITAL) program partially funded through CANARIE [12]. It was this level of provincial activity that led the Institute for Health Research (IHR) to recognize the need to evaluate local telehealth initiatives in a structured and standardized fashion. In response, and in the absence of any recognized standard, the IHR developed the Telehealth Integrated Research Model.

In concert with other authors, TIRM emphasizes the need that evaluation be an integral part of any telehealth program design (i.e. establishing the ***Context*** of the program); execution (i.e. ***Implementation*** of the study); and review (i.e. ***Reassessment*** of the program), to inform other initiatives.

Context :

Broad and ongoing implementation should be the goal for telehealth programs. To maximize the likelihood of long-term implementation of successful telehealth programs, careful design must address a wide variety of issues.

➢ *Draw from experience*

Similar or comparable initiatives in other jurisdictions or countries can inform, providing a perspective on strategy, policy, and assessment criteria.

➢ *Understand policy implications*

Analysis of formal (legislative) and informal (administrative) structures is essential to understand local and broader implementation needs.

➢ *Assess barriers and receptors*

Broad implementation requires a clear understanding of potential barriers and receptors. Social science research, often neglected, can satisfy this need.

➢ *Set evaluation priorities*

The program will be evaluated on the basis of criteria set out during this phase. Broad input is essential if any program is to satisfy the expectations of all stakeholders, since the desire is to provide an assessment of overall effects on all significant parties. As a minimum, the elements recommended in the literature must be addressed, i.e. clinical equivalency, quality of care, health outcomes, access to care, health care costs, cost-effectiveness, patient perceptions, and clinician perceptions.

Implementation :

- *Data elements.* As with all research, ethical standards require that data elements be clearly defined, and restricted to those essential for the intended purpose.
- *Data collection.* Throughout the program it is essential that the required data be collected consistently. Development of highly structured Case Report Forms, as is done in clinical trials, can satisfy this need.

Reassessment :

Regular reporting of outcomes and any side effects should be carried out after the initial assessment, and reassessment should rapidly follow the evolving health care technology [10].

6. Moving Evaluation to Center-Stage

By providing an accepted, standardized evaluation framework, those familiar with the telehealth evaluation process can provide an important service. With the shift of telehealth to network-based activity, the framework will have to reflect a network evaluation approach.

The literature is repleat with statements of the need for appropriate evaluation of telehealth applications, and with recommendations for components of such a process. Yet at this time there is no standardized framework or set of tools to allow „the systematic application of the best available evidence to the evaluation of options and to decision making in clinical, management and policy settings" in relation to telehealth.

The lack of sound evaluations, even in the simplest form, coupled with the dramatic increase in demand for such information by health insurers, patients, clinicians, and policymakers, dictates that the proponents of telehealth provide better evaluations of their programs. In an international environment striving for 'interoperability', it makes sense to follow current examples and develop a mechanism whereby a standardized evaluation framework and set of tools can be provided to those individuals, groups, or agencies implementing telehealth initiatives. We are hopeful that this presentation will stimulate pursuit of such an option.

References

[1] Picot, Jocelyn. Industry Canada. *Sector Competitiveness Frameworks, Telehealth Industry, Part 1- Overview and Prospects*, 1998 http://strategis.ic.gc.ca/SSG/hs01322e.html

[2] Association of Telemedicine Service Providers (ATSP) http://www.atsp.org/survey/regFrame.html

[3] Global Healthcare Applications, G8 Pilot Projects, Telehealth, Health Canada, International Health. http://strategis.ic.gc.ca/SSG/in02287e.html

[4] Telemedicine: A Guide to Assessing Telecommunications in Health Care http://www.quasar.org/21698/textfodder/summary.html

[5] Proceedings of the Mayo Telemedicine Symposium, A Consensus Conference to Explore Telemedicine as a Vehicle for Expanding Access to Cost Effective Health Care. 1993, Rochester, MN: Mayo Clinic.

[6] http://joint.mccaig...evaluation/field.html

[7] Perednia D A. *Telemedicine System Evaluation and a Collaborative Model for Multi-Centered Research* 1995;**19(3)**:287-294

[8] John Mitchell & Associates, Telemedicine Evaluation Workshop http://www.jma.com.au/telemEv.htm

[9] Telehealth in Canada: Clinical Networking, Eliminating Distances http://strategis.ic.gc.ca/SSG/it04134e.html

[10] Mowatt G, *et al.* *When and How to Assess Fast Changing Technologies: A Comparative Study of Medical Applications of Four Generic Technologies* 1997;1(14), i-vi:1-149
[11] National Forum on Health, Canadian Health Action: Building on the Legacy, Vol. 1 http://wwwnfh.hc-sc.gc.ca/publicat/finvol1/1trans.htm
[12] CANARIE Inc., http://www.canarie.ca/

Address for correspondence

Richard E. Scott
Institute for Health Research
c/o 5DN Saint John Regional Hospital
400 University Avenue
Saint John, New Brunswick, Canada E2L 4L2
E-mail: ihr@health.nb.ca

The Impact of Telemedicine on Health Care Management
M. Nerlich and R. Kretschmer (Eds.)
IOS Press, 1999

Assessing the Impact of Telemedicine on Health Care Management

Rainer KRETSCHMER[1,2], Michael NERLICH[2]
[1] *Center for Health Care Quality, University of Missouri – Columbia, USA*
[2] *Department of Trauma Surgery, University of Regensburg, Germany*

Abstract: Telemedicine is undoubtedly one of the most dynamic developing fields of IT-technologies in health care. From research and development to routine clinical use of telemedicine applications, decision-makers demand information on the impact that widespread use will have on structures and processes in health care.

To date published evaluations have mostly focused on technical core functions. Future evaluation concepts have to consider side-effects the use of telematic systems in health care might have. The report of effects should consider the 4 major interest groups: patients, providers, third-party payers, and society.

Learning from experiences in other IT-fields, system developers can avoid pitfalls that might lead to a poor acceptance of their systems or the discontinuation of their R&D project at an immature stage.

1. Introduction

Research and development efforts to use telematic applications to support the delivery of health care have been increasing for over 30 years. Today this research field has its own name - Telemedicine - and around the world applications are slowly crossing the line from pilot projects in experimental settings to integrated systems in the clinical routine of health care management.

Naturally associated with the increased clinical importance of telematic applications, a growing interest in the commercial use of the information technology (IT) systems can be observed. For example in Teleradiology , there are more than a dozen service providers in the USA, Japan, and Norway that derive a significant portion of their revenues from providing teleradiology interpretations [1].

The enormous achievements in the field of IT and telecommunications in the last years have opened up fantastic perspectives for health care: Improvement of the quality of health care and better access to the system as well as an optimization of the cost-efficiency of certain segments. However, several major problems have to be solved before the full potential of telematics in health care can be realized:

- The integration of new information technologies into the complex structures and processes in health care is still considerably under-developed compared to the rapid progress in technical development.
- Standards on the interoperability of telemedical systems are still confusing and have not yet led to an easy, flawless use and interoperation of applications.
- Currently developed solutions for confidentiality and legal problems still need to be integrated in the applications.

- Seemingly as soon as users have purchased an application and integrated it into their environment, a new still more promising, powerful, attractive (and costly?) system becomes available. Keeping pace with the technology at present requires very short amortization intervals. However, economic analyses are hardly available.
- Concepts for reimbursement procedures are still indistinct.
- Decision-makers should understand that there are players who fear the adverse affects of the broad use of telemedicine. As long as they regard themselves as potential losers threatened by new technology, they will impede the implementation of these systems.
- Little information is available about the overall impact of health telematics on the health care sector, both on the institutional level and on society in general,[2,3] allowing decision-makers to postpone decisions to apply telemedicine.

However, experts representing all perspectives in the health care systems agree that telemedicine is not simply a trend and that it has the potential to significantly influence the delivery of health care in many environments and medical specialties.

But what will be the *impact*? Decision-makers will increasingly demand from developers and vendors more complete and relevant information, not only on the general effectiveness and efficiency of the applications, but also more specifically on the impact the use of the system might have from their perspective in their own environment.

2. Lessons learned from the Field of Expert Systems/Artificial Intelligence in Medicine

The explosive growth of knowledge in all scientific fields, in medicine in particular, is overwhelming. Today it is simply impossible for human experts in medicine to have a comprehensive and up-to-date knowledge on a whole clinical field; at best they can keep pace with a specialized segment of it. The half-life of medical knowledge is as short as 2½ years in some medical specialties[4]. On the other hand patients expect to be informed and treated with the up-to-date expert knowledge, irrespective of time,place, and resources.

A promising way out of this dilemma was suggested by the rapid development of computer technology in the last decades. Scientists worked on the use of *artificial, computer-based intelligence* to support decision making in medicine by making expert knowledge available through the use of computer systems. Numerous projects evolved, many of them providing scientific evidence from lab tests demonstrating the high potential of expert systems to imitate the performance of human experts. Nonetheless very few applications found their way into routine medical use.

Some reasons for this have been identified and discussed, the most important possibly being that the development of the system had been dominated by engineers and computer specialists,whereas the future users have not been adequately involved in the development process. This has had two serious consequences:

- the applications have been poorly adopted to the clinical needs and the structural and process environments
- physicians perceived the intelligent systems as a threat to their status and not as the intended means for supporting and expanding their decision processes.

Many other problems have hampered the widespread use of expert systems, e.g. responsibilities for system maintenance and legal issues, but the most important factor in the failure of expert systems in medical decision making seems to have been an insufficient acceptance by the users. All of these issues are also critical to the use of telemedicine systems: "Technical systems still may be poorly adapted to the human infrastructure of health care, that is, the work environment, needs, and preferences of clinicians, patients, and other decision-makers [5]."

Today still a few scientists continue the development of artificial intelligence in medicine, but the great enthusiasm of past days has given way to a certain disillusionment. System developers in telemedicine should therefore pay attention to mistakes and lessons learned from the past artificial intelligence development efforts to preserve their own projects from preventable setbacks and increase the chances of a user acceptance.

3. Effectiveness vs. Impact

It is still a long way from effectiveness to impact. Today growing numbers of reports on the effectiveness (though very rarely the *efficiency*) of telemedicine systems become available. Most of them find that telematic applications, at least in some respects, are effectively helping to solve certain problems in the delivery of healthcare better than existing procedures do. However, much of the currently evaluated telematic applications are still in the form of experimental or pilot projects. The interim report of the EU Directorate General XIII on the impact of telemedicine rated only 17% of all known applications as "established" (Fig 1.).

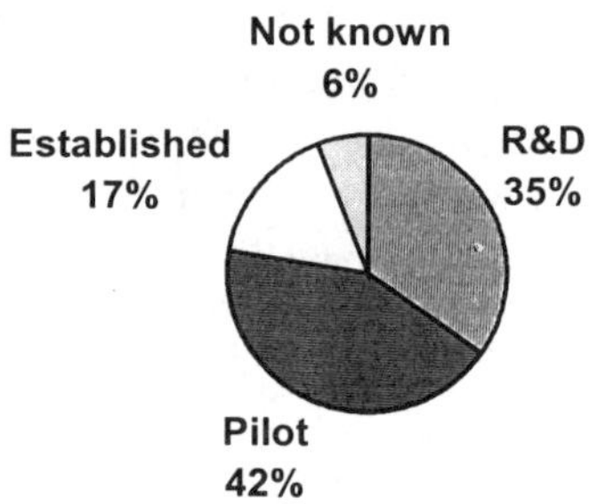

Fig. 1: Status of Telematic Applications for Healthcare in Europe in June 1996[3]

Decision-makers have to consider that evaluations of system performance and effectiveness that have been done in a research and development (R&D) or pilot environment frequently are seriously biased:

- Systems are tested by the developers and people that have somehow been involved in the development process and therefore are highly motivated to use the system.
- Systems are usually tested in locations very close to the system developers which ensures exceptional technical support by the developers.
- Weak points are frequently not made public in order to ensure the project survival.

For these and other reasons it is not at all clear that the systems' effectiveness can be reproduced in other than the R&D or pilot environments; in other words, systems might be effective but may not have a significant impact.

The impact will further depend on the degree to which telematic applications will help to solve frequent, widespread everyday problems [5]. Dazzled by new technical possibilities, decision-makers' attention is frequently diverted from more relevant issues by demonstrations showing how telemedicine helps to manage spectacular cases or problems.

Findings from analyses in industrial processes have shown that [6]

- systems supporting decision making processes should not aim at solving only the most complex, demanding problems, but
- should focus on the elimination of poor decisions in everyday situations that account for large parts of risky and costly errors.

Break-even analyses can be very helpful here to come to an economically well justified decision for which purposes telemedicine should be used or not (see also: Walz, M.: *Economic Analysis of Teleradiology Applications with KAMEDIN*, in this volume) .

4. Consequences for Evaluating Telemedicine Applications

Evaluations of telemedicine systems to date mostly focus on clinical objectives. Many other important aspects frequently do not attract the attention of the researchers as much. The situation is analogous to developing a painkiller, focusing on its analgesic effect but not caring for the side effects. These side effects can arise in areas the developers might not think of. Therefore the perspective from which the analysis is performed is critical and should consider 4 major interest groups: patients, providers, third-party payers, society.

Customers do not want to buy the pig in a poke. Therefore it seems essential to include evaluation issues that go far beyond the technical core measurements, e.g.

- acceptance measures of the system from the point of view of the user and the patients
- effects on the qualification of professional system users in both horizontal and vertical communication
- identification of impediments: causes for personal resistance (e.g. anticipated loss of status, job rationalization, skepticism towards new technologies etc.)
- Scenarios showing the effects of possible reimbursement mechanisms

At this point the impact of telemedicine on health care management can only be estimated. Impact will be achieved if developers succeed in establishing their systems in clinical routine use. Only then can the potential of telemedicine applications be fully exploited, since in a R&D phase of system development traditional clinical structures and procedures will not yet be changed and adapted to the new functionalities. Therefore theoretical anticipation of changes in *technical, clinical, and administrative processes* (see Chart 1) seems to be essential.

Finally, it should be stated clearly: conscientious evaluations serve to distinguish qualified concepts and systems from those less suitable. This will result in the discontinuance of some projects and the suspension of funds for certain research lines. Although this might sober some individuals, the discipline of telemedicine will benefit.

Elements of an Evaluation Plan

Project description and research question(s):
the application or program to be evaluated and the basic questions to be answered by the evaluation

Strategic objectives:
how the project is intended to serve the sponsor or parent organization's purposes.

Clinical objectives:
how the telemedicine project is intended to affect individual or population health by changing the quality, accessibility, or cost of care.

Business plan or project management plan:
a formal statement of how the evaluation will help decision-makers judge whether and when the application will be a financially and otherwise sustainable enterprise or, less formally, what the project's management, work plan, schedule, and budget will be.

Level and perspective of evaluation:
whether the focus of the research question(s) and objectives is clinical, institutional, societal, or some combination thereof.

Research design and analysis plan:
the strategy and steps for developing valid comparative information and analyzing it.

- *Experimental and comparison groups:*
  characteristics of (a) the group or groups that will be involved in testing the target telemedicine application and (b) the group or groups that will receive alternative services for purposes of comparison.
- *Technical, clinical, and administrative processes:*
  as planned and actually implemented, the communications and information systems, the methods for providing medical care, and the supportive organizational processes.
- *Measurable outcomes:*
  the variables and the data to be collected to determine whether the project is meeting its clinical and strategic objectives.
- *Sensitivity analysis:*
  the inclusion of techniques to assess to what extent conclusions may change if assumptions or values of key variables change.

Documentation:
the explicit reporting of the methods employed in the evaluation and the findings so that others can determine how the results were established.

Chart 1: Proposal for Evaluation Plans of Telemedicine Applications, compiled by the Committee on Evaluating Clinical Applications of Telemedicine[5]

5. Conclusion

Clinicians, patients and third party payers' increasing interest in telemedicine demands a much improved adaptation of existing systems to the human infrastructure of health care. Evaluations accompanying the research and development phases should stress these issues to impart to decision-makers that their perspectives are anticipated. Only a widespread use of telemedicine in clinical practice will allow for a measurement of the true impact, which can only be estimated at this point.

Applications poorly adapted to the clinical setting will also have an impact - they confirm prejudices of skeptics, waste resources, and contribute to the diversion of research and industry interest towards other promising IT-sectors.

Telemedicine evaluations should examine the needs of the users and make clear that telematic applications have got the potential to be beneficial to all parties. If this can be demonstrated, the line from effectiveness to impact will be crossed.

References

[1] Allen A, Stein S. *Cost Effectiveness of Telemedicine*. Internet: http://www.telemedtoday.com/articles/cost_effectiveness_of_telemedici.htm, 1998.

[2] European Health Telematics Observatory. [downloadable slides at http://www.ehto.be], 1996.

[3] Cullen J, et al. *TELMED - The Impact of Telematics on the Healthcare Sector*: European Commission, Directorate General XIII, DELIVERABLE No. 02: Interim Report, http://www.ehto.be, 1996.

[4] Poliwoda H. *MEDKOM - Vom Konsilium zu Pferde zur kooperativen Visite per Videokonferenz*. Kabelmetal-Treff, 12. November 1991 1991, Bonn.

[5] Committee on Evaluating Clinical Applications of Telemedicine. *Telemedicine - A Guide to Assessing Telecommunications in Health Care*. National Academy Press, 1996.

[6] Harris LR. *Woran erkennen Sie eine Anwendung künstlicher Intelligenz?* Chip Professional 1990;Programmieren 9(1. Auflage):30-8.

Address for correspondence

Rainer Kretschmer
Center for Health Care Quality
University of Missouri- Columbia
313 Clark Hall, Columbia, Missouri 65211, USA
Voice: +1 – 573 – 882 – 8905
Fax: +1 – 573 – 884 – 0474
E-mail: CHCQ@health.missouri.edu

The Impact of Telemedicine on Health Care Management
M. Nerlich and R. Kretschmer (Eds.)
IOS Press, 1999

A Review of Japanese Telemedicine Research and Global Co-Operation

Yoshikazu OKADA, Yoichi OGUSHI, Yasuo HARUKI
Department of Medical Informatics, Tokai University, School of Medicine, Isehara, Kanagawa, JAPAN 259-1193

Abstract. We can trace 229 telemedicine trials in Japan. Of these, 150 were active in 1998, including 73 in radiology, 24 in home care, 22 in medical imaging, 20 in pathology, 5 in ophthalmology, and 3 in dentistry. Some of them have been reformed into practical daily activities. However, activities using the same method work in some local areas but not in others. Typical successful cases will be presented and discussed.

We are constructing Japan-Canada cooperation in numerous areas using several communicative methods: ordinary telephone, ordinary Internet, ISDN (2B/6B), and an offline network using optical memory cards (which patients carry). We have introduced successful domestic cases into global cooperation. Some of them will be useful for exchanging medical information among developing countries.

1. Introduction

There are many telemedicine trials in Japan, and some of them have been reformed into practical activities. However, because information technology has become so widespread and economically defined, we have found it difficult to collect exhaustive data on telemedicine activities. So we will introduce a report about current telemedicine activities from the Japanese Ministry of Health and Welfare, as well as offer some additional examples of domestic and global telemedicine activities in Japan.

2. Materials and Methods

The report on telemedicine activities in Japan is introduced in the following chapter. Even though more than 200 telemedicine activities are gathered into this report, we cannot trace all of the projects. We also introduce some typical Japanese domestic and global telemedicine trials.

3. Results

3.1. "Telemedicine in Japan"

There is a well-summarized report about telemedicine studies in Japan [1]. Dr. S. Kaihara, formerly a professor at the University of Tokyo, reported on the status of Japanese telemedicine to the Japanese Ministry of Health and Welfare in March 1997. This "Kaihara Report" is available (note, in Japanese only) at the following URL:

http://square.umin.ac.jp/enkaku/96/Enkaku-RepSoukatu-nof-eng.html

In this report, each application considered uses medical images; applications using only ordinary telephones or TV-phones have omitted. The report list includes 20 telepathology, 73 teleradiology, 24 home care, 5 ophthalmology, 3 dental, 22 medical imaging and 3 other applications.

Dr. Kaihara defines telemedicine as: "Medical care and health supporting practices based on patient information derived from images transmitted from a remote site". He finds some benefits of Japanese telemedicine, including: leveling of regional differences, improvement of efficiency, enhancement of patient services, and overcoming of distance.

He also points out some barriers to popularizing telemedicine applications due to ambiguous positions in the Japanese medical system.

3.2. Examples of domestic telemedicine applications in Japan

3.2.1. Example 1

An ISDN (6B/T1) network for ophthalmology which includes Asahikawa Medical College and 14 local hospitals has been established since 1994 [3]. Terminals have been installed in outpatient offices. Each terminal has an ordinary TV-camera, a slit-lamp microscope, and an ophthalmoscope that can offer moving pictures to another station. The terminals have other displays to hold still medical images. Each terminal has an additional camera in an operating room. The system is usually used for teleconsultation in severe cases.

3.2.2. Example 2

A teleradiology network on ISDN (T1/2B) involving Kyoto Prefectural University of Medicine and 5 hospitals was started in 1994 [4]. The system is used for preliminary diagnosis with MR, CT or RI images. It uses standard method (DICOM 3.0), and many medical devices can be connected.

3.2.3. Example 3

A telepathology system [5] using ISDN (2B) between Kyoto Prefectural University of Medicine and a provincial hospital has been established since 1992. It contains a robotic microscope and special non-interlace image displays. It is practical and economical for daily consultations.

3.2.4. Example 4

Tokai University School of Medicine gave 37 one-hour lectures for continuing medical education to 19 general practitioners using telecommunications in 1997 and 1998 [8].

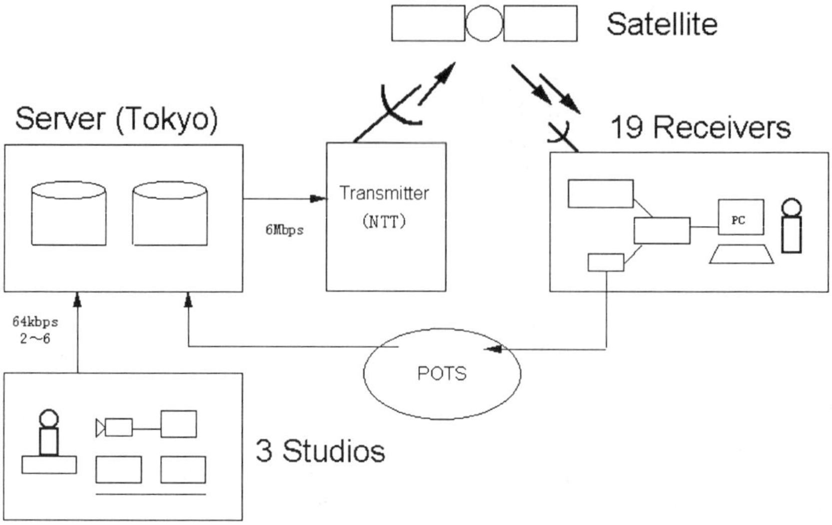

Figure 1: Satellite-based Internet.

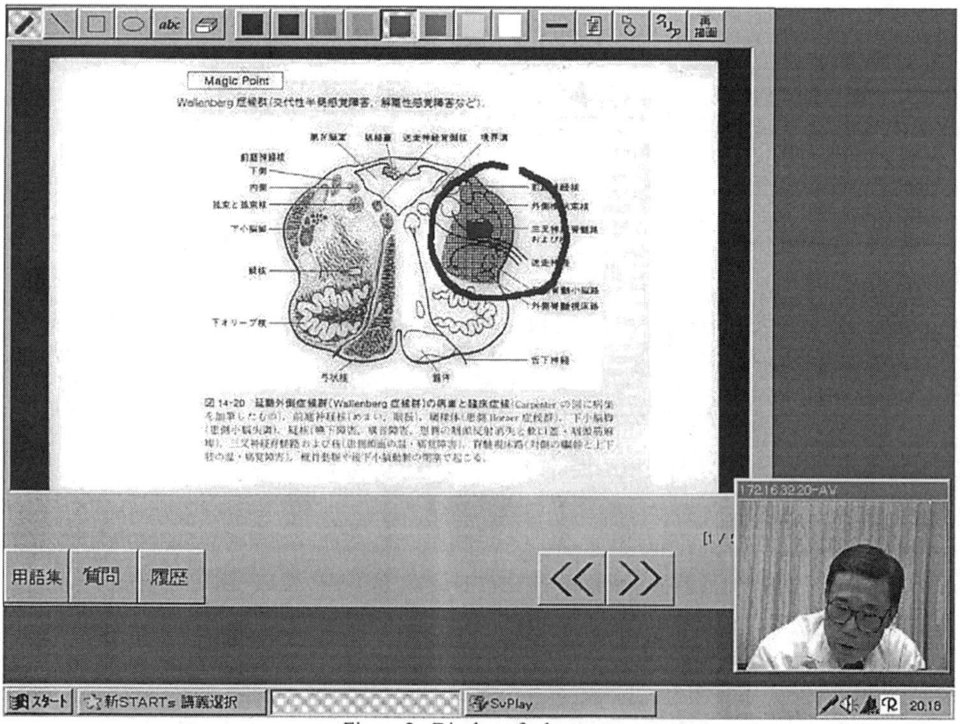

Figure 2: Display of a lecture.

This system uses satellite-based Internet to distribute still slide images and the voices of lecturers. Each lecturer can download images from a database any time *via* a satellite line. Students can type and send questions *via* ordinary telephone line to the lecturer. The terminals and studios are economic, and we were able to have three studios and more than 100 terminals at Tokai University. We also used the line for emergency practices [7].

3.3. Global Cooperation

3.3.1. Example 1

Dr. I. Nakajima, lecturer from the Tokai University School of Medicine, established the Asia-Pacific Medical Information Network via ETS-V (AMINE) in 1992. It contains a communications satellite and 25 earth stations: 5 in Papua New Guinea, 4 in Cambodia, 4 in Fiji, 1 in China, 5 in Thai, and 6 in Japan. It can exchange voice and color still images between any two stations without hub stations. The system has been used for teleconferences more than 50 times per year.

3.3.2. Example 2

We had point-to-point HDTV conferences between Ottawa University Heart Institute and Tokai University twice in 1998. Two national institutes, CRC (Industry Canada) and CRL (Japanese Ministry of Posts and Telecommunications), offered the line and studios to us as a project of G7 Global Interoperability for Broadband Networks (GIBN). We exchanged movie data of heart surgeries online. Although this system has extremely high quality medical moving images, it is very expensive for daily practices.

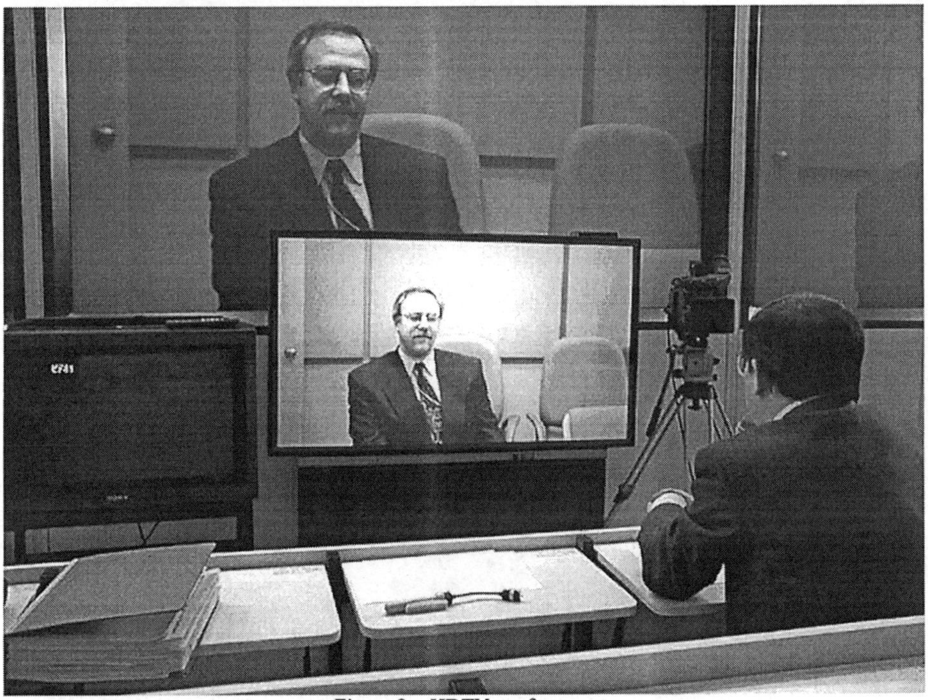

Figure 3: HDTV conference.

3.3.3. G7 GHAP SP4 IMPACT project

We have started to evaluate a global telemedicine network between Canada and Japan as a part of the G7 Global Healthcare Application (GHAP) / Sub-Project 4. It includes a feasibility study on global multipoint tele-education programmes and teleconferences using TV-phone with PC application sharing (T120). Two or three meetings will be held before the end of March 1999.

It also includes a feasibility study about exchanging and storing clinical data *via* Internet with encryption methods. We will use the clinical data that are derived from a medical record system with a Graphical User Interface (GUI). The data are exchangeable with optical memory cards as an offline network by patients [6, 9].

We will use standardized elements for these studies, and many groups may be able to join the project easily.

4. Discussion

There are several definitions of telemedicine [2]. The definition in the "Kaihara report" seems to be typical. Medical images-- still images or movies-- are important in Japan. However, because the report includes home care applications which are called "telecare" or "telehealth", but does not include telemedicine activities using POTS or simple TV phone systems, the actual number of telemedicine activities in Japan is actually greater than reported.

The report points out several barriers against popularizing telemedicine activities. These barriers may exist; however, many physicians use information equipment daily. Multipoint TV conferences are held regularly by the Saitama Medical Association (a local medical association in Saitama prefecture), for example.

The typical telemedicine cases included in the report often used special equipment. Using general-purpose equipment, including personal computers, becomes popular gradually. This means that the number of large telemedicine activities without any publication will increase.

Acknowledgments

I thank Dr. Kaihara Sigesato (National Okura Hospital), Professor Akitoshi Yoshida (Department of Ophthalmology, Asahikawa Medical University), Dr. Yasutomi Kinosada (Kyoto Prefectural University of Medicine), Dr. Isao Nakajima (Tokai University, School of Medicine) and Mr. Yoshiyuki Matsumoto (Japanese Ministry of Health and Welfare) for making this paper.

References

[1] S. Kaihara, Telemedicine in Japan, 1997.
http://square.umin.ac.jp/enkaku/96/Enkaku-RepSoukatu-nof-eng.html

[2] J. Picot, Sector Competitiveness Frameworks Series, Telehealth Industry, 1998. http://strategis.ic.gc.ca/SSG/hs01324e.html

[3] A. Yoshida and H. Hirokawa, Telemedicine and Telescience in the Field of Ophthalmology at Asahikawa Medical University, Proceedings of the 78th Hokkaido Medical Congress, 1998.

[4] Y. Kinosada *et al.*, Real Time Radiology in Kyoto. In: Proceedings of the 17th Japan Congress of Medical Informatics, 1997, pp. 530-531.

[5] H. Nagata *et al.*, Remote Control Method of Microscope in Still Image Telepathology System. In: Proceedings of the 16th Japan Congress of Medical Informatics, 1996, pp. 674-675.

[6] Y. Ogushi, Y. Haruki, Y. Okada, S. Shiraokawa, and H. Hirai, Development of a Clinical Information System Using Optical Memory Cards. In: Health Cards '97, IOS Press, Amsterdam, 1997, pp. 181-183.

[7] Y. Haruki, Y. Ogushi, Y. Okada Y, *et al.,* Emergency Medical system in a Great Disaster Using Communications Satellite. In: Proceedings of the 2nd Conference of Asia Pacific Association of Medical Informatics, 1997, pp. 874-878.

[8] Y. Okada, Y. Haruki, Y. Ogushi Y, *et al.,* A Multimedia Medical Textbook on a Satellitic Network System, *Journal of the American Medical Informatics Association*, Symposium Supplement, 1997, 882.

[9] Y. Okada, Y. Haruki, Y. Ogushi, M. Horie. Personal Health Data on Optical Memory Cards in Isehara City. In: Personal Medical Information, Springer-Verlag Berlin Heidelberg, 1997, pp. 195-198.

Address for correspondence

Yoshikazu Okada
Department of Medical Informatics
Tokai University, School of Medicine
Isehara, Kanagawa
JAPAN 259-1193
Tel: +81-463-93-1121, Fax: +81-463-96-4301
E-mail: yoshikaz@is.icc.u-tokai.ac.jp

The Impact of Telemedicine on Health Care Management
M. Nerlich and R. Kretschmer (Eds.)
IOS Press, 1999

Telehealth in British Columbia: From Design to Delivery

Barry R. WIGGS
University of British Columbia - St.Paul's Hospital, Vancouver, Canada

Telehealth initiatives are notoriously difficult to fund due to a lack of evidence in the cost effectiveness of expensive, difficult to deploy technology. British Columbia, as other provinces, has been wrestling with how to use advanced technologies in a manner, which maintains BC's lead for state of the art health care, and yet also ensure financially stable solutions.

The BC Provincial Government, through the Information, Technology and Science Division, has deployed a network connectivity system in BC (HealthNet BC) which interconnects 100% of all health professional institutions. The network is an open standards architecture also available to for profit corporations that obey strict security and information privacy regulations. HealthNet is the primary and preferred method for sharing patients related information in British Columbia. Two key value added services were deployed early on the HealthNet system. Teleplan is an electronic billing system first established in 1985 and through which all Medical Services Plan reimbursements are made. PharmaNet is a Provincial access and deployment system for pharmaceuticals. The system tracks dangerous drug interactions, enforces a valuable reference based pricing scheme and serves as a user point of contact to update Provincial Health ID's and basic patient information. With these key features, an electronic prescription system, a unique patient identifier and a ubiquitous health information network British Columbia is clearly grasping the capabilities of advanced technologies in a rational manner for the benefit of their residents.

Apart from Provincial efforts individual health regions are further striving to use advanced technologies in their specific health regions (20 such regions exist in British Columbia). Providence Health Care is a conglomeration of eight facilities in urban Vancouver, over 5,000 employees, numerous affiliated clinics and physicians offices all with an annual operating budget of approximately ½ billion dollars. St. Paul's Hospital, the largest member of the cluster is also the BC Heart Centre as well as a key resource site for projects in renal, ICU, emergency, cardiac, utilisation management and other health information areas. As a new feature Providence Health Care has an aggressive senior leadership team with a specific goal of achieving a seamless single operating environment. With a strong focus on staff education and cost containment the role of technology in aiding these goals was seen as pivotal.

Health facilities run on paper, lots and lots of paper. In fact we are not satisfied with just one piece of paper, we insist on numerous copies of the same form. Focusing for now on technology friendly areas like radiology and biomedical engineering we are exploring using CrossPad devices from the Cross-Pen Computing Group and IBM. These devices allow standard paper forms to be completed using normal pen and ink and yet record an electronic copy of the form in the tablet for computer to read. Using IBM's hand writing recognition software these sheets and forms are translated automatically saving technician time and dramatically increasing the time to deliver the form to its needed locations. Zero training time, deployment cost 1/5 that of a PC, using technology to achieve valuable cost effective solution that aid information flow.

An important goal, at this conference and others, is the achievement of an electronic lab information system. To date no health institution has achieved this objective, at least until Friday November 13th. On that date St. Paul's hospital successfully deployed a full feature lab information system containing lab test collection data, available of lab tests, information on test interpretation. The system is scheduled for a full role out in Jan-Mar of 1999 to numerous BC facilities. The financial focus for this project was to reduce lab help calls and to reduce retest requests due to information errors. Again, using information technology to meet a need that can aid all British Columbian health professionals and patients.

In one of BC's largest health regions, Simon Fraser Health Region, the nursing professionals have placed their manuals online in a web-based manner. These manuals have been received with enthusiasm from the nurses. While a basically simple task again, we have British Columbians working to deploy valuable information services for British Columbians. Keeping with the Simon Fraser Health Region they soon realised that once skill manuals were deployed, users would need interactive based training to help increase their skill level when needed. In addition, large health regions like Simon Fraser have government-mandated training required for areas such as hazardous material handling and infection control measures. Given that most regions already had extensive training materials in video or paper based forms Simon Fraser approached a BC firm called CanCoach which helps educators develop self paced, interactive, multimedia training CDs with testing that could be user driven and yet educator monitored. In only a few hours a deployable infection control module was available for regional use. Again, British Columbian technology is being used to aid British Columbians.

What about broadband, the high-end level of networking that makes everyone wonder as each application is deployed and demonstrated? Well at St. Paul's Hospital we haven't been ignoring this exciting network option! We looked at telepathology, but our studies clearly showed that near HDTV resolution would be needed for clinical accuracy. Teleradiology taught us the need for PAVS system, which we are now deploying (a self-built Canadian solution by the way at a cost of just 10% of commercial packages!). Cardiology was a voracious eater of bandwidth and is one where we hope to deploy services beyond OC3 in the near future.

Where do we sit with our brightest lights, our most cherished moments that show us the true future that technology can offer both health professionals and health service users alike? Our brightest lights exist in the youth of British Columbia, in young professionals like, the soon to be, Dr. Robin Verhaege. As one of BC's new candidates, a second year medical student, she represents the goals of BC's new medical education program. Based on problem based learning with a focus on self-directed skills she has taken up the additional challenge to learn and understand the technology of telehealth. Using systems from StarVision, a BC company specialising in high quality medical health systems. By involving people like Robin British Columbia is ensuring that the next generation of medical professionals will be well prepared to use advanced technologies in their daily practice.

As a facility, St. Paul's Hospital has elected to remove its existing data communications infrastructure and replace it with an ATM based technology from a world leader in advanced network devices, Newbridge Networks. Deploying a fully redundant broadband network has allowed a vast reduction in trouble calls, ability of a reduced staff to manage a vastly larger network and to begin investigation into voice via IP technology.

Where does the future lie for those willing to study and deploy these cost effective and enabling technologies? The future lies in the realisation of contracts for service delivery to nations across the globe on a for profit basis. The future further lies in delivering a higher standard of care to our own provincial members so they can benefit from better care, closer to home. The key is better health, the tool is simply technology.

Address for correspondence

Barry R. Wiggs
Providence Health Care, St. Paul´s Site
1081 Burrard Street
Vancouver, BC V6Z 1Y6, Canada
Phone: +1-604-631-5518
Fax: +1-604-631-5302
E-mail: bwiggs@stpaulshosp.bc.ca

The Impact of Telemedicine on Health Care Management
M. Nerlich and R. Kretschmer (Eds.)
IOS Press, 1999

The SIREN Legal Workshops: List of Urgent Legal Actions for Telemedicine

Otto RIENHOFF
Medical Informatics, University of Göttingen, Göttingen, Germany

1. Security and its Legal Basis

The EU funded Accompanying Measure SIREN was designed for the dissemination of relevant information about security in regional health networks to as many European Health Telematics projects as possible. In addition, health policy makers, users, and specialists on the international level should be informed about the results of European research and development projects dealing with security under the specific conditions of the healthcare systems. Furthermore, SIREN contained a small legal work-package, which was designed to bring together the experience from various projects and legal initiatives to embed technical security options into a legal framework which, in the long run, will give health telematics a sound and comfortable legal basis.

In consequence to this mission statement, most of the SIREN experts were selected according to the links they had to other projects or national/regional activities in that field. Of specific interest in this context were several other studies financed by the European Union, e.g. in DG XV, several national legislation (e.g. Italy and Germany), and a couple of implementation plans for so-called health professional cards (e.g. France, Slovenia, etc.). SIREN is addressing security in regional networks. In this context „security“ is defined as:

> *safeguarding the confidentiality, integrity, availability and accountability of data through the implementation of appropriate and effective security measures, guaranteeing thus the freedom and integrity of individuals in a potentially harmful health telematics environment.*
> *According to the Oxford Dictionary: security is something that provides safety, freedom from danger or anxiety.*

In this respect, digital signatures and cryptography are measures to guarantee security in networked healthcare systems. Regarding legal aspects of security one has to remember that the medical document is the centrepiece of all medical documentation which takes place in the context of a given patient-provider contract.

When SIREN started in 1996, harmonisation and standardisation activities were already on their way within CEN, ISO, and the spectrum of the so-called G7 Projects. Therefore specific attention has been paid to these issues.

In addition, one SIREN work-package (overseas relations) was orientated towards security developments in countries or regions to which the European Union has specific relationships (e.g. Canada, Latin America, South Africa and Central Asia). These SIREN related activities provided further information about the international approaches to security in health related

networks and to the various national and international plans for legislation regarding telemedicine in healthcare.
A state-of-the-art analysis prior to the SIREN project proposal in 1996 had led to the conclusion that the diversity of the legal aspects of security may be difficult to harmonise if not a general description of the medical documentation process framed into a kind of metamodel of the legal aspects can be formulated. After two years of work and numerous contacts in the European Union and globally, it can be concluded that this assumption was not only valid, but that the situation regarding a possible legal harmonisation has become less favourable in the meantime. The latter is due to the fact that because of pressing legal questions, specifically regarding liability issues, several countries have started to regulate the issue on national level. This leaves a perspective that in the rather short time of two to three years, national rules and regulations will be so diverse, that cross-border telematics applications in healthcare cannot develop.

2. Current Status

It can be stated that during the last fifteen years players in given healthcare systems have traditionally focussed on various issues other than communication security with the exception of the limited area of data protection. In addition, the cost containment discussion has become overwhelming for most health administrations focussing on public health oriented national health systems with the intention, to keep costly technological innovations in the patient care area as low as possible. In this school of thought, every new care provider produces a new market and new costs. Therefore, technical developments able to raise the numbers of providers (e.g. through consultation services) have been greeted with scepticism.

Security technology is perceived as another element of highly developed technological infrastructure. Therefore plans for effective introduction of health telematic systems to prepare the sector for the so-called information age are perceived as causing a new stream of high-tech equipment into the provider arena with a resulting rise in overall health care costs.

This situation has resulted in a lack of confidence into telemedical work, specifically regarding liability consequences.

3. Bottom-up Approach

The bottom-up approach of SIREN started with the analysis of the most relevant scenarios. From extensive discussions in the G7 Sub-Project 6 (Health Professional Cards) as well as in TRUSTHEALTH I and in SIREN, it is to be expected that two main telemedicine scenarios are the most likely to be of relevance in the next decade:

- A patient moves to a different region or country and needs medical support there. The health professional treating him contacts a healthcare institution which has relevant patient data for the treatment episode. A communication is thus established in relation to medical data in which authentification of both sides and communication security is of utmost importance.
- The health professional is treating a patient in one country and requires tele-consultation with health professionals in other countries. In this case, the same requirements for authentification and security apply as in the first example. In addition, the legal framework for the consultation purpose has to be defined.

There is an agreement that tele-assistance will also become an important issue within the next decade, but it will take some years for this to gain same relevance as the first two points.

Because of the extensive work which has been published already on data protection, and as the current discussion is focussing on liability issues and intellectual property rights, SIREN analysis is limited to the liability aspects. Nine topics were identified which play a role in this context:

- Medical liability
- Organisational liability
- Product liability
- Service liability
- Criminal liability
- Contract liability
- Patient liability
- Patient safety
- Data protection principles.

The final report of SIREN gives many details to these headings and information about the legal situation in the EU member states. It will be available for the 5th Framework Programme as a book to help project tenders in this issue. Some conclusions are summarised below.

4. Conclusion

1. To support the development of cross-border health telematic systems, systematic research as well as the development of European or global codes of good practice and ethics is urgently needed.

2. The most common solutions which can be expected in telemedicine within the next two to three years urgently necessitate the development of a set of model contracts which can be used between patients and service providers or between different service providers in the field of tele-consultancy.

3. A strong promotion of collaboration between health professional societies in the European Union is of vital interest to start harmonisation of professional regulations and specifically of authentification procedures in the different member countries. In addition, a harmonisation of the professional registration procedures would be extremely helpful as they would be the basis for smooth operation of Trusted Third Parties services.

4. Research into the new legal issues raised by the future developments in medicine and health telematics technology is urgently required, specifically in relation to the consequences of molecular medicine and virtual reality systems.

5. The complexity of the issues as well as the scarcity of senior professionals in the field able to integrate knowledge about health telematics, law and medicine defy easy solutions put forward by many individual technically oriented projects for their specific purpose only. Instead, it is necessary for future research and development programmes of the European Union to address this matter with substantial specialised legal projects which link closely to technical projects. However, the experiences of SIREN teaches that the link to other projects has to be contractually built into their projects programmes.

6. The high interest which the SIREN work found in many European countries and overseas makes it clear that there is an urgent need to know more about the issues addressed. As many overseas countries are interested in tele-collaboration with European institutions in the healthcare area and as international tele-consulting on a global level may become reality in a few years, all European projects should address the matter on a global scale following early developments in the so-called G7 / G8 projects.

Reference

[1] Rienhoff et al. (Eds.): A Legal Framework for Security in European Healthcare Telematics. IOS, Amsterdam 1999 (in preparation)

Address for correspondence

Prof. Dr. Otto Rienhoff
Medical Informatics
University of Göttingen
Robert-Koch-Strasse 40
D-37075 Göttingen
Tel.: +49-551-39 34 31, Fax: +49-551-39 24 93
E-mail: haegar@med.uni-goettingen.de

The Impact of Telemedicine on Health Care Management
M. Nerlich and R. Kretschmer (Eds.)
IOS Press, 1999

Health Care Professionals Protocol for Secure Online Transmission of Patient Data

Christoph F-J GOETZ
Projekbuero Telemedizin, Kassenaerztliche Vereinigung Bayerns, Munich, Germany

Abstract: One of the results of the 49th Bavarian Physician's Conference was that in 1996 the Bavarian Statutory Health Care Administration (Kassenärztliche Vereinigung Bayerns, KVB) and the Bavarian Medical Association (Bayerische Landesärztekammer, BLÄK) jointly suggested a project for the development and verification of a security infrastructure for the online transmission of medical patient data. This Project, the so-called "Health Care Professionals Protocol" (HCP-Protokoll), was designed to establish the first consensus standard for a secure and provably open system to be used in the health care system operating under the constraints of the diverse and heterogeneous IT-infrastructure in Bavaria, with a view towards utilization in all of Germany.

In January 1997, the HCP-Protocol was accepted as the strategic mainline project for telematics applications in medicine by the State of Bavaria and endowed with more than 1.3 million DM in the framework of "Bavaria Online II".

In the meantime, various national organizations of the German medical community as well as important industrial partners have expressed support for this initiative. Mention in the Roland-Berger study "Telematics in Health Care, Perspectives of Telemedicine in Germany", designation as an "exemplary scenario" in the final report of the Working Group 7 of the *Forum Info 2000* "Telematics Applications in Health Care", as well as integration of the new German health professional card, make the HCP-Protocol the most promising candidate for a *de facto* standard in the security infrastructure for all participants in health care telecommunication in Germany.

Since the middle of 1998, an expert group under the guidance of the joint "Projektbüro Telemedizin" of the KVB and BLÄK has been working on the definition of this protocol, taking into consideration the current legal framework of the German medical profession (Berufsordnung), the German signature law (SigG), and the national data security laws (BDSG), as well as today's technical possibilities and existing components.

The results of this definition will be published at the first opportunity (sometime during the first half of 1999) and then placed into public domain, so that any solution provider can reference this source to create secure and mutually interoperable application programs for health care professionals in Germany.

1. Health-Telematics Infrastructure in Germany

The abstract promise of telemedicine is very much in the front of every health professional's mind as he tries to decide how one or more of the suggestions presented at this conference can be implemented in his daily work. Presumably, it is a moot point to emphasize that one of the major effects for which all investors in telematics applications hope is a reduction of costs in our health care systems. In this context, it becomes clear that the vision which moves us all is that of a qualified, secure, and provable health telematics application for the transmission all of the data which physicians need in their offices or in hospital settings. The hopes are the same in Germany; however, the situation is very complex here and so it is probably necessary to give a short indication of where the major aspects of the inherent problems lie.

This diagram is intended as a schematic representation of communication channels in German health care. The left apex of this hexagram ("Prx") represents one of the doctors' offices, while the small circles grouped around it represent the remainder of the over 120 thousand offices in Germany. The next circles ("KV") represent the 23 public health care administrations and the ones at right ("ÄK") represent the 18 medical associations on a state level. There are numerous insurance companies ("Ks"), both statutory and commercial, pharmacies ("Apo"), and hospitals ("Kl"), to name only a few of the most important partners in our health care system. Generally speaking, each of these has a potential need to communicate with any or all of the other partners.

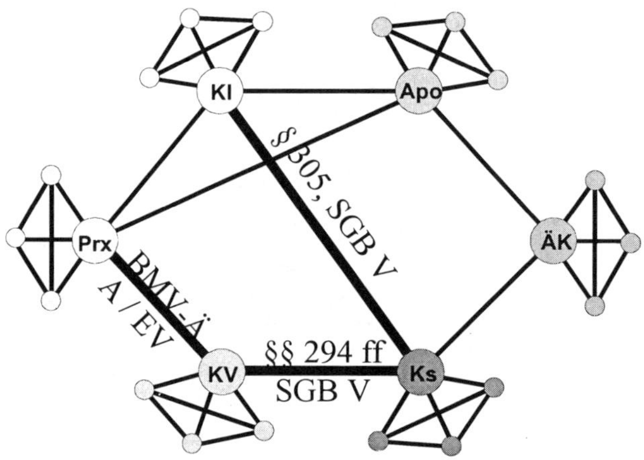

Figure 1: Exemplary Topology of Major German Health Communication

At this time, three major routes of electronic communication are firmly established in German health care. The first route transports statutory health care billing information from the doctors' offices to the public health care administrations ("BMV-Ä"). The forwarding of this data to statutory insurance companies ("§294") constitutes the second route, and the forwarding of comparable information from hospitals ("§301") directly to insurers is the third route of established information transfer. All three together transport on the order of a terabyte of data each quarter.

When considering the future potential for communication, however, it is necessary to face up to the fact that the communication needs between physicians among one another far outweigh these routes in terms of data volume as tomorrow's primary information mainlines. Physicians' communication with hospitals is expected to come in as a close second in future data volume, with perhaps information transfer between doctors and pharmacies in third place. While this ranking is speculative, it is certain that today's established communication lines will fade into the background in comparison with future data transfer volumes.

2. The Standardization Challenge

It is a fact that in health care almost every player has potential communication needs with any other participant, and therefore the question arises as to how this can be realized. Classically there are two methods: on the one hand, everyone can begin on their own, but the result of a Babylonian chatter of different systems is obvious; on the other hand, everybody can wait for nationally standardized components, or maybe even internationally standardized methods. In this case, experts would still be sitting around talking in ten years, without ever having transmitted a single byte of information. A different method therefore has to be found to avoid both extremes.

What the user in health care needs is a single, transparent, operable, and secure communication tool for the transfer of all potentially patient-related data-- almost in the sense of a "fire and forget" situation, in which the user never has to worry as to which network his intended addressee is connected, which communication application his partner will be using to receive the transferred data, or which security system the other has installed.

This implies that three levels of standardization are necessary for the postulated data transfer and that each of these has to be considered in the development of future projects.

- The first level is that of *addressing standards*. It is expected that this will be solved by the communications industry in terms of Internet compatibility. This means that the participants of health care will have to take this as a "given". Specifically, each physician will decide on his own provider for networking purposes, on the individual basis of cost, availability, and many other subjective factors. A single centralized communications network for health care is not a realistic concept for the future.
- The second necessary level of communication concerns the *security standards* used for authentication, etc. This is the level for which the Health Care Professionals Protocol is suggesting a solution.
- No security is necessary if there is no communicable content, or if the transmitted data cannot be interpreted or "understood" by the recipient. The third level therefore concerns *content standards*, and there are a number of different standards currently being used here in Germany which have an international potential. Among these is the originally national "xDT" standard, used here by all doctors' office computer systems (at least for statutory health care billing purposes) and which is currently being migrated towards the international XML standard, as it is known from Internet communications.

The salient point is that none of these necessary standardizations can be imposed or ordered by any single institution in German health care. The diversely organized groups in the German health care system previously mentioned are not united by a single institution which can implement methods or standards by directive. This means that major standards must be established here *via* the so-called *de facto* standardization which comes from widespread use of published or public domain standards.

3. The HCP-Protocol Concept

The HCP-Protocol project aims to address the four major security issues entailed in the online transmission of patient data for health care professionals. The *authentication* aspect will be solved by the introduction of an official physician's ID as the first implementation of a health professional card here in Germany. This card will also be a basis for delivering the *cryptography* methods used for hybrid model (asymmetric-symmetric) communication of transport data. Other security aspects include the *non-repudiation* of origin and receipt, as well as the verifiable implementation of a *time-to-live* scheme for transmitted data.

An example may clarify what is meant with by a "time-to-live scheme". During daily work, a physician or health professional does not have time to check on the receipt of each important transmitted message, and therefore must be automatically notified by the system whenever a receipt is not received within a specified period of time.

It is obvious that such a protocol definition cannot be created without taking into consideration standards or methods which already exist. The official German electronic physician's ID will be one of the cornerstones of the planned security infrastructure. The specification is currently being developed by a joint working group of the German Statutory Health Care Administration (Kassenärztliche Bundesvereinigung, KBV) and the German Medical Association (Bundesärztekammer, BÄK). Also necessary are card reader terminals which will conform to the already established "MKT" standard. These card readers are already in production. Finally, other established methods can also give valuable aid in developing a consensus standard for needed security protocol.

A look beyond the reaches of the HCP Protocol shows how the activities of other online projects are progressing. Table 1 shows only a small portion of major online projects as they exist in Germany. Currently at least 15 major groups are trying to provide communication services for the medical community and therefore all of them have to find a method to produce interoperability.

- Multimedica (HOS): Bertelsmann-Springer
- TeleMED Datennetz: TeleMED
- SEDI-Health (§ 301): Siemens
- T-Mart. Global Healthcare: Telekom
- Health Net: Inter Medical
- D/G/N: Deutsches Gesundheitsnetz
- (Networked Doctors' Offices . . .)

Table 1: Major Network Projects in Germany

The Health Care Professionals Protocol Project intends to provide security for asynchronous point-to-point and/or server-based communication using a container standard as a black box for all currently used content standards. The black box concept ensures that a developer does not have to worry about how the data is encrypted here for each type of message, using the keys from the electronic physician's ID. The project participants expect to achieve a consensus on this standard by placing the specification into public domain and by specifying only the minimal necessary implementation procedures so that encryption as well as decryption can be realized using both software and hardware options.

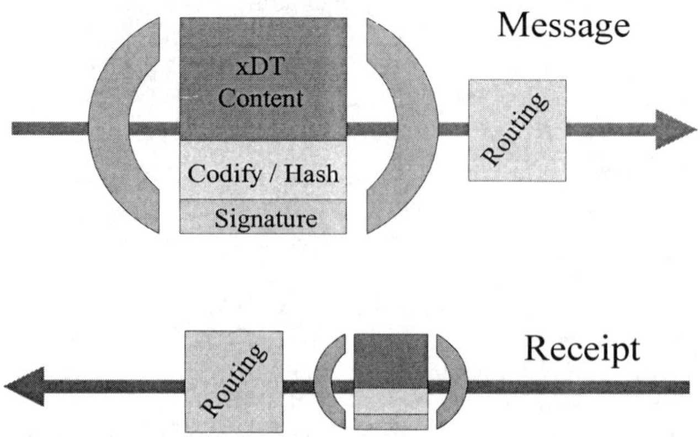

Figure 2: HCP-Protocol Black-Box Container Model

It should be emphasized that even potentially personalized data in health care should be included in this security context. The reasoning behind this is that a health professional generally does not have time to determine if each bit of clinically relevant data is completely anonymous; or even if not, re-identification of a patient may be possible from a specific combination of otherwise non-personalized data. Because of this, medical data acquired in a clinical setting should always be considered personalized and treated as such.

Basically, the HCP-Protocol specifies a cryptographically secured block of data with a hash and digital signature to prove its authorship and completeness which can be transmitted *via* any open-routed network. The Protocol itself will require certain types of receipts as answers to specific types of transmitted message contents; ensuring that non-repudiation of origin, a receipt can be securely implemented.

Why is it that such a security infrastructure has to be specified as an open protocol in the public domain and cannot be realized using a single piece of commercial software? The fact of the matter is, that more than 68% of the more than 120 thousand privately practicing physicians in Germany already use computers in their offices and the software used comes from more than 200 different companies. Adding the fact that more than 15 network providers are currently offering their services, the health telematics situation in Germany must be described as enormously diverse and heterogeneous-- and yet it has been possible to establish a single, standardized interface for the transmission of billing data in statutory health care by its consequent publishing and rigorous certification. This method is also to be used for the implementation of a security infrastructure.

The HCP-Protocol implementation specification will therefore have to define a "plug-in" which any software company can program. This plug-in will have to protect the client system from attacks outside of the telecommunication network in the sense of a fire-wall, and at the same time cipher and decipher transmitted messages as necessary. Functionally, it has a connection to the generic network system, accepts and generates the necessary control data, and passes patient data through a protocol engine which ciphers or deciphers in accordance with the security state provided by health professional cards in the MKT reader.

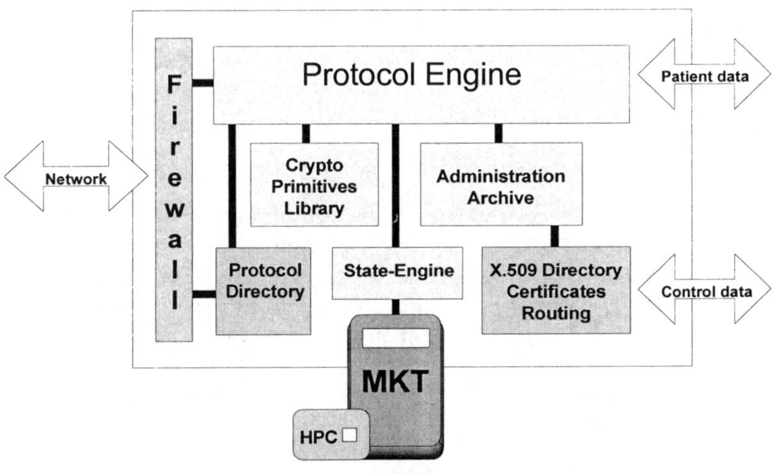

Figure 3: HCP-Protocol Functional Block Diagram

The Health Care Professionals Protocol will be specified in a public domain paper which will be called the "White-Blue Book". Any institution, company, or individual wishing to implement this protocol in their software will have access to this specification and can learn how to create functionally compatible and interoperable software.

This project is publicly funded through "Bavaria Online II" by the State of Bavaria, with more than 1.3 million DM; work was officially begun on the 18th of June, 1998. This means that the planning stage has been successfully finished and first facts are beginning to emerge. Currently, available standard components and methods are being screened for possible implementation. Two dedicated positions will ensure that the work proceeds at the pace necessary for this rapidly developing technology.

Finally, to give an impression of the seriousness with which this project is being taken by its participants, all experts have signed a waiver of commercial rights to the contents of the White-Blue Book, ensuring that the results of the definition phase will be available to everybody without cost. This can be interpreted as clear and unequivocal industry support for the project, since it quickly proved obvious to all participants that only a unified, interoperable, and realistic security infrastructure can result in real "traffic" between the telecommunication partners in German health care.

4. The HCP-Protocol Work Items

The Project has already considered necessary legal issues and is currently addressing the identification of possible components for this protocol; therefore, they still have a lot of work cut out for them. The practical application is expected to be in place towards the middle of 1999. At first, patient data will only be transmitted in a closed shop setting, so that the efficiency of the method can be realistically tested before the interim report is published. After this proves successful, patient data will be transmitted over other open networks-- even to the point of allowing open Internet connections to be used, something that is currently not permitted in Germany.

- **National**
  - German Ministry of Health
  - Central Research Institute of Ambulatory Care in Germany
  - WG Health Professional Cards
  - WG Chip Cards in Medicine
  - TeleTrusT e.V.
- **State**
  - Bavarian Ministry of Health and Social Care
  - Bavarian Data Protection Commissioner
  - MEDIS-Institute of the GSF

Table 2: HCP-P Consensus Institutions

The project enjoys a consensus on the state and national levels by a large number of institutions. It should be emphasized that the major work in this project is not the selection of the correct technology, but the achievement of a consensus between the diverse institutions and partners in German health care telecommunication.

The perspectives of the project have been published by independent experts as exemplary. Among these was the so-called Roland-Berger Study, "Telematics in Health Care, Perspectives of Telemedicine in Germany" [1] funded by the national Finance and Health ministries, and the final report "Telematic Applications in Health Care" of the *Forum Info 2000* [2], an initiative of the German Federal Government together with the Ministries of Finance and Development.

5. The German Physician's ID

A first coordination of all major potential partners in a future German trust center for health care already took place on the 18th of December, 1997-- specifying that the first implementation of a Health Professional Card here in Germany is to be the Physician's ID. This will be a cornerstone of cryptographic methods and it is expected to be available for pilot projects in the beginning of 1999.

The specification is currently undergoing last consensus meetings, but the major points have already been finalized. Starting with a master file, three different asymmetric keys will be implemented, one for the legally binding and official German digital signature, one for the management of hybrid transport cryptography, and a third for enciphering local patient data. In addition, there will be a variable number of attribute certificates, divided into two groups: one for medical association specializations, and the other for health care administration authorizations. Each of these certificates will be implemented as an open tuple of attribute type and content, thereby ensuring that other partners in health care can implement their own institutional structure, thus preserving basic interoperability.

For the introduction of a German Health Professional Card for physicians, a specific organizational structure will be needed. The current model may seem somewhat complicated, but is definitely necessary to take into account all of the legal aspects now in force after the passing of the German digital signature law [3] on the one hand, and on the other hand, be in accordance with the policy specified by the German medical association. Each in their own right governs how Physician's ID's will be used in the future.

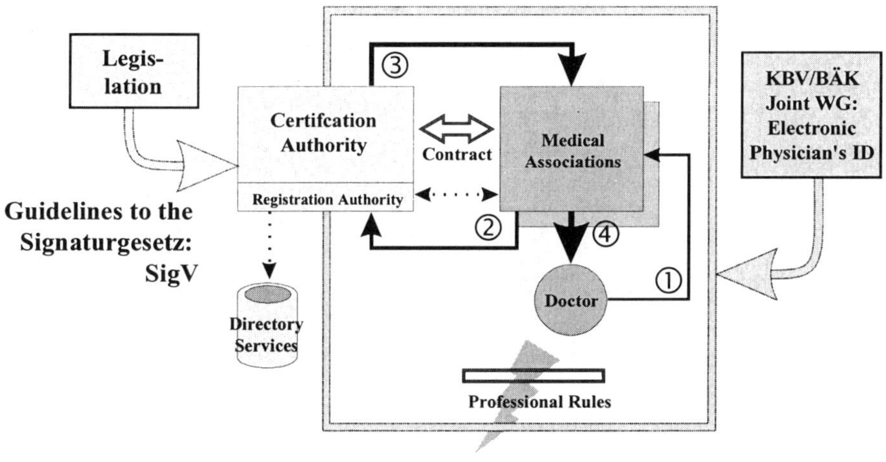

Figure 4: Organization of Physicians' ID Distribution

Specifically, it is planned to have the physician apply for a Health Professional Card with the State Medical Association, which will pass the application, HPC data, and certification data to the trust center; this center will charge the card and deliver it back to the State Medical Association, which will then send it to the applying physician. This somewhat roundabout scheme for HPC delivery is necessary to take into regard all of the current legislation concerning the official German digital signature and the medical profession regulations.

As a last thought, it may be good to keep in mind the final goal which this technology is setting about to achieve: the goal of the Health Professional Protocol is to provide a secure and interoperable platform, so that every physician and other health professional can exchange patient data with any other participant in the health care system here in Germany, and thereby take advantage of the cost reduction expected from the rapid and easy availability of medical data.

References

[1] Roland Berger and Partners, Telematik im Gesundheitswesen - Perspektiven der Telemedizin in Deutschland. Roland Berger Publishing, Munich, August 1997. http://www.iid.de/forschung/studien/telematik/

[2] Bundesminister für Gesundheit (Ed.), Telematik-Anwendungen im Gesundheitswesen: Nutzungsfelder, Verbesserungspotentiale und Handlungsempfehlungen. Schlußbericht der Arbeitsgruppe 7, Forum Info 2000, ISBN: 3-7890-5508-5. Nomos Publishing House, Baden-Baden, pp. 19-32.

[3] N.N., Gesetz zur Regelung der Rahmenbedingungen für Informations - und Kommunikationsdienste (Informations - und Kommunikationsdienste-Gesetz - IuKDG), Bundesgesetzblatt, 1997, Part I of the 28th of July 1997, pp. 1870 ff.

Address for correspondence

Christoph F-J Goetz
Projekbuero Telemedizin
Kassenaerztliche Vereinigung Bayerns
Arabellastrasse 30
81925 Munich, Germany
E-mail: christoph.goetz@kvb.de

The Impact of Telemedicine on Health Care Management
M. Nerlich and R. Kretschmer (Eds.)
IOS Press, 1999

Results of European Projects Enabling Secure Regional, National and International Health Care Networks

Bernd BLOBEL
Otto-von-Guericke University, Magdeburg, Germany

Abstract: Based on the work of the ISHTAR, the TRUSTHEALTH1, the EUROMED-ETS and the MEDSEC project funded by the European Commission, the synergetic results of these different projects in providing a security infrastructure for the test environment of an oncological network will be demonstrated.

The ISHTAR project investigated security issues in Health Care Establishments (HCE). It provides guidance for threat and risk analysis, and defines a schema for specification and implementation of appropriate security services and mechanisms to respond to the HCE security requirements of both communication and application security concepts.

The TRUSTHEALTH1 project dealt with specification and test implementation of basic security services and mechanisms based on Health Professional Cards (HPC) and Trusted Third Party (TTP) services.

Within the EUROMED-ETS project, the security solution has been extended to the Internet environment and WWW tools, successfully creating an Internet-based international TTP structure between the universities of Athens, Calabria, and Magdeburg.

Finally, in the MEDSEC project the specification and implementation of a generic EDI security solution has been delivered to provide secure communication between applications and sites.

In the ongoing TRUSTHEALTH2 project, the results of all these projects will be implemented in a real environment of cancer care.

1. Introduction

In all countries around the world, societal domains including the health care sector are changing due to important changes in political, social, organisational, and technological constraints and circumstances. This movement is characterised by increasing quality and efficiency of systems and procedures, as well as by extending or integrating their underlying structures regionally, nationally, or even internationally. Considering the health care domain, the specialisation and decentralisation of service providers is inseparably connected with the enforcement of communication and co-operation between all parties directly or indirectly involved in patients' care or citizens' health in the future [1]. The current development is also called the movement towards shared care and the establishment of health (care) networks. In that context, shared care is defined as "a continuous and co-ordinated activity of

- different persons in
- different institutions under
- employment of different methods at
- different times

in order to be able to help patients optimally with respect to their

- medical,
- psychological and
- social being" [2].

The structural changes mentioned above must be accompanied by communication and co-operation at the level of underlying information systems (IS). To enable communications and co-operation between systems from different vendors with different environments in hardware and software, middleware concepts are the appropriate way to realise open integration of the systems involved. The common middleware approaches in health information systems are EDI[1] (HL7[2], XDT[3], EDIFACT[4]), open interoperable systems (RICHE, DHE, SYNAPSE[5]), or component systems (CORBA[6], COM/DCOM/ActiveX[7]). For the first time, the most important middleware solutions during the last two or three years, such as HL7, DHE and CORBA, have been discussed and compared in [3]. The resulting systems are networks of health care providers (direct and indirect) with networking IS (health networks).

2. Communication and Information Services in Health Networks

Medical Networks provide communication services, information services, and interactive services. These services might be common, domain-specific, area-specific, or group-specific. Electronic mail and file transfer are examples of communication services. Non-specific information services are search engines for intelligent information retrieval (e.g. LYCOS). Well-known examples of common information services are timetables, phone directories, city maps, etc. Traffic IS, environment IS, and geographical IS are domain-specific. Area-specific information services are, e.g., regional IS (e.g., citizen IS). Examples of group-specific IS are patient IS, doctors' profiles, etc. Examples of interactive services are teleteaching, electronic commerce (virtual mall), and teleworking.

For the creation of health networks, we need an appropriate infrastructure to provide the physical net and security, methods, and solutions (World Wide Web = WWW, video conferencing), and adequate IS (doctor's IS, HIS, pharmacist's IS, patient's IS). Network security responding to the results of threat and risk analysis is dependent upon the communication partner involved, communication content to be exchanged, communication services used, and communication infrastructure available or applied, respectively [1]. Essential fundamentals for trustworthy health networks are legal, professional, and personal consent between all partners involved or influenced, and an appropriate policy.

Security policy consists of a complex of legal, organisational, functional, social, ethical and technological aspects, which has to be considered in the context of data security and data protection. Policy defines the framework, rights and duties, but also penalties for the involved and/or responsible individuals and organisations [1, 4, 5]. In Germany, data protection concerns the individuals' rights and data security specifies the services needed. In the USA,

[1] Electronic Data Interchange.
[2] Health Industry Level Seven Communication Standard.
[3] German EDI protocol enabling communications between doctor's office systems and between them and other parties in the health care system.
[4] EDI for Finance, Administration, Commerce and Transport.
[5] European projects dealing with health information systems architecture (see, e.g., www.ehto.be).
[6] Common Object Request Broker Architecture, the OMG's middleware concept.
[7] Component Object Model, Distributed Component Object Model and ActiveX are Microsoft's middelware solutions.

privacy is separately mentioned. But in common use, the term "security" covers protection and privacy issues.

Looking at access rights, in general more detailed and comprehensive information is restricted for communication between fewer persons, as principally shown in Figure 1.

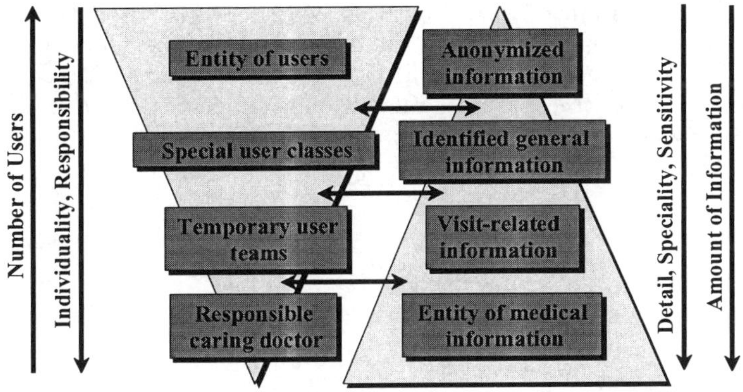

Figure 1: General relationship between access rights on the one hand and sensitivity and comprehensiveness on the other.

3. The Magdeburg Pilot of an EHR in Oncology

Among others in the German new federal states, the registry in the Magdeburg Cancer Centre was founded in 1992. Contrary to other German registries, this registry was designed and implemented from the beginning as a regional Electronic Health Record System supporting the shared care of cancer patients. Therefore, the cancer registry has been developed as a pilot with the first advanced security solution in German health care. 1993, the first German secure real time connections were established in routine, using analogous lines with the Modem Access Control device to provide strong system authentication, integrity proof, and DES encryption. 1995, the connections were replaced and extended by a secure ISDN line, providing systems security with strong authentication, digital signature, and confidentiality by an hybrid algorithm (RSA for session key exchange and 3DES for the plain text encryption). To realise real time behaviour, this solution is based on hardware, too. Because health care establishments cannot be considered internally as secure environments (about 70 % or more of attacks are caused by insiders) and due to legal requirements (there is a need for mutual authentication and accountability on the users' level), the security services must be user-centred or user-related. Therefore in 1996, specifications for an open solution of user-related (and additionally also system-related) security were developed, based on the European projects described in this paper. In that context, the first European implementation of the TrustHealth (Trustworthy Health Telematics) [6] Health Professional Card (HPC) was achieved in January 1997. Within the EUROMED-ETS (Trusted Third Party Services for Health Care in Europe) project [7], in September 1997 the first Internet-based Trusted Third Party (TTP) was installed, including the universities of Athens (Greece), Calabria (Italy), and Magdeburg (Germany) [8]. In April 1998, the first secure HL7 communication was demonstrated and is now routinely in use in the Magdeburg cancer registry. The activities described are also part of German initiatives like the German HPC model trial "Deutscher

Modellversuch Health Professional Cards" [9]. The detailed solution and ongoing work will be presented in the following sections.

Currently, 57 clinics and the Oncological After Care Organisation of the Kassenärztliche Vereinigung in our federal state Saxony-Anhalt-- representing about 250 GPs specialising in oncology-- are covered in the Clinical Cancer Register Magdeburg, which includes a catchment area of about 1.2 million inhabitants. Half of the partners (clinics of the university hospitals, public hospitals, private hospitals, ecclesiastical hospitals, and some GPs) are actually online. Until the end of 1999, all partners will be securely online by connection to our registry. Figure 2 gives an overview of the Saxony-Anhalt locations involved into the oncological network, also mentioning the two other registries which are not distributed like the Magdeburg facilities.

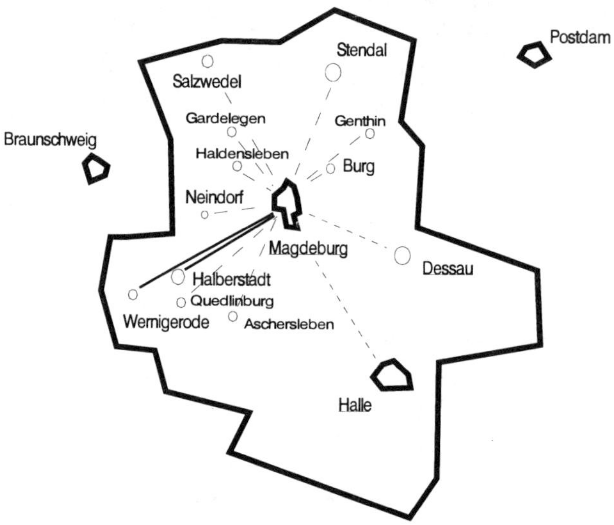

Figure 2: The Clinical Cancer Registry Magdeburg in the German federal state Saxony-Anhalt.

4. Security Model

The conceptual model for security in health information systems distinguishes the concepts of quality, safety, and security. All of them are fundamental for secure communications and co-operation between information systems. The latter concept contains also the very complex issues of security policy. Looking at the security concept only, we can distinguish the application security concept, describing the security services needed for secure applications and their trustworthy environment, from the communication security concept, dealing with security services for trustworthy communications (Figure 3). For references see, e.g., [1].

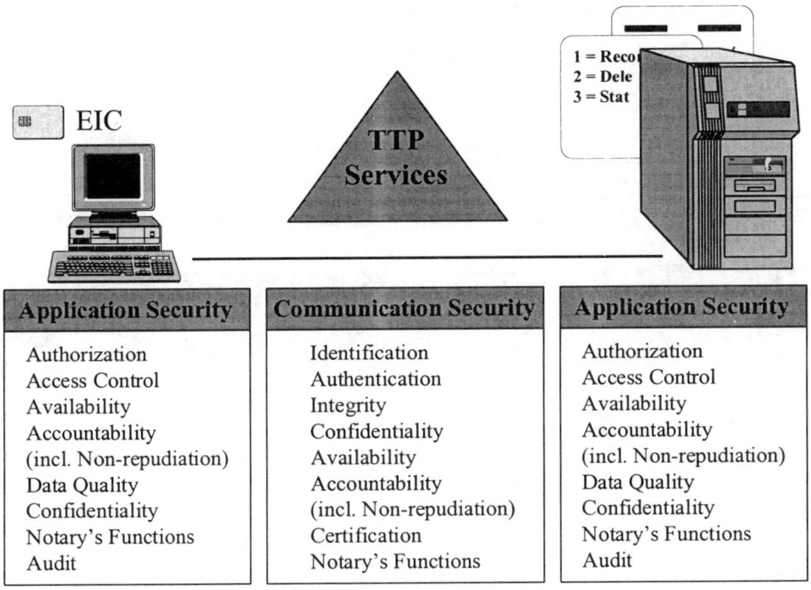

Figure 3: General security model

5. Threat and Risk Analysis

Within the ISHTAR (Implementing Secure Health Telematics Applications in Europe) project, a comprehensive threat and risk analysis has been performed using the SIDERO toolset developed by the Leiden University [10]. This toolset reflects the ITSEC criteria, the CRAMM methodology widely used in the U. K., and further skills [4].

To support different users' views, at the Magdeburg Medical Informatics Department an additional and universal methodology has been developed for information systems security analysis, systems specification, design, and implementation [11].

6. Security Services and Mechanisms

To define the security services needed and the security mechanisms required to implement them, an UML-based methodology has been developed within the ISHTAR project to analyse, define, design, and implement security solutions in health care [11]. Using different diagrams describing systems and their behaviour as class diagrams, use cases, state diagrams, sequence diagrams, collaboration diagrams, and development diagrams for the aforementioned concepts, a concept-services-mechanisms-algorithms-data scheme may be provided to respond to specified requirements with appropriate solutions. Figure 4 gives an example of communication security essentially for health networks. (Networks are also requesting specific application security not discussed in this paper.)

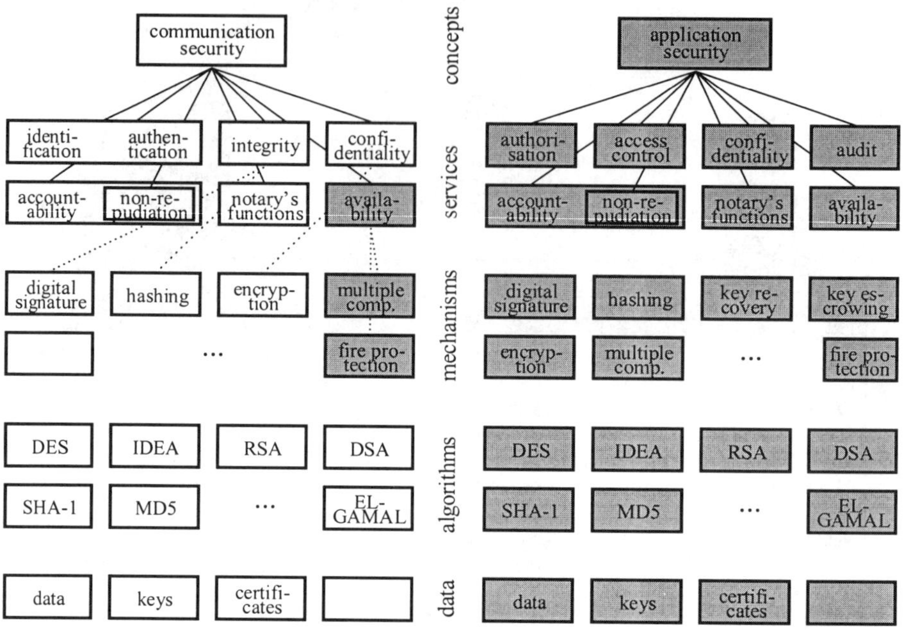

Figure 4: Security concepts-services-mechanisms-algorithms-data scheme.

7. Secure Communications and Secure Internet

To realise a trustworthy regional oncological network, first of all the communication security issues are the important challenges. The additionally required secure application has been provided for our routinely used distributed EHR in oncology, but the present paper does not concern this problem.

The security solution provided has to fit into the underlying middleware concept of the communicating and co-operating systems involved. According to the results of threat and risk analysis, the security concepts-services-mechanisms-algorithms-data relationship must be defined. Available standards have to be considered for specifying and implementing a practical solution. Table 1 describes the security threat and services needed for communication security.

Threats	Security Services
masquerading (unauthorised use of authorised services)	principal identification and authentication
data manipulation	integrity
concealment or manipulation of data origin	accountability in the sense of non-repudiation of origin
repudiation of receipt	accountability in the sense of non-repudiation of receipt
disclosure of data	confidentiality

Table 1: Security threats and services for communication security

Regarding the provision of services mentioned in Table 1 within the ISO OSI model for open systems interconnection and the protocols and products for fulfilling these requirements, two groups of communication security solutions may be distinguished (Table 2) [12, 13]:

- security solutions on the application level which provide object or message security in the sense of (user-related) end-to-end security, and
- security solutions of lower layers served to the upper layers which provide channel security in the sense of secure connections between systems.

Different protocols like MOSS, SSL, S/MIME, etc., combine different security services and related mechanisms at different levels according to their conceptual framework. For instance, SSL above TCP provides authentication, integrity, and confidentiality on a lower layer transparently to the applications. SSL Record Protocol encapsulates other higher level protocols like the SSL Handshake Protocol for two-way authentication between client and server, as well as for negotiation of algorithms and keys used at data transmission.

Security Services / OSI Layers	Confidentiality	Integrity	Entity Authentication	Data Origin Authentication	Non-Repudiation of Origin	Non-Repudiation of Receipt
Data Link	SILS/SDE, PPTP[8], L2TP	SILS/SDE, L2TP	PPTP, L2TP, L2F	SILS/SDE, L2TP	–	–
Network	IPSEC, NLSP	IPSEC, NLSP	IPSEC, NLSP	IPSEC, NLSP	–	–
Transport	SOCKS, TLSP, SSL, TLS, PCT, SSH	SOCKS, TLSP, SSL, TLS, PCT, SSH	SOCKS, TLSP, SSL, TLS, PCT, SSH	TLSP	–	–
Application	SHTTP, SPKM, MHS, MSP, PEM, SFTP, PGP/MIME, MOSS, S/MIME, PKCS#7	SHTTP, SPKM, MHS, MSP, PEM, SFTP, PGP/MIME, MOSS, S/MIME, PKCS#7	SHTTP[9], SPKM, SFTP	SHTTP, SPKM, MHS, MSP, PEM, SFTP, PGP/MIME, MOSS, S/MIME, PKCS#7	SHTTP, SPKM, MHS, MSP, PEM, SFTP, S/MIME, ESS	SPKM, MHS, MSP, SFTP, S/MIME, ESS

Table 2: Placement of security services

Within the MEDSEC (Health Care Security and Privacy in the Information Society) project-- which investigated available security standards in health care-- several specific standards, such as the CEN prENV "Security Categorisation and Protection of Health Information Systems", the "Digital Signature Standard", the DICOM standard, and the EDI standard HL7, which are important for the health care environment have been analysed and evaluated in the context of specific demonstration environments at the test sites involved in [14].

Finally, proposals for the security improvement of these standards have been made and validated. Within our oncological network, the HL7 standard has been explored. Any

[8] PPTP does not address any security issues in the current version, but end-to-end security is addressed by PPP which is tunnelled by PPTP through an IP network.

[9] Only the client is authenticated to the server by showing that he is able to apply message enhancement according to the security requirements of the server.

solutions have to be agreed upon internationally. To use these solutions routinely in our heterogeneous environment and to provide input for different international standardisation bodies, the investigations have been extended and the solutions have been generalised to include different EDI protocols and even channel security issues [12, 13]. The security solutions are based solely on standards or Publicly Available Specifications (PAS), e.g., CEN and ISO standards, Internet Engineering Task Force (IETF) RFCs, and cross-industrial standards such as Public Key Cryptography Standards (PKCS). Solutions have to be open and flexible (negotiable), fulfilling multi-protocol conditions by multi-protocol Application Programming Interfaces (APIs). Thus, the results comprise secure mailing (e.g., [15]) and secure FTP, but also other EDI protocols such as EDIFACT, XML, or the German XDT standard for communication between doctors' office systems and between these systems and the systems of other providers directly or indirectly involved in the health system.

For structuring messages and applied security mechanisms, Secure/Multipurpose Internet Mail Extensions (S/MIME) with PKCS#7 security enhancement is a preferred solution, but other protocols such as MOSS (MIME Object Security Services), PGP (Pretty Good Privacy), MSP (Message Security Protocol), PGP/MIME, etc., are also usable. The principals' authentication is provided by the ISO mutual three-way strong authentication procedure. Different use cases request open procedures for strong authentication not only for different principals such as systems or applications (e.g., HL7), but also for different users (e.g., XDT). To meet such flexible challenges, not only software solutions and plug-in-card solutions, but also user-related authentication "tokens" such as Health Professional Cards (HPCs) and their corresponding Trusted Third Party (TTP) services, are needed as defined in TRUSTHEALTH1 [16].

The underlying generic mechanism is based upon wrapping the communicated information. Reflecting the results of the EUROMED-ETS project funded by the European Commission and dealing with the security infrastructure for a pan-European health care network based on the WWW environment of the Internet, the secure channel solution could also be included in implementation. Within this project, the secure communication between EUROMED-PCs and EUROMED-Servers is provided *via* SSL [8].

8. Security Infrastructure

To realise security services based on cryptographic algorithms, a security infrastructure is needed for key generation, registration, naming, certification, directory services (including the management of certificate revocation lists), time stamping, etc. [16]. The entity of authorities providing such services are called Trusted Third Party (TTP). The German Digital Signature Law and its accompanying legislation are defining the German security infrastructure to support the future German smartcard-based electronic doctor's licence as the doctors' HPC. In the TRUSTHEALTH2 regional pilot for a secure oncological network, any type of health professional will be included. Therefore, besides a public TTP, a private one will also be used, mirroring certificates and thus reducing communication fees. Additionally, such a private TTP also supports international communications which are not covered by the legally bound TTP.

Some fundamentals for international communication and co-operation have been practically provided as of 1997 by the EUROMED-ETS project: as naming schemes, TTP structures, and cross-certificates. The corresponding pilot of cross-referencing TTPs has been established between the University of Athens (Greece) as root TTP and the universities of Calabria (Italy) and Magdeburg (Germany) (Figure 5) [8, 17].

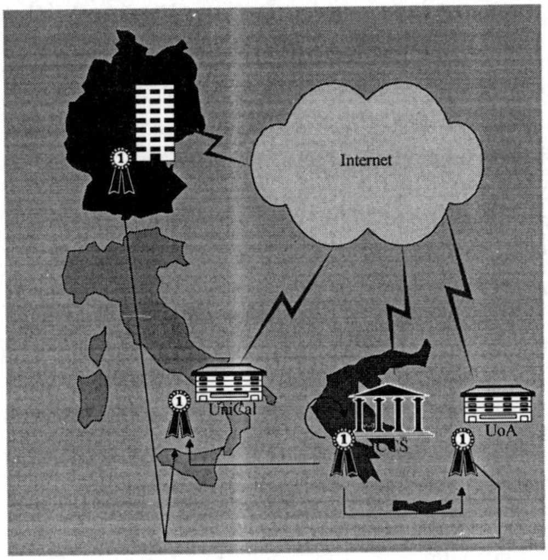

Figure 5: Internet-based International TTP Structure.

9. Conclusions

As a result of different projects funded by the European Commission, a secure distributed Electronic Health Record has been specified, developed, and implemented which supports scientific challenges, epidemiological requirements, and the practical needs of cancer patients' care. This small-scale pilot provides the basis for establishing a regional oncological network within the TRUSTHEALTH2 project. To meet the different requirements for such a system solution, the results of other projects dealing with

- the High Level Security Policy, threat and risk analysis, and tools which specify solutions in the sense of concepts, services, mechanisms, algorithms, and needed data (ISHTAR),
- the analysis and security enhancement of health informatics standards (MEDSEC),
- the security infrastructure for security services based on cryptographic algorithms as HPC and TTP services (TRUSTHEALTH1 and TRUSTHEALTH2), and
- the security requirements and solutions for European Internet-based health networks (EUROMED-ETS) have been combined to realise complex and practical solutions.

Unfortunately, the necessary added values could not be established without personal participation in results collection and integration. In summary, the appropriate technical services for secure health information systems and networks are available. However, there are huge legal, political, social, and organisational efforts needed. The involvement, education, and increased security awareness of future users are important challenges which must be met in order to fulfil the task of trustworthiness provision. Security is a legal, organisational, ethical, social, and psychological issue-- and a continuous task of management.

Acknowledgement

The author is in debt to the European Commission and to the Ministry of Education and Science of the German Federal State Saxony-Anhalt for funding, as well as to the partners of the projects mentioned for their kind co-operation.

References

[1] B. Blobel, G. Bleumer, A. Müller, E. Flikkenschild, and F. Ottes, Current Security Issues Faced by Health Care Establishments. *Deliverable of the HC1028 Telematics Project ISHTAR*, October 1996.

[2] K.-H. Ellsässer and C.O. Köhler, Shared Care: Konzept einer Verteilten Pflege-Kurz und Langfristige Perspektiven in Europa, *Informatik, Biometrie und Epidemiologie in Medizin und Biologie* **24** H.4, S. (1993) 188-198.

[3] B. Blobel and M. Holena, Comparing Middleware Concepts for Advanced Healthcare System Architectures, *International Journal of Medical Informatics* **46** (1997) 69-85.

[4] The SEISMED Consortium (eds.), Data Security for Health Care, Volume I-III. Studies in Health Technology and Informatics, Vol. 31-33. IOS Press, Amsterdam, 1996.

[5] B. Barber, A. Treacher, and K. Louwerse, Towards Security in Medical Telematics. IOS Press, Amsterdam, 1996.

[6] TrustHealth Consortium, Trustworthy Health Telematics 1. Project of the Fourth EU Health Telematics Applications Programme.http://www.ehto.be/projects/trusthealth/

[7] ETS Consortium, EUROMED - European Trust Structure. Information Society Standardisation Programme.
http://euromed.iccs.ntua.gr/

[8] S.K. Katsikas, D.D. Spinellis, J. Iliadis, and B. Blobel, Using Trusted Third Parties for Secure Telemedical Applications over the WWW: The EUROMED-ETS Approach, *International Journal of Medical Informatics* **49** (1998) 59-68.

[9] Arbeitskreis Health Professional Card, Deutscher Modellversuch - Health Professional Card. Arbeitspapier der Arbeitsgemeinschaft Karten im Gesundheitswesen, Universität Göttingen, Göttingen, Oktober 1996.

[10] ISHTAR Consortium, Implementation of Secure Health Telematics Applications in Europe. Project of the Fourth EU Health Telematics Applications Programme.
http://www.ehto.be/projects/ishtar/

[11] B. Blobel and F. Roger-France, Healthcare Security View Based on the Security Services Concept. ISHTAR Project HC 1028, Deliverable, August 1998.

[12] B. Blobel, V. Spiegel, R. Krohn, P. Pharow, and K. Engel, Standard Guide for HL7 Communication Security. ISIS MEDSEC Project, Deliverable 30, August 1998.

[13] B. Blobel, V. Spiegel, R. Krohn, P. Pharow, and K. Engel, Standard Guide for Implementing EDI Communication Security. ISIS MEDSEC Project, Deliverable 31, August 1998.

[14] MEDSEC Consortium, Health Care Security and Privacy in the Information Society. Project of the EU ISIS Programme.

[15] G. Schadow, M. Tucker, and W. Rishel, Secure HL7 Transactions using Internet Mail (draft-ietf-ediint-hl7). Internet Draft (EDIINT Working Group), July 21, 1998.
http://www.ietf.org/internet -drafts

[16] B. Blobel and P. Pharow, Security Infrastructure of an Oncological Network Using Health Professional Cards. In: L. Van den Broek and A.J. Sikkel (Eds.), Health Cards '97. Series in Health Technology and Informatics, Vol. 49. IOS Press, Amsterdam, 1997, pp. 323-334.

[17] B. Blobel and P. Pharow, Results of European Projects Improving Security of Distributed Health Information Systems. In: B. Cesnik, A.T. McCray, J.R. Scherrer (Eds.), MEDINFO '98,. IOS Press, Amsterdam, 1998, pp. 1119-1123.

Address for correspondence

Bernd Blobel
Otto-von-Guericke University Magdeburg
Institute of Biometrics and Medical Informatics
Leipziger Str. 44
D-39120 Magdeburg, Germany
Phone: +49-391-6713542, Fax: +49-391-6713536
E-mail: Bernd.Blobel@mrz.uni-magdeburg.de

Telemedicine Applications For Clinical Practice

NOAH
A Mobile Emergency Care System

Ulrich SCHÄCHINGER, Rainer KRETSCHMER, Carsten NEUMANN, Michael NERLICH
University of Regensburg Medical Centre, Dept. of Trauma Surgery, Regensburg, Germany

Abstract: Experiencing communication problems in our emergency services, we developed an innovative communication network and system (NOAH, which stands for Notfall-Organisations-und Arbeitshilfe, or Emergency-Organisation Active Aide System). In contrast with the currently established emergency services communication in Germany by radio wave, data is transferred from the scene in the form of an electronic record on a notepad-computer by means of the wireless data communication network Modacom (Mobile Data Communication), which is provided by German Telekom. It is received at the dispatch-centre in mentioned format and transferred to the admitting hospital without any loss of data.

In a prospective study, the technical and conceptual suitability of this system was investigated. It was shown that an admitting hospital was informed more than 20 minutes in advance about the admittance of a patient. To assure the quality of transferred data, information was ranked by different criteria. This further demonstrated that much more precise information about a patient's condition was already available upon admittance to the hospital.

1. Introduction

Emergencies occur anywhere, at any location, at any time, and in various different ways-- thus making any one of us susceptible.

Although the structure of the emergency care systems differ across nations, the aims in applying emergency medical services are worldwide the same:

- to save life,
- to limit damage to individual health,
- to initiate recovery procedures ensuring the best possible quality of life.

To reach these aims, the Federal Republic of Germany affords a very sophisticated emergency care system. The emergency medical services in Germany are provided by ambulance cars, vehicular emergency life support, and by helicopter-- making it one of the best systems world- wide [1]. In almost all serious medical emergencies, an emergency physician on-scene is alerted in addition to paramedics. The paramedics and on-scene physician are specially trained regarding emergency medicine and their medical equipment is highly advanced; this is why a German ambulance car or helicopter is sometimes dubbed a "Mobile Intensive Care Unit".

Due to technical and medical progress during the last few years and continued efforts to increase educational guidance for emergency physicians, emergency medical services have significantly improved. Despite good overall medical care, however, we have identified some weak points and points of non-conformance in the single phase of the rescue course which subject the patient to avoidable life-threatening situations. As an example, we find that an inadequate shock treatment facilitates development of post-traumatic multiple-organ-dysfunction, which threatens the patient's life even days after an accident. On the other hand, an improperly attended injury can lead to a life-long disability with secondary effects in reference to social and economical problems.

Therefore, the demands placed upon any rescue system are to reduce the therapy-free time intervals as much as possible, and to provide the emergency physician with the means required to foster optimal care.

Whereas physicians in the hospital environment are used to working on a team and can cross-reference with others, the emergency physician on the scene is confined to make his decision without the usual diagnostics. His basic knowledge has to handle specific emergencies on various specialities from gynaecology and obstetrics, to paediatrics, internal medicine, surgery, and others. In case of an accident, the physician additionally has to cover managerial functions, from the initial scene analysis to timely requests for additional rescue devices, as well as the choice for the proper hospital.

This procedure must be accompanied by complete, easy to evaluate, and transparent documentation [2].

While the medical and technical progress in the field of emergency medicine has been developed (e.g., lyse-therapy on acute myocardial infarctions or a new defibrillator) with considerable financial and investigative efforts, data communication and scene handling, as well as managerial functions, are comparatively underdeveloped. Primarily in the area of data communication, technical and managerial functions seem to be nearly unexplored.

We must therefore make an effort to optimise the information flow from the initial emergency call to the admitting hospital. Currently, communication between the emergency physician or ambulance and the dispatch-centre occurs wireless, using reserved radio frequencies (BOS-radio). Experienced communication problems are due to technical and system-related inadequacies, such as radio shadows (communication dead space), or the simultaneous use of different frequencies by the emergency physician/ambulance, fire-brigade, and police. While the use of existing direct frequencies has improved data communication regionally, this method entails considerable financial and technical efforts, and is therefore not widely used. It is the case now, as it has been before, that only one operator can communicate on any given channel at one time. The information flow also remains unchanged, dispersing unscreened and unstructured information to the operator in the dispatch-centre. This will inform the operator of the emergency physician's/ambulance location and their status, as well as additional information about other required rescue systems or special fire-brigades. This condition may foster the loss of information, or cause a delay in passing the medical condition to the admitting hospital, as experienced in the children's game "silent mail". At the present time, it is very difficult for the on-scene rescue team to obtain quick and secure information in selecting the most advantageous hospital. This also means that the admitting hospital is not properly informed about the incoming patient.

Upon admission to the hospital, the patient should be treated carefully, effectively, and spontaneously by a pre-informed and thoroughly prepared team in the shock room.

Incomplete (or lack of) incoming patient information for the admitting hospital leads to uneconomical usage of resources in cases of overestimation, and to damage to the patient in cases of underestimation.

Time loss in data communication in reference to time-sensitive situations-- such as severely injured patients, inter-cerebral haemorrhaging, myocardial infarction, or poisoning-- are not acceptable. These evident deficits in the intersection between rescue system and hospital have sparked headlines declaring "tourism of emergencies".

Our primary effort should therefore be concentrated on optimising the information-flow for all links within the rescue chain, starting at the emergency call and proceeding to the admitting hospital. Our goals are to specifically control available rescue-devices by means of improved communication technology, to inform the on-scene emergency physician of the availability of free regional capabilities, and lastly to standardise patient reporting.

Solution-approaches for improving the rescue system:

Given those negative headlines and problems encountered daily based in practical experience, (e.g., having no or false information about the injuries of an incoming patient), prompted our Department of Trauma-Surgery at Regensburg University and the Rescue-Centre Regensburg to develop an innovative communication network and co-ordination system called the Emergency-Organisation Active Aide System (NOAH, Notfall-Organisations- und Arbeitshilfe).

NOAH's solution approach focuses on improving the communication link from the emergency ambulance to the hospital and dispatch-centre by electronic data transfer.

2. Materials and Methods

The requirements for the new communication technology encompass the following merits: easy handling, consideration of all participants, integration of existing systems, optimised information flow during emergency missions, and avoidance of repetitive data collection [3,4].

This means: using notepad-generated patient identification cards, making individual data accessible prior to admission, and negating repeated record creation and processing.

The notepad-computer currently used is the "FORTÉ Wireless CommPad" from Motorola, Israel. It features a backlit VGA-compatible LCD display with a pen-based interface, an internal radio-modem for data-networks using the RD-LAP (Radio Data Link Access Protocol) protocol, an exchangeable internal battery providing 4 to 8 hours of operation, a 486DX processor, and a vehicle docking station. It is operational in wide temperature/humidity range and has a shock-proof, water-resistant design (e.g., withstands a four-foot drop). A close-up under winter conditions is shown in Figure 1.

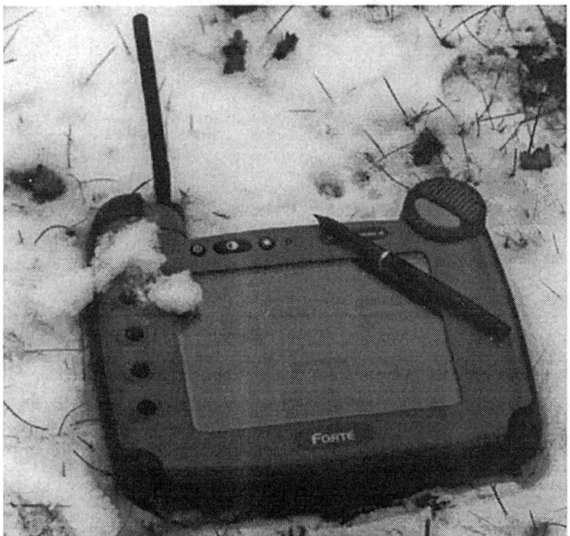

Fig. 1: FORTÉ Wireless CommPad in the Snow

Specifically, improvement of the pre-hospital to hospital process is achieved by using the notepad loaded with an electronic version of the German Society of Intensive Care and Emergency Medicine (DIVI) standardised emergency report [5], and the use of mobile data transfer *via* the wireless data communication network Modacom (Mobile Data Communication), which is provided by German Telekom and employs the RD-LAP 9.6 protocol.

The NOAH software has been developed by an interdisciplinary team consisting of on-scene physicians, trauma surgeons, MIS faculty members, and programmers from the company "Kratzer Communications, Munich" (an expert in wireless vehicle management solutions). The software has been developed for a standard PC platform and runs under Windows 3.1 or Windows 95/98.

The two methods mentioned above assist in improving the communication flow between the on-scene occurrence and the dispatch-centre. Within a few seconds, bi-directional data transfer and synchronisation with up to 1,000 other participants is possible.

After an emergency call reaches the dispatch centre, the dispatcher feeds the emergency instructions (e.g., the kind of emergency, location, and so on) to the dispatch centre's computer system; the NOAH communication-terminal at the dispatch centre will automatically forward this information to the notepad-computer of the alerted EMS. The respective actual EMS-status, e.g., departure or arrival at the scene, is transferred to the dispatch centre by using the notepad's shortcut EMS-status-messaging buttons.

Upon arrival at the scene, the emergency physician feeds the notepad-computer with important information linking age, sex, emergency category, and initiated corrective action (such as intubation) and sends this data to the dispatch-centre by a "fire and forget" method. Figure 2 shows the screen interface which is used to put the so-called “first information” into the computer.

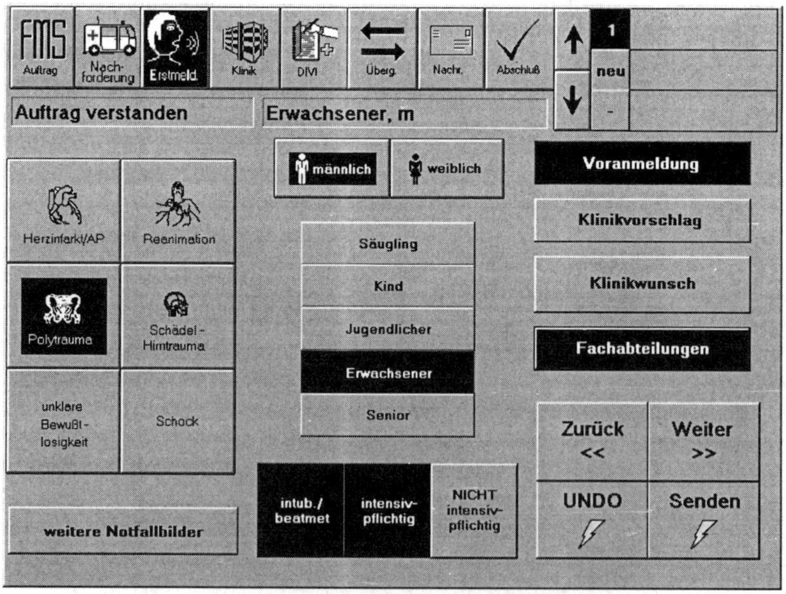

Fig. 2: First Information Interface.
Important information is fed into the notepad-computer upon arrival at the scene.

With this data, the dispatch-centre can pre-select the admitting hospital in advance by submitting significant details. Another advantage is provided through automatic documentation recording and its selective information flow. This can be especially helpful during disasters, when hopeless communication confusion on different radio waves channels is experienced.

3. Results

The results of our studies can be summarised as follows. The use of the NOAH system is practicable. First-sight information can be fed in less than 15 seconds, and entirely submitted within the first three minutes after arrival at the scene. This data is available at the dispatch-centre only a few seconds after its initial submission, and is available only a few minutes later at the admitting hospital. Practical application of this system showed a significant improvement in time (Figure 3) and information processing, and was achieved through quantified information ranking (Figure 4).

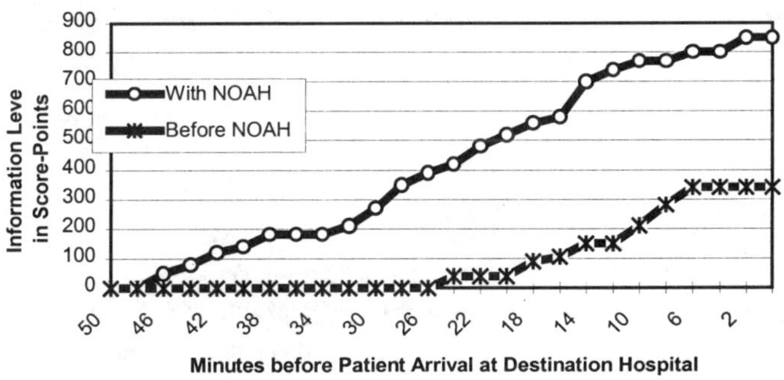

Fig. 3: Information level at the admitting hospital during emergency treatment at the scene and patient transfer

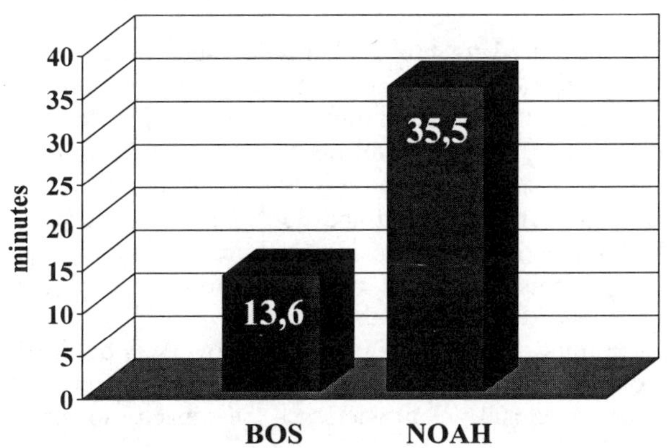

Fig. 4: Comparison of preparation time in the admitting hospital with BOS and NOAH

The admitting hospital was immediately and thoroughly informed of the incoming patient. There was an average time saving of more than 20 minutes in comparison to conventional data transfer (BOS-radio), a distinct-- and most likely life-saving-- advantage.

4. Discussion

Using the NOAH system first of all involves quite a different way of information management handling during an emergency (Figure 5). Because of the well-structured data transfer (first information) to the dispatch centre only a short time after arrival on the scene, the dispatch centre is able to pre-select and inform an admitting hospital while the emergency patient is being treated at the scene (parallel information management). Using conventional data transmission *via* BOS-radio involves serial information management, because transferring information to the dispatch centre happens after finishing initial treatment of the patient normally.

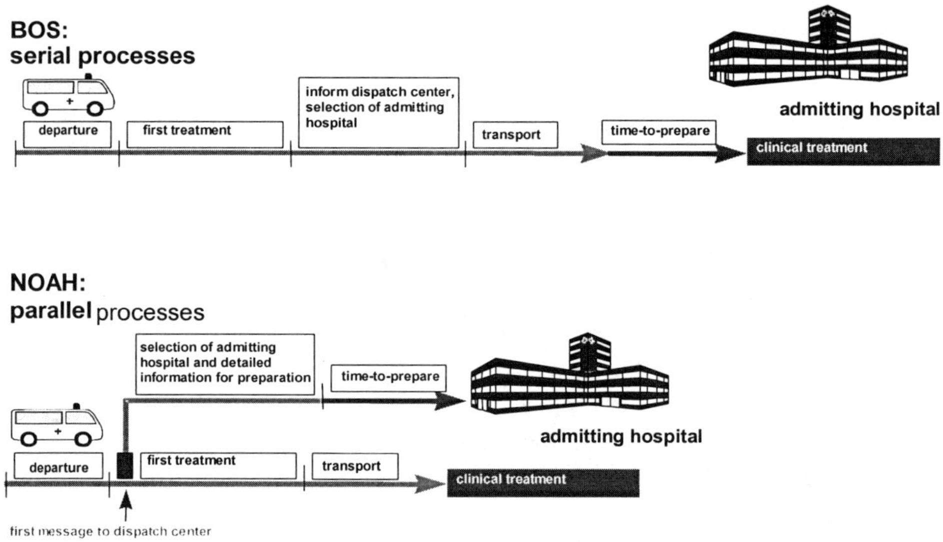

Fig. 5: Emergency Management – Information Management

This additional time may be used to inform all needed specialists in the hospital, and to prepare for the following situations: preparation of the operating room, transfer of patients from the intensive care unit, and information transfer to on-call physicians. High quality pre-information and high accuracy of this information reduce the wait, and see strategies consequently leading to time conformance and properly taken action.

In addition to communication facilitation and documentation, the properly programmed notepad-computer enables the flawless deposit of medical information and algorithms for specific emergencies (e.g., poisoning), and could lead to additional improvement in the quality of medical service provided on the scene.

The total concept of a multi-media communication network is outlined in Figure 6. The concept is not limited only to emergency care, but also includes aspects of telemedicine. The expanding network of hospitals and practitioners has the capacity to increase the quality of health care.

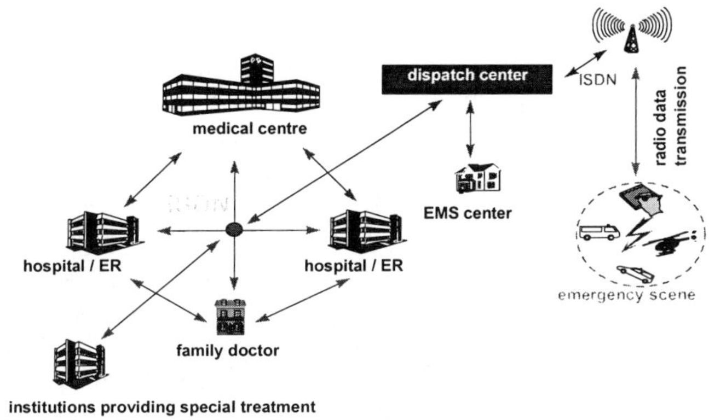

Fig. 6: Eastern Bavaria Telemedicine and Emergency Care Communication Network

Opportunity link of outcome research:

This project could impressively demonstrate the effectiveness of the NOAH concept, which reduces the pre-clinical interval and improves the flow and content of information, *via*:

- mobile data communication using a wearable notepad computer with integrated modem and smart card reader (import/export of data),
- shortcut EMS-status messaging,
- "fire and forget" data transmission (First Message),
- time gained by parallel information management,
- access to emergency algorithms and databases of dangerous chemicals or rare emergencies,
- medical documentation.

It is most important to define the medical advantage produced by this innovative application. This innovative concept shows ways to save lives, to prevent invalidity, and to improve quality of life. Statistics measuring reduction of deaths and invalidity are constantly recorded in extensive analysis projects. The NOAH concept is currently undergoing a scientific and statistical validation program in Eastern Bavaria. It is necessary to measure its direct, indirect, and intermediate use [6].

References

[1] D.D. Trunkey, Society of Universal Surgeons Presidential Address: On the Nature of Things That Go Bang in the Night, *Surgery* **92:2** (1982): 123-132.

[2] A. Donabedian, The Quality of Medical Care: Methods of Assessing and Monitoring the Quality of Care for Research and Quality Assurance Programs, *Science* **200** (1978) 856-864.

[3] M.F. Collen, The Use of Documents for Computer-Based Patient Records (Editorial Commentary), *Methods of Information in Medicine* **32:4** (1993): 269.

[4] D.J. Essin and C.D. Essin, Computerized Medical Records: Software Criteria for Systems to Document Patient Encounters, *Critical Care Medicine* **18** (1990) 100-102.

[5] DIVI. Das Bundeseinheitliche Notarzteinsatzprotokoll der Deutschen Interdisziplinären Vereinigung für Intensiv- and Notfallmedizin (DIVI), *Notarzt* **5** (1989) 91-93.

[6] D. Lobley, The Economics of Telemedicine, *Journal of Telemedicine and Telecare* **3:3** (1997) 117-125.

Address for correspondence

U. Schächinger
Dept. of Trauma Surgery
University of Regensburg Medical Centre
Franz-Josef-Strauß-Allee 11
93042 Regensburg, Germany
E-mail: ulrich.schaechinger@klinik.uni-regensburg.de

The Impact of Telemedicine on Health Care Management
M. Nerlich and R. Kretschmer (Eds.)
IOS Press, 1999

MediLink: A Wearable Telemedicine System for Emergency and Mobile Applications

Tamara KOVAL[1], Martin DUDZIAK[2]
[1]*Medical College of Virginia, Richmond, Virginia, USA*
[2]*Silicon Dominion Computing, Inc., Richmond, Virginia, USA*

Abstract: The practical needs of the medical professional faced with critical care or emergency situations differ from those working in many environments where telemedicine and mobile computing have been introduced and tested. One constructive criticism of the telemedicine initiative has been to question what positive benefits are gained from videoconferencing, paperless transactions, and online access to patient record. With a goal of producing a positive answer to such questions an architecture for multipurpose mobile telemedicine applications has been developed. The core technology is based upon a wearable personal computer with a smart-card interface coupled with speech, pen, video input and wireless intranet connectivity. The TransPAC system with the MediLink software system is designed to provide an integrated solution for a broad range of health care functions where mobile and hands-free or limited-access systems are preferred or necessary and where the capabilities of other mobile devices are insufficient or inappropriate. Structured and noise-resistant speech-to-text interfacing plus the use of a web browser-like display, accessible through either a flatpanel, standard, or headset monitor, gives the beltpack TransPAC computer the functions of a complete desktop including PCMCIA card interfaces for internet connectivity and a secure smartcard with 16-bit microprocessor and upwards of 64K memory. The card acts to provide user access control for security, user custom configuration of applications and display and vocabulary, and memory to diminish the need for PC-server communications while in an active session. TransPAC is being implemented for EMT and ER staff usage.

1. Introduction

In the last several years, the confluence of large-scale database technology, coupled with high-speed communications, data compression, and the overwhelming need to address larger populations with limited staff and resources has been a driving force for telemedicine applications in many medical institutions and regional provider networks. Perhaps the most dramatic factors from the technology perspective have been the ability to provide more data, including large image files in lossless or low-loss compressed formats, [1] at speeds that are commensurate with the needs of physicians, nurses, and other health care practitioners. However the increasing speeds and shrinking sizes of computing and telecommunications technology is in itself not a guarantee, nor even a strong convincing argument, that the elaborate and sophisticated techno-structure available today is improving health care management on a global or even regional level. The technology may be enabling the environment and the mechanisms for many improvements but there are questions about the adequacy for many service sectors and population groups. The fundamental question may be raised as to *whether many of the telemedicine undertakings and initiatives are today as successful and further ahead as they*

[1] Foremost are wavelet and enhanced JPEG techniques, but also ePIC and JBIG

could be, given the resources that have been employed and the energies expended by persons in the health care community at all levels – practitioners, administrators, and infrastructure support personnel.

The objectives of our consortium in the field of telemedicine since 1994 has been to identify the ways and means of improving the service and management of the medical process through sensible application of communications that will enhance response, diagnosis, treatment, and recovery. To mitigate the technology demand while providing better access to patient data and other health care providers during an "off-site" or "in-field" procedure has been the overriding goal in designing TransPAC and MediLink. One area of health care where there have long been perceived needs for faster and improved quality of information exchange, and where the telemedicine field has been viewed as a possible avenue for major leaps forward, is in emergency medical response, in the field and in the hospital or clinic. "Emergency" is used here in a very broad sense, referring not only to immediate life-threatening conditions that merit rapid transportation to a receiving hospital, but also conditions that may arise without expectation, including those that may be discovered or hinted-at during the course of a routine visit. These situations bring about questions that can best be answered by either of two general situations: (1) having additional patient medical data from the past, such as records on file in a hospital or clinic database server, or (2) having dialogue and additional interpretation and heuristic advice from other medical practitioners that cannot easily be present at the patient site. The use of a physically unobtrusive, low-maintenance, low-care communications device that allows for speech interface as well as traditional I/O and which provides unemcumbered wireless access to large databases and image servers, plus security measures for data – this is how TransPAC and the MediLink software can serve such emergency and non-routine medical situations.

2. The TRANSPAC™ WEARABLE COMmunications SYSTEM

The TransPAC system is a full-function wearable PC capable of running the Windows95/98 operating system as a portable unit or as a desktop system. It was originally designed in order to provide a platform for mobile engineering applications requiring real-time internet connectivity for transmission and reception of photos, video, CAD, and GIS data. TransPAC is illustrated schematically by Figure 1 below which shows the basic organization of components. The base hardware system is platform independent but in the prototype development TransPAC is built around a commercially available wearable PC unit. [2] This unit is capable of being worn on the body through a convenient beltpack, over the shoulder, or in a backpack or chest harness. However, TransPAC is designed to accommodate other hardware platforms from other manufacturers that meet the same basic specifications for providing a fully wearable PC platform, and a future ultralight PC core unit is currently in the design stage, specifically for TransPAC, which will provide a much smaller and lighter platform than any wearable PC currently on the market. [3]

The Mentis PC platform, illustrated in Figure 2 below, has a base system unit that contains the system board, hard drive, plus all PC card slots and interfaces including for peripherals (serial, parallel, mouse, keyboard, display) and for extended module packs that plus into the base unit. This component measures approximately 14 x 19 x 3.8 cm, weighing approximately 1.9 kg.

[2] The Mentis, from Interactive Solutions, a division of Teltronics, Inc. (www.teltronics.com/is)

[3] The basis of the TransPAC core hardware is a technology developed by Silicon Dominion Computing, Inc. that makes use of conductive polymer inks for circuit board design and which enables a high-density of three-dimensional circuit layering. Entirely RAM-based for memory and involving no hard drive, this core unit is essentially a thin-client machine that will weight less than 1 lb. (without battery or peripherals) and be extremely unobtrusive when worn in a beltpack or chestpack configuration, with microphone, speakers, and display built directly into the core unit.

A large heat dissipation plate handles cooling of the electronics which are based upon Tape-Carrier-Package technology from Intel.

The base system unit may be operated as a desktop with AC power unit through an adapter module or it can be entirely portable using a snap-on battery pack that attaches easily and quickly to the base unit. This operation can be performed while the system is operational. A third extension pack which snaps on between the base unit and the battery pack enables the user to have one or more removable I/O units – CD-ROM, DVD, tape, or additional hard drive. These snap into the extension pack bay and communicate through connectors that link the top of the extension pack and bottom of the base unit. The specifications for the current Mentis PC base system unit are summarized in Table 1 below:

Feature	Specification	In Base Unit	Optional
CPU	166 MHz MMX Pentium	X	
	200MHz MMX Pentium		X
Input/Output	2 serial ports	X	
	1 parallel port (enhanced)	X	
*	2 infrared ports	X	
	Keyboard (PS/2 style)	X	
	Mouse (PS/2 style)	X	
	Enhanced IDE	X	
	Floppy drive	X	
	Audio headset	X	
	External LCD display	X	
DRAM	32 MB to 128MB	X	
Cache	256K to 512K	X	
BIOS	Phoenix (Flash, 256K)	X	
Video	VGA, SVGA, XGA for CRT or LCD; color 16-bit (hi-color)	X	
Sound	Full duplex, 16 bit 44.1KHz sampling and playback	X	
MPEG	Full-screen, full-motion, up to 30 fps at all resolutions	X	
Network	32-bit PCI		X
PC Card	1 Type II or 1 Type III slot	X	
Hard Drive	2.1 to 8GB enhanced IDE drive	X	
Power Mgt.	Full power mgt. Plus battery recharging circuitry	X	

Table 1 : Mentis Base System Unit Specifications

TransPAC accommodates any input form – keyboard, mouse, pen, touch screen, and voice – with the ability to be converted easily from one medium to another depending upon the user and the situation. Multiple forms of communication and control by the user are possible in parallel, as described in Table 2. There is no requirement for extensive manipulation of software menus or configuration panels, nor of hardware reconfiguration, in order to switch protocols.

Display	Application Control & Command	Data Entry	User-to-User Communications	Internet / Intranet Access
Headset LCD	Voice	Voice (special user-independent command vocabulary)	Cell phone	Wireless modem
6-in. flat panel (wrist-wearable)	Touch screen	Voice (general vocabulary)	Email	Standard modem
10-in. flat panel (universal-mountable)	Pen (for screen)	Pen	Internet phone	NIC and LAN
Standard CRT	Mouse Wrist-worn keyboard Standard keyboard	Mouse Wrist-worn keyboard Standard keyboard	Paging Fax Web postings	Prior downloads Prior CD write

Table 2: TransPAC Communication and Control Protocols

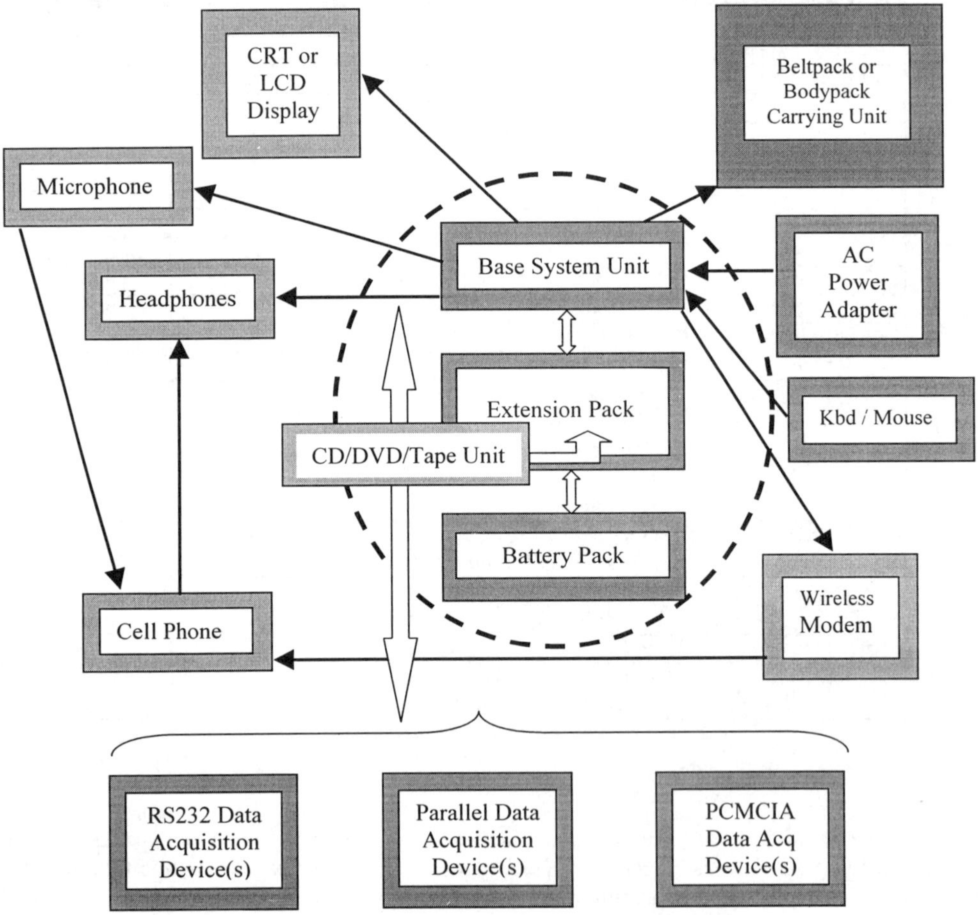

Figure 1: TransPAC System Architecture

Several wireless modem designs are currently being evaluated for providing the main data communications link for TransPAC to the outside world. These are discussed further in Section 4. Once again, the governing design philosophy is to enhance user functions without overloading the user in learning, remembrance of special techniques and codes, special "four-hand" dexterity, a maze of plugs and wires, and all the other demands that often turn a great technological idea into an impractical albatross in the "field" (whether that be outdoors, in an ambulance, in the patient's home, or in a hospital ward). Therefore, when it comes to maintaining communications that for the medical user may be real-time voice or real-time video or database access, TransPAC combines multiple channels into one pipe, so to speak, and offers the user what they are accustomed to having, but simply smaller, faster, and with less gadgetry about which to be concerned, even though the complex circuitry and logic is physically present, albeit invisible to the average user. A cell phone can be attached and used for voice communications, a wireless modem for the data, and either one or two lines can be dedicated to the tasks.

TransPAC has several modifications that set it apart from the basic Mentis or any other wearable or portable PC. These include the availability of more than one speech interface component for both speaker-independent command and control (navigation) of menus and forms- driven data entry that is derived from a speech-to-text-to-database software toolset pre-

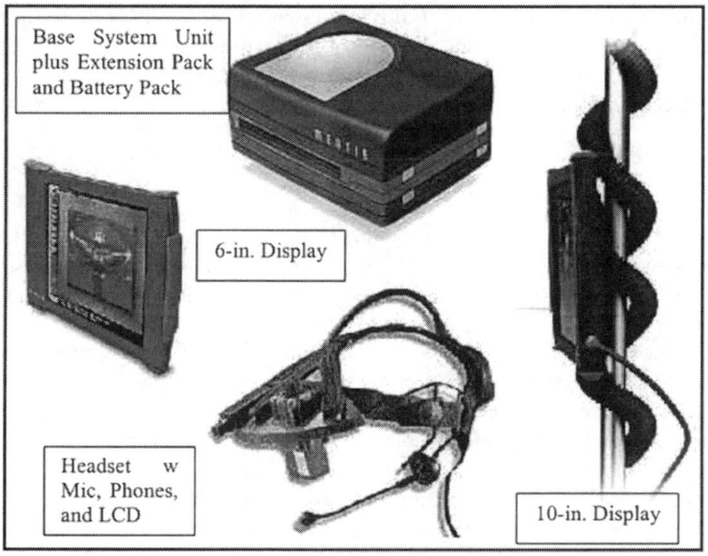

Figure 2 : Basic Mentis Components

viously developed and rigorously tested in the transportation engineering field. There is also for speaker-tailored voice recognition to be used in custom note-taking and document composition, kept separate from the former in order to limit both the scope of training as well as the possibilities for errors in speech recognition of basic keywords and command paths. There is a third form of speech processing, available for the navigation of Interactive Manuals that can be used for training or reference. These Manuals are documents composed in a web-type framework, with active links accessible through voice, mouse, or pen response, leading the user to documents consisting of multimedia content – text, graphics, animation, or full-motion video. The Interactive Manuals are created through the RTMEditor software and accessed through the RTMNavigator. Both software applications are tools developed by Interactive Solutions, producers of the Mentis hardware platform, and are in the process of being customized for use in the TransPAC.

In addition there is employed within TransPAC a unique feature bv which a microprocessor-based smart card provides simultaneously user access control and security plus the ability to pack densely compressed patient and session information including URL and database record reference links. These speech and smart card features are described in Section 4 and the overall functional diagram of the TransPAC is illustrated in Figure 3.

3. MEDILINK™ Application

MediLink is the main application that runs on the TransPAC under Windows95 and Windows98, for medical applications. It is designed to be a common application useable by an emergency medical technician operating under adverse time demands and spatial constraints including physical and temperature constraints that may be faced at highway accident scenes, industrial locations, mines, at sea, or in the air. A MediLink system, for instance, equipped with a full Interactive Manual for standard cardio-vascular, childbirth, and other common emergency conditions and placed on every commercial passenger aircraft, could help to save lives and limit the dangers of emergency flight re-routing in order to respond to onboard situations.

MediLink's main screen is shown in Figure 4 below. All functions operate in the background of a main window that is the "workspace" for both data input and ouput over the internet and locally. The application makes use of common browser technology to keep most interaction steps and sequences familiar to the way common browsers such as Internet Explorer and Netscape Navigator operate.

Writing Pad

The main application window is the *Writing Pad* that can be used to produce ordinary handwritten text and sketch graphics that are stored as a set of pages in a predefined folder on the PC as Windows BitMap (.BMP) images, or a collection of text and graphic objects that are stored with reference locations on the coordinate space of the Pad. Upon storage the bitmapped portions are also automatically compressed using Multi-Resolution Seamless Image Database (MrSID) wavelet compression to enable rapid transmission if so desired. The Writing Pad pages can be processed on a receiving server or desktop "base station" using software that extracts character-stream image data and performs optical character recognition on the text, converting it into a standard ascii text file, one per page or else one text file for all pages in a given session. The main .SID or .BMP files remain unaltered with graphics and character script, and a user can subsequently cut-and-paste graphic regions into other documents using any standard image editor such as Microsoft PhotoEditor or ImageComposer. Most of the elements in the Writing Pad space are, however, text boxes (bound or unbound) and pictures that have been dragged and dropped from elsewhere (e.g., online patient record, or data acquisition device.)

The main menu has several key functions that the user can activate at will, and all of these are intended to be voice-activated. Some selections are familiar to the typical PC user and this is intentionally so in the design, in order, once again, to minimize special training. TransPAC is more like the ordinary desktop PC than it is not, and in fact it can be used as a regular desktop for virtually any PC operation. With a keyboard, mouse, and standard CRT display, the main difference between the TransPAC and the typical desktop is that the former occupies only approximately 30% of the footprint and less than 8% of the volume of the typical mini-tower desktop.

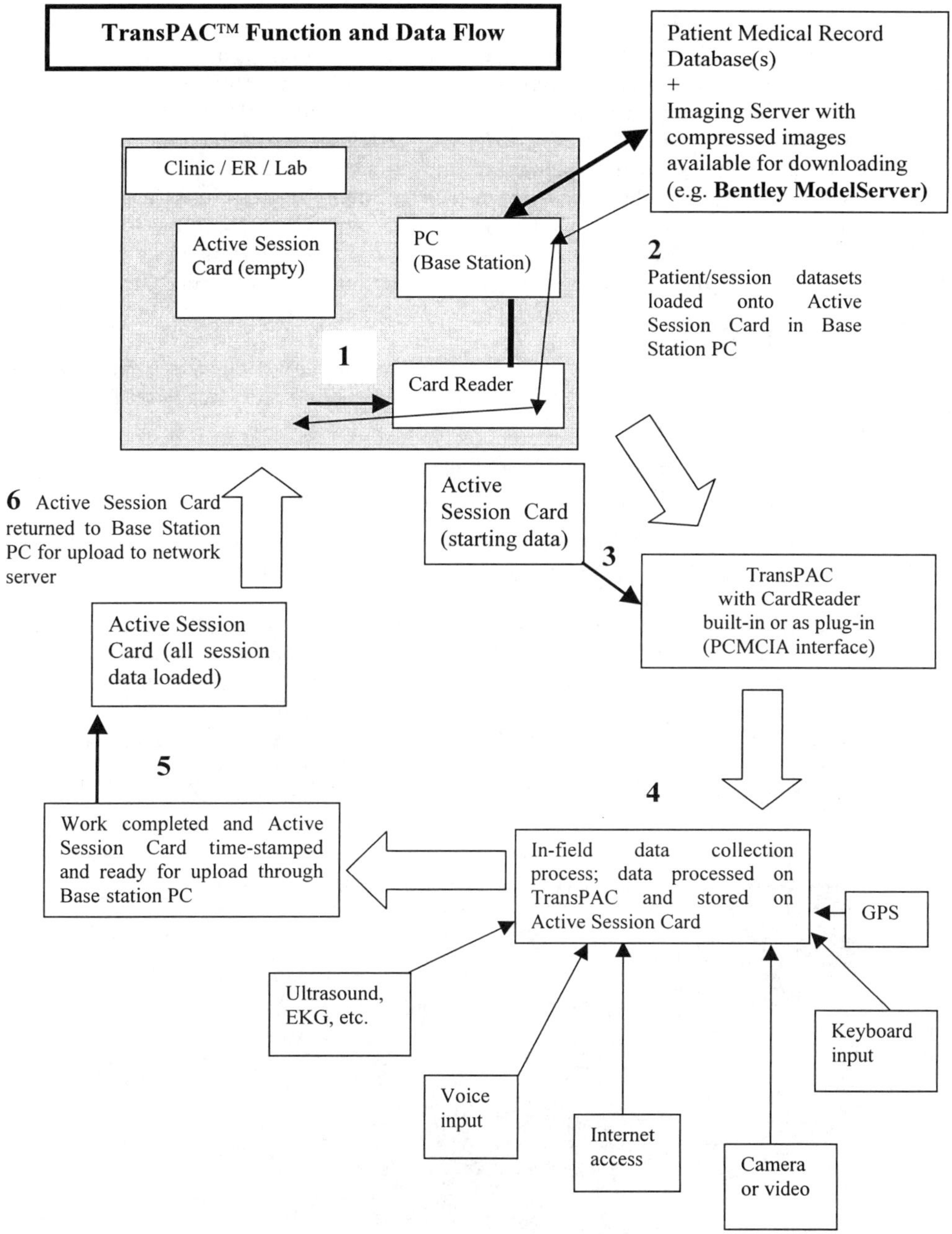

Figure 3: TransPAC™ Functional Design

Sessions

MediLink operates with patient sessions. A session is a collection of tasks that may involve several different applications and files, all tied together with one common denominator – a particular patient whose Patient-ID is the connecting link. The Patient-ID originates in a hospital or clinic database or it is assigned by the MediLink operator as a new ID which subsequently may be processed to match up with a standard ID such as a social security number. The Patient-ID, if supplied from a hospital database in the instance of a physician or nurse using MediLink to conduct home visits, nursing home rounds, etc., will be entered first into the Active Session Card, the 16-bit smart card that contains all start-up data about the patients, tasks, services, and other requirements that the user will want prior to starting a set of rounds and visits (cf. Section 4).

A dynamic HTML page is created and updated during the entire session process, so that when a provider is finished with a given patient session, this main page contains all the links to all other documents created or modified during the session. A new session instantiated by the user generates automatically the following:

- new folder on the hard drive, c:\medilink\newsession
- new dynamic HTML session page, c:\medilink\newsession\new_session.htm

The user fills out requisite patient information and during the course of the session generates new files either directly from the TransPAC and perhaps through data acquired from attached instrumentation (e.g., EKG, ultrasound), or through downloads from an internet or intranet server. All files that are saved during a session, unless specifically noted otherwise by the user, are automatically part of the new (current) session. When the session is saved on hard drive or via the internet on a server, the folder "newsession", now automatically renamed after the identified patient (e.g., "jgsmythe-243-67-9631") contains the session header "new_session.htm", now automatically renamed also after the patient (e.g., "jgsmythe-243-67-9631_session.htm") and a variety of forms, images, notes, URLs, etc. that have been compiled, created, modified, and downloaded by the medical practitioner as part of his or her duties in the session. Figure 5 below illustrates the data flow. The user is freed of about 90% of the headache tasks of managing and manipulating file and folder names.

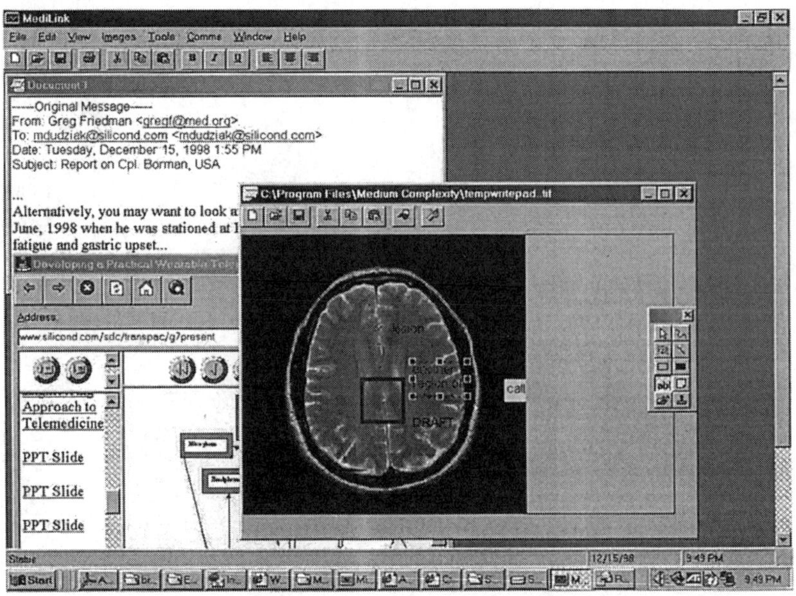

Figure 4 : MediLink Main Application Screen (‡ - cf. Section 7)

The *Writing Pad* was described above and it constitutes the most generic and commonplace interface for the medical professional, the equivalent of the paper notepad for making any form of notes during a patient session. If it can be done with a pen, it can be saved and later processed – or simply printed in exact replica form. The advantages of the wavelet compression algorithms for Writing Pad page bitmap-portion storage are to enable not only fast transmission to a waiting server but to enable anyone to zoom and view the document at multiple scales. The wavelet methods enable image reconstruction that eliminates many of the problems with zooming that are difficulties for JPEG and other formats. Writing Pad was designed to provide some of the features found in applications like Microsoft Word as well as Adobe PhotoShop and even the archetypal Microsoft Paint, for the benefit of the user who wants to PUT things onto a blackboard and WRITE notes. Simple. Direct. Plain.

Body Map

The *Body Map* is another application feature of MediLink. It operates as a browser that brings up a series of overlaid image maps each of which pertains to a system or layer of the human body. The user can set the parameters of the Body Map to be oriented to all generic anatomical and physiological systems or only to certain ones pertaining to the patient of the current session. In the former case, all possible links to different anatomical systems will be displayed or reachable through page navigation, by mouse/pen or voice command. Once at a terminal link level, the user can activate a search of the patient medical records for those records – in database form format or as images, notes, reports, etc. that are maintained as separate files – which exist for that patient. In the latter case, only those links for which there is data existing for the given patient of the current session will be displayed as active links. All of this activity is managed "behind the scenes" by the MediLink software and its gateway to different ODBC compliant databases (Microsoft Access and Oracle being the most common and for which MediLink is initially targeted).

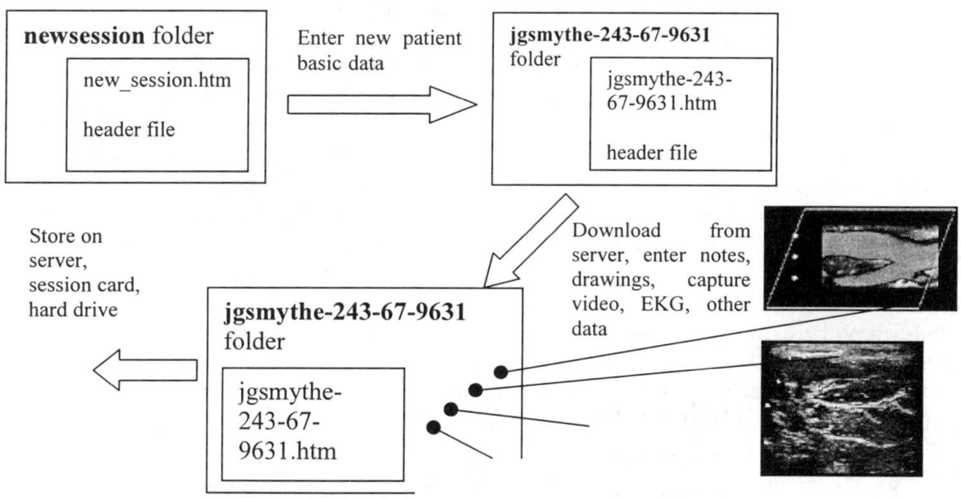

Figure 5: Session Data Flow and Data Structure Buildup (‡)

A very early prototype of the Body Map uses an image map that originated in the web-based medical informatics system, *CommonHealthNet*[4]. By either mouse/pen click or verbal command, the user can activate one of the particular links that are displayed. If the cardiac system is selected, then a dynamic web page will appear in the Body Map browser window showing a list, of text and icons, for all accessible records and files pertaining to the cardiac system for the specified patient (X). The requisite indexing operation is performed at the database server level when each new record is added for (X) and no special search procedure is required of the MediLink user when accessing records in this manner. Similarly, activating the link for neurology would produce a different page of dynamically generated text and icon links, although clearly some records and files could appear through both paths. This is not the only interface method that a user can employ to get patient information, but it is one of the most direct and visual, reducing entirely the need for the user to think and search about file names, folders, query expressions, and other computer terminology that detract from the process of performing medicine and healing, the true business at hand.

The *Data Table*, *Reference*, and *Internet* services are other means that the medical professional can employ to obtain patient data, communicate with other professionals on a case, or enter new data into the system. The Data Table provides a standard form which can be customized to suit the needs of any given institutional patient database format. An example is provided in Figure 7 below. Using the form, the practitioner can rapidly browse through lists of files, records, or folders according to established set categories. The emphasis is upon minimizing the search, deliberation, and decision-making process steps wherever possible. Naturally this requires substantial coordination on the data server end of the channel connecting MediLink to the medical histories, images, and other data objects. However, the bulk of the task is accomplished through standard software gateways that exist on the MediLink side for connecting to Oracle, SQLServer, or Access databases through the web. It is a matter of configuration and demands less change on the part of hospital or clinic database administrators than may at first be imagined. What serves for data access also serves to allow the user to make new records, submit notes (including Write Pad not pages), and enter photos or biomedical instrumentation results into a patient database.

The Internet services within MediLink per se are to enable the practitioner to access more than just the resources of a given hospital intranet or database system. The intent is that in a dialogue with other health care providers connected by cell phone, radio link, or internet, the user can have at his or her disposal whatever may be needed that is a resource accessible through the web. This could include reference materials or live video feeds – for instance, to demonstrate a technique to be performed with a patient. Not everything may be in the manual and sometimes a demonstration of technique is in order. With wavelet compression of video it is possible to obtain relatively real-time full-motion video over a high-speed modem connection, or reduced 8-15 fps streaming over a fast wireless modem link. Without question this type of communications demands that there be a sufficient network in place for supporting and maximizing the bandwidth, but even over a standard telephone connection the performance for general non-video transfer is adequate for most conceivable applications, especially if the real-time voice dialogue is handled through a cell phone and not also loaded onto the requirements of the TransPAC and its modem.

The Reference feature of MediLink is a dynamic, self-indexing note system that the user can build on the TransPAC hard drive, with online links to intranet or internet resources, as a personal or group medical help system. It is designed to be a growing compendium of commonly accessed notes and documents, generated by the user as well as drawn in from

[4] The image in Fig. 6 was produced for the CommonHealthNet web site and not for MediLink, therefore there are several variations, but it is presented only as a conceptual illustration and testing tool.

outside sources, about techniques, pharmaceuticals, case histories, etc. It can be accessed in the usual manners – mouse, pen, keyboard, voice.

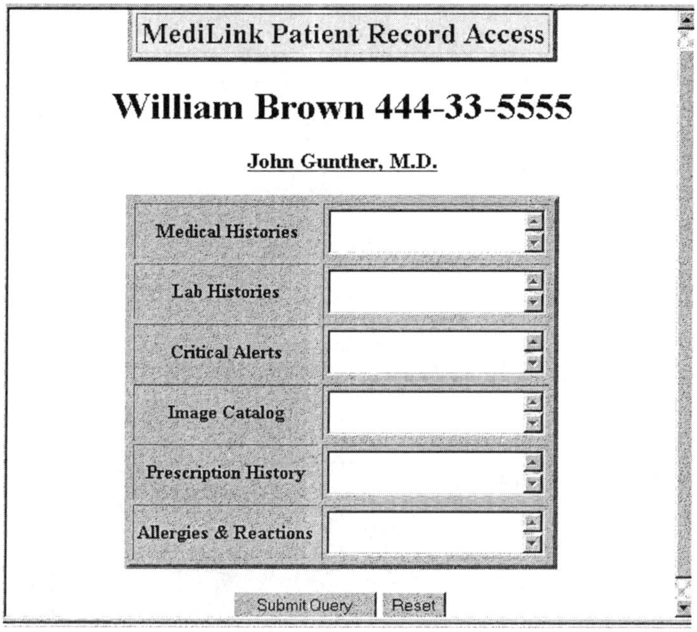

Figure 7 : MediLink Data Table (prototype)

4. Imaging, speech, security and OTHER ENHANCEMENTS

4.1 Imaging

Figure 8 provides an illustration of the Verité image comparison module that is one of the Tools available in the MediLink application. Verité was designed as a specialized image comparison and recognition tool to be used for real-time high-resolution work with images in multiple formats and itself incorporates both compression and recognition algorithms, the latter being drawn principally from neural networks and conventional image processing. A pen input scheme is currently being designed to enable a user to select regions of interest in two images that are side by side and to make comparisons visually and with software functions. For instance, two possible tumor regions or lesions may be compared – patient MRI (today) with patient MRI (six months previous) or patient MRI (recent) with other known case image(s).

The operator has the capability of viewing a maximum of four separate images that can derive from either the active scanner, disk file, or internet sources. Any one image can be compared with another by using a variety of user-configurable algorithms built in to the application – edge enhancement, area texture analysis, Fourier, Gabor, wavelet, and neural network tools are available for use with the image as a whole or for a user-selected rectangular region. The primary use of this tool is to enable the operator to rapidly isolate and identify interesting features and to bring out highlights in images while the medical procedure is ongoing. Once again, the tool can be used with new images that have been acquired at the point of current medical service, and this is not limited to images that are already in some large database.

A simple example illustrates the value of having in-field, real-time analytical tools for image comparison. Consider a victim of acute anterior wall myocardial infarction who is being cared for first by EMT, then in a small hospital or clinic ER, then in an ICU, then moved to a larger regional hospital for bypass surgery. During any time interval of interest, ranging from a few hours after onset to the entire period from t0 (last visit to physician) to t5 (pre-surgery) there may be benefits from viewing two or more EKG readings together, side by side. It may difficult to manage physically to obtain the desired EKGs at a moment's notice, and especially difficult to work with them as physical pieces of paper.

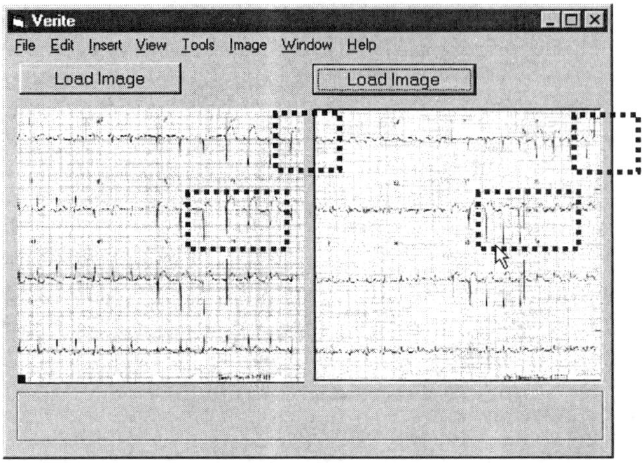

Figure 8 : 2-day Interval EKG, Acute Myocardial Infarction (‡)

However, consider that all these EKGs have been input (direct-digital or by scanning) into a database. Using MediLink, the physician can call up arbitrary EKGs and drag-and-drop them into the Verité windows, set up as two or four to the screen, as shown in Figure 8 above. Interactive testing windows can be moved over two or more images and a comparison of signal patterns can be generated, with graphical results visible to the user in the "base" window of choice. In Figure 9 two comparison regions are being employed simultaneously, indicated by red and blue dashed-line boxes. In the final release version of Verité, the user will be able to obtain a pop-up table comparing selected regions by histogram analysis, wavelet, FFT, Gabor, and other measures and also will be able to overlay one signal segment over another for visual comparison of similarities and differences.

4.2 Speech

TransPAC uses a complete speech-to-text-to-database command interface that supplements rather than replaces the pen/keyboard/mouse channel. This speech interface provides for a trained vocabulary of approximately 100 words that are speaker-independent and resilient to external noise and in particular speaker accent, tone, and volume variations and also non-verbal noise such as that from operating machinery. The software is used within a widely-accepted transportation data collection product for highway and urban roadside asset data collection [5] and has demonstrated the rigors of tests with variable speakers and noise levels.

[5] VoCarta by Datria Systems, Inc. For further information refer to www.datria.com or contact Datria Systems, 7211 S. Peoria St., Englewood, CO 80112

Commands include both single words and phrases, and include amongst the vocabulary the following elements (besides menu items):

> Go Up, Go Back, Go Down, Next Page, Go Ahead, Previous Page, Stop, Take Photo, Take Video, Take Temp, Take Pulse, Take Pressure, Take Ultrasound, Enter Prescription, Cancel, New, Old, List, Undo, Zoom In, Zoom Out, plus a user-modifiable set of standard diagnostic and prescriptive codes.

All of these are intended to be speaker-independent and use a different speech algorithm than the generic speech tool for data entry, also included in the repertoire of MediLink tools. The latter requires individual training and is intended for when the medical practitioner wants to make extended notes or document entry by speech. Its functions are quite similar to those of many commercial speech recognition tools.

4.3 Global Positioning

For certain remote or emergency contexts, it may be necessary to engage the use of a global positioning system or GPS. TransPAC is designed to accommodate any one of several units, and the command speech interface software is already established to handle GPS inputs. The role of the GPS depends upon the medical application. For certain outdoor inspection tasks it may be necessary to reference the location of the patient and other objects. This could be the case in several accident or disaster related situations. A variety of GPS units with as much as sub-meter accuracy may be employed with TransPAC. One such system is the Trimble Pro XRS 1m real-time or post-process 12-channel GPS/DGPS receiver and antenna which is typically worn by the operator in a convenient backpack with no interference to physical movement or the operation of the TransPAC and other modules.

4.4 Security

The role of the 16-bit 16K microprocessor smart card within TransPAC is twofold. First it serves as a compact and reliable form of access security for the system, identifying the operator and thereby setting up all access parameters for online network or internet linkages while the TransPAC is being used on an assignment. The issue of security and traceability is of paramount importance from the larger-scale systems engineering and business process perspective. A widely-deployed, operator-intensive medical activity puts more weight and responsibility on the persons doing the tests and demands more accountability than activities which heretofore may have depended upon special planning and a special team of experts. Currently the TransPAC has an industry-standard PCMCIA Type II interface for the smart card device. The card remains in the unit during all times of operation and its removal would constitute a security violation for which MediLink could, if desired by the hospital administrators and physicians, shut itself down automatically to prevent data security violations.

There is a second role to the smart card, again one of enhancing the system of operation. The 16K of application-accessible memory on the card is divided into two sections: (1) Upload and (2) Download. The Upload section acts as a memo pad for instructional data and pointers for the operator regarding the specific testing assignment at hand. It stores the URLs of reference files, generally large (> 1 MB) files that may need to be accessed by the operator while performing procedures in the field. These can be obtained through either modem, LAN, or more often that not, the wireless connectivity over the internet to a central server. TransPAC is designed to interface specifically with Bentley Systems' ModelServer Discovery, an application expressly designed for managing the retrieval and use of Microstation and other CAD format files over intranets and the commercial internet. However, TransPAC will also interface to any standard web server that will provide natively or through plug-ins JPEG, CGM, SVF and other format files for display, without application interaction, on a web browser provided as part of the MediLink software.

This capability of accessing a large MRI or Ultrasound file that is either already loaded onto TransPAC's hard disk or else obtained ad hoc during a task via the internet allows the care provider to have a remarkably more versatile control over how tests are performed. If it is necessary to refer to a particular x-ray or MRI image while performing a procedure, it is only a matter of seconds away. LAN-based access tests show a response time averaging 5 sec. for drawings obtained via ModelServer Discovery. Wireless connectivity has come of age for the purposes needed by mobile medicine. Operators can make annotations to an image file for reference by other real-time or at a future date. A user makes use of reference points that are accessible in tabular form to the operator and can be entered, through the speech interface, into the transaction database recording all inspection activity. The reference points are read by the operator from the TransPAC display and appropriate entered verbally (or by pen input) into the data record for each imaging task.

Whereas the Upload section of the smart card memory serves to bring useful data to the operator during a task, the Download section is reserved for transaction recording that will preserve on the card with without possible erasure [6] during a session. Each session record that is entered into the database on the TransPAC with images, location data, operator comments, and so forth, has an encapsulated summary record created at the time the MediLink application writes the record into its onboard database. This encapsulation includes a time stamp, location information, and a compressed-text summary of the recorded information about the action performed by the care provider but without any actual large text or image data. Each transaction record will on average occupy less than 50 bytes due to the encoding scheme employed that uses one-byte and two-byte codes for a variety of words and strings. There is only one primary transaction record (PTR) per work session. Numeric data is accommodated by integer and real representation. Future smart cards will have additional memory of upwards of 64K for Upload and Download purposes.

There are two main purposes underlying the Download operation of encapsulated data. First this provides a secure record of the work performed which cannot be altered on the smart card once entered, except by an optional override that itself stamps the smart card with a recording of that override. This is for data security and consistency. Second this offers a fast-track access for a colleague or expert who may be evaluating the tests and procedures done in the field on a real-time basis. A fast and concise record of what was inspected can be gained by anyone connected via a network to a server receiving the primary transaction and transaction content records from the inspector's smart card once it is entered into the reader at the hospital or clinic. An evaluating physician could easily browse through this data to ascertain if all tests were performed and if additional data should be collected, even before examining in detail the images collected. Such a quick review could determine if it is necessary to look at all images, or which ones should be reviewed or forwarded.

5. Future Directions

TransPAC and MediLink have been designed and both are in the implementation and testing stages. Custom-tailored systems based upon the Mentis and ViA platforms along with some components of MediLink are being developed for clients. A survey concerning the use of different elements found in the TransPAC and MediLink designs within the global medical community is planned for 1999, and availability of MediLink, Version 1.0 for beta testing is targeted for the second quarter of 1999. There are several studies that can be performed to

[6] Override is possible but it inserts a record of the override action that cannot be erased by the card user and only after authorized transcribing of the card session data can this be cleared for future use

evaluate the effectiveness of the TransPAC-MediLink system in particular for emergency medicine, military medicine, home health care, travelers' medical emergencies, and rural medical practice. It has been an aim of the present undertaking to lay the groundwork for a collaborative project involving medical practitioners from several disciplines and regions, worldwide. The aim of this project will be to evaluate the use of such mobile technology under diverse population and cultural conditions in order to refine the functions and the devices, including both hardware and software, for more convenient and practical use by the maximum number of medical professionals.

Acknowledgements

Sample MRI image in figure 4:
Courtesy Harvard Medical School, Whole Brain Atlas, www.med.harvard.edu/AANLIB/home.html. Site administered by Drs. Keith Johnson, M.D. (Harvard) and J. Alex Becker (MIT).

Sample EKG images in figures 5, 9:
Courtesy Emergency Medicine and Primary Care web site, www.embbs.com. Images contributed by Dr. H. Nussbaum and Dr. G. Fink; site administered by Drs. Ash Nashed, M.D. and Glenn Fink, M.D.

Sample ultrasound images in Figure 5:
Courtesy General Electric Ultrasound. Produced with the LOGIQ 700 MR 3D Ultrasound. www.ge.com/medical/ultrasound/msul7im3.htm. Site maintained by GE Medical Systems.

This work was conducted as an internal research and development project by Silicon Dominion Computing, Inc. of Richmond, Virginia.

References

[1] Allen, A., Cristoferi, A., Campana, S., and Grimaldi, A. (Dec. 1997) *An Italian telephone-mediated home monitoring service*, TeSAN personal emergency response system & teleservices : 25,33

[2] Dudziak, M. and Koval, T. (July 1996) *CommonHealthNet as an Architecture for Practical Global Medicine*, Global Telemedicine and Federal Technologies Conference, Williamsburg, VA

[3] Dudziak, M. and Koval, T. (Oct. 1995), *IMEDNET : Information Gateways and Smart Databases for Telemedicine and Distance-Based Learning Using the Internet and the WWW*, Internet Medicine Conference, Chicago, Oct. 23-24, 1995

[4] Grad, O., Hassol, A., Gaumer, G., Mintzer, C., Puskin, D., and Grigsby, J. (Apr/May 1997) *Rural teleradiology: a snapshot*, Administrative Radiology 16(4-6) : 28-33

[5] Kukkonen, C.A. (June 1995) *NASA high performance computing, communications, image processing, and data visualization-potential applications to medicine*, Journal of Medical Systems 19(3) : 263-273.

[6] Nordberg, M. (1996) *Remote control. Telemedicine revolutionizes EMS in rural America*, Emergency Medical Services 25(8) : 39,41,43-45.

[7] Otto, C., and Pipe, A. (1997) *Remote, mobile telemedicine: The satellite transmission of medical data from Mount Logan*, Journal of Telemedicine and Telecare 3(Suppl 1): 84-85

[8] Rosen, E. (Oct 1997) *Mobile telemedicine arrives*, Telemedicine Today 5(5) : 14, 42,44

[9] Takizawa, M., Sone, S., Takashima, S., Feng, L., Maruyama, Y., Hasegawa, M., Hanamura, K., and Asakura, K. (1998) *The mobile hospital--an experimental telemedicine system for the early detection of disease*, Journal of Telemedicine and Telecare 4(3) : 146-51

[10] Thorborg, S. (1990) *Mobimed; a telemedicine system for mobile monitoring of physiological parameters*, Proceedings of SPIE; The International Society for Optical Engineering 1355 : 32-33

[11] Shimizu, K., Matsuda, S., and Miyanaga, T. (1994) Optical biotelemetry.(Yamamoto K , ed.) IEEE Instrumentation and Measurement Technology Conference, IEEE Press, New York, NY: 579-582

[12] Stevens, L. (Apr 1998) *Has Internet-based telemedicine finally come of age?*, Medicine on the Net : 8-14

Address for correspondence

Tamara Koval
Dept. Family Practice
Medical College of Virginia
Richmond, Virginia, USA
E-mail: tkoval@silicond.com, tkoval@visi.net

The Impact of Telemedicine on Health Care Management
M. Nerlich and R. Kretschmer (Eds.)
IOS Press, 1999

Integration of Quality Programs by Telemedicine in Surgical Services

Ronald MERRELL, James ROSSER
Department of Surgery, Yale University
New Haven, Connecticut, USA

Abstract: Surgical procedures can be performed and monitored in operating rooms physically isolated, but electronically linked to a parent medical center, and certainly from distant consultation. Quality of surgical care has been measured in retrospect rather than in real time, and outcomes have generally not had the benefit of immediate consultation and group analysis. However, telemedicine can connect consultants, surgeons, patients, and databases. The Yale Telemedicine Center has developed network schemes, which connect the OR of trainees with the laboratory of the teacher, and has opened a continuum between pedagogy and product. The program has connected regional hospitals, connected components of hospital systems, and has been used in international testbeds. The particular operative procedures studied have been laparoscopic procedures. The consultant is based at Yale and is connected with the distant OR to share the laparoscopic surgical field. Connection includes real time video, audio and the ability to draw instruction on the OR screen. Bandwidths as low as 12kbs(POTS) have been employed with modification with effective intervention. The potential for quality improvement is substantial, and inclusion in quality programs is strongly recommended.

1. Introduction

Programs for surveillance of quality have a long history in surgery. The tradition of Mortality and Morbidity conferences has been highly developed for most of this century. Whenever a surgical outcome deviates from the expected, the case should be analyzed to determine the cause of the complication or poor outcome. The analysis then relates the problem to an error in technique, an error in diagnosis, an error in judgment, a delay in diagnosis, or patient disease. Surgeons individually or as working groups in departments are accountable for the outcomes and closely monitor such metrics as infection rate, days for recovery, and mortality rate for specific procedures. This tradition of quality assurance is by definition retrospective since problems are reported after the fact and analyzed. Improvement in outcomes is the response to quality assurance [1,2]. In other words, future patients may benefit from the recognition and correction of past problems.

It would be better to look for problems in prospect rather than retrospect, as complications could then be anticipated through a surveillance tool [3]. This has not been possible in the past because surgeons worked in relative isolation in operating rooms physically separated from one another. In fact, surgeons have been specifically trained to work independently because the likelihood of receiving help in the course of an operation was generally low. The operating surgeon needed to be competent to work in isolation while achieving excellent outcomes. This approach has been strained in recent years by two factors. First, the expectations of patients and of our profession are for near perfect outcomes. Second, surgical innovation has brought vast new areas of technology to the surgeon, and there is therefore a steady need to retrain in new skills. This latter reality implied a slow acquisition of complete competence during the early independent application of new skills after being trained. This phenomenon, termed the learning curve, is not accepted with enthusiasm by patients or physicians.

Until recently, new technology and skills required training, obtaining a credential to perform the procedure, and a period of monitoring in transit to full independent practice. Monitoring was done by having a surgeon with substantial experience with the new technique physically present in the operating room. This monitor could intervene at any time to support the surgeon. The objective of monitoring was to assure colleagues that the surgeon was ready to practice the technique alone. It was critical that the surgeon be ready for independent application. However, the learning curve persisted. Real time assistance to the surgeon applying a new technique in an isolated operating room was not practical. Therefore, the learning curve was the rule. It would be preferable to train and credential a surgeon, and after a period of monitoring with another surgeon present, to continue the support by trainers through electronic mentoring during early independent application.

A clear example of the problems of learning and new technology is the problem of common bile duct injury in the course of laparoscopic cholecystectomy [4]. This approach involves a new technology and set of skills for even the most experienced surgeon. Scores of thousands of general surgeons were trained in the early 1990's to perform this procedure, and great concern was given to instruction, quality assurance, and credentialling [5]. The procedure was so much preferred over open cholecystectomy that surgery for gallstones changed over in a very few years. In some areas of the US, the changes occurred in a matter of weeks. There was a great deal of motion and frenzy, and the transition phase to generalized competence was associated with many complications. The most characteristic complication was common duct injury [6,7] and even now it seems that injury to this structure continues to be a problem even after surgeons have extensive experience with the technique. Yet review of films of procedures that resulted in such injuries can almost always demonstrate to the trained eye the steps leading to the injury.

Another feature of the learning curve was anatomical variants or technical challenges which lead to consternation on the part of the surgeon and conversion of the minimally invasive laparoscopic procedure to an open cholecystectomy with all the increasing pain, disability, and prolonged recovery. If real time consultation were available, these injuries and conversions could probably be avoided. Thus the learning curve could be truncated, and especially difficult cases could receive the benefit of more experienced consultation. Since the laparoscope is used with a camera and television monitor, it is possible to transmit the image to another site for surveillance, mentoring and consultation. The laparoscopic image need not be isolated in the operating room with the lonely surgeon. New procedures are being regularly designed for the laparoscope. The need for continued training remains, and the matter of learning curve persists [8].

2. Materials and Methods

We have designed three programs to share the operating room images of laparoscopy with training and consulting center. We report on the organizational aspects of such real time mentoring programs. One project served as outreach from Yale and one of its peripatetic professors to a community hospital where a surgeon had been trained by our faculty. Another program involved expansion of this concept to an entire health care system of 13 hospitals, and the last involved mentoring via POTS to the rainforest of eastern Ecuador to test the limits of infrastructure in delivering this support.

Laparoscopic surgery is performed with a puncture in the abdomen through which a short rigid tube is placed. Several of these punctures allow introduction of a camera and surgical instruments. The operating field in the abdomen is seen on a TV monitor. The surgeon must follow events in the abdomen by the image on the monitor. This image can be transmitted to a distant site and shared with a colleague. The consultant can interact with the surgeon by voice or by transmission of review images which remind the surgeon of certain aspects of the operation or which demonstrate rare anatomical variants that may confound the surgeon. Also, the consulting surgeon can draw on the screen to amplify verbal instructions. Further, the consultant could use a robotic arm to physically intervene, but that has not been scripted into these three programs. In all three programs the surgeons seeking consultation or mentoring had been trained in the Yale curriculum for laparoscopic surgery as developed by Dr. Rosser [9]. The metrics for the success would include a reduction in the expected rate of bile duct injuries, a reduction in complications related to abnormal anatomy and a reduced frequency of conversion of laparoscopic to open cholecystectomy. This presentation describes the logistics of the three programs and not the clinical outcomes.

Program 1: Regional Hospital. After full training and full monitoring in a new laparoscopic procedure, a surgeon at a regional hospital sought mentoring and consultative support from Dr. Rosser. It was clear that the trainer could not always be available for the trainee. Whenever Dr. Rosser was on campus at Yale, contact was readily achieved by ISDN from the operating room at the regional hospital to the telemedicine center at Yale. The laparoscopic camera fed into a Picture-Tel unit (H.320 compliant). The image was easily shared and discussed, and a marker was used (Figure 1). The absence of the trainer from campus is fairly frequent. Therefore, far distant connections were tested by connecting Dr. Rosser at a conference in Zimbabwe to the trainee in his operating room back at the regional hospital in Connecticut. A satellite connection was utilized with 384 KBS and the same Picture-Tel equipment. (Figure 1)

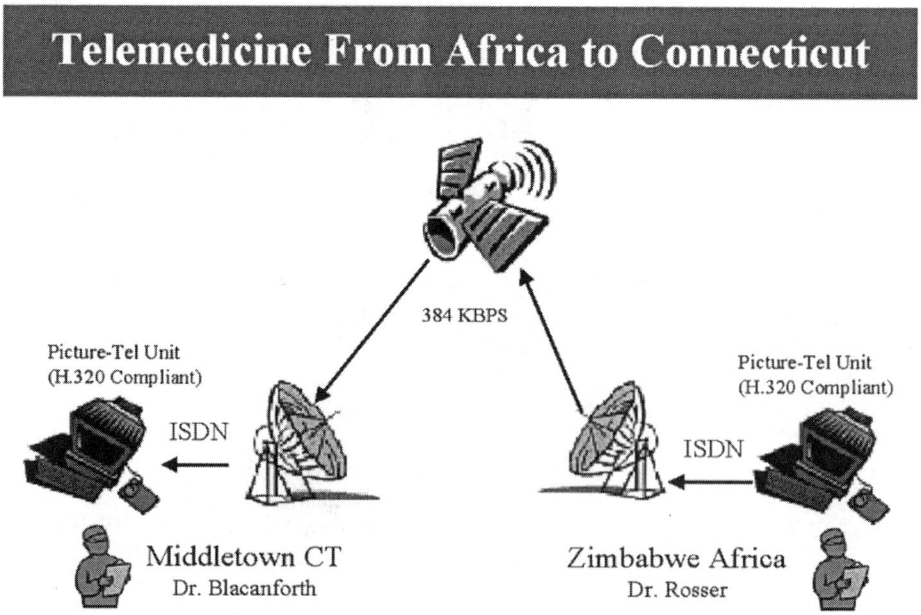

Figure 1. Schematic for telemedicine connection from Zimbabwe to a regional hospital in Connecticut

Program 2: The expansion of Program 1 to a hospital system has required much more logistical effort. First, the surgeons at thirteen hospitals have been enrolled in training courses in laparoscopy. Even those well experienced need to use the same terms and orientation as well as OR set-up in order to communicate effectively by image and voice for effective consultation. The courses cover laparoscopic skill development as well as cognitive matters related to laparoscopic surgery. Those surgeons identified as having less than expected results are enrolled in remedial education. The managers of the operating rooms at the various sites are enrolled in tactical leadership programs to make the performance of these procedures logistically sound at the site of services. They are also involved in the technical connection aspect of the program to effectively access mentoring and consultative services. Further, there is a nursing program to develop and maintain critical pathways for patients having laparoscopic surgery. All units share a common quality program, and each has access to Yale through Picture-Tel ISDN. The shared image is joined to voice, drawing, and the possibility to introduce educational material onto the working screen at one of the member hospitals from the media laboratory at Yale. (Figure 2). This program is set up as one of quality improvement and data are reviewed monthly. After full credentials for independence, every tenth procedure is reviewed on tape and a critique is made. The skill credentials of the surgeons are renewed every year much like flight credentials. In the quality improvement program, outcomes are reviewed and benchmarks set for metrics. (Figure 2)

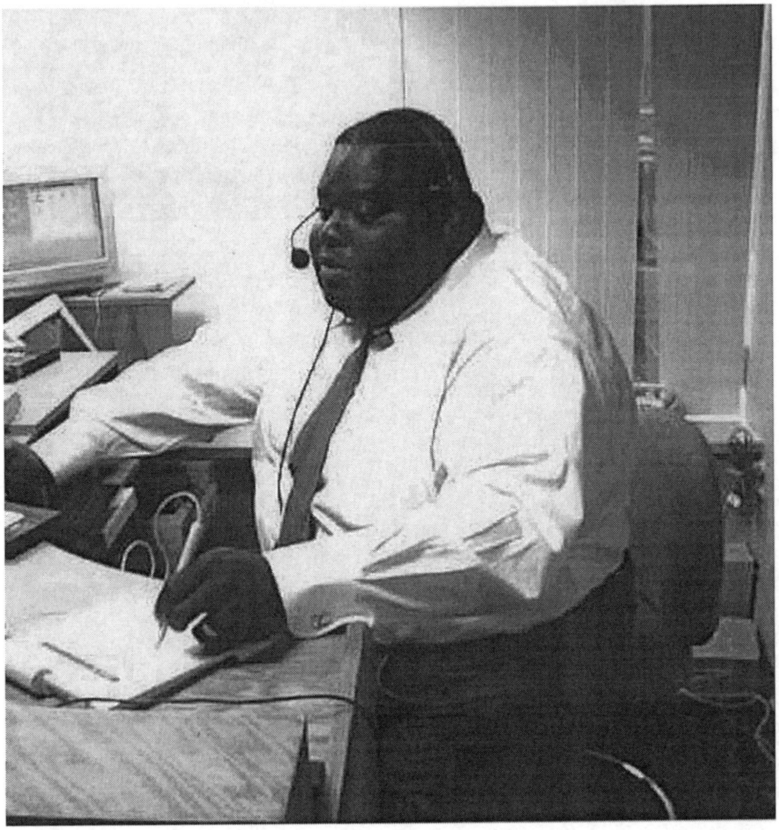

Figure 2. Use of the telestrator to interact in real time with surgeons at a distant site.

Program 3: In a remote clinic in Ecuador on the banks of the Ipuna River, surgical services are intermittent and provided by a mobile van. The only connection to the outside world is a copper wire phone line (POTS) which transmits at about 12KBS. A direct phone line to Yale was established and connected to the computer, which was feeding from the laparoscopic camera. Freeze frame allowed transmission of excellent images of the laparoscopic field. Two surgeons trained in the Yale curriculum by Dr. Rosser were operating in Ecuador to perform a laparoscopic cholecystectomy. Each was fully credentialled to perform the procedure. The consultant was asked to identify critical elements of the surgical anatomy and to make the decision as to the application of surgical clips and to guide the resection.

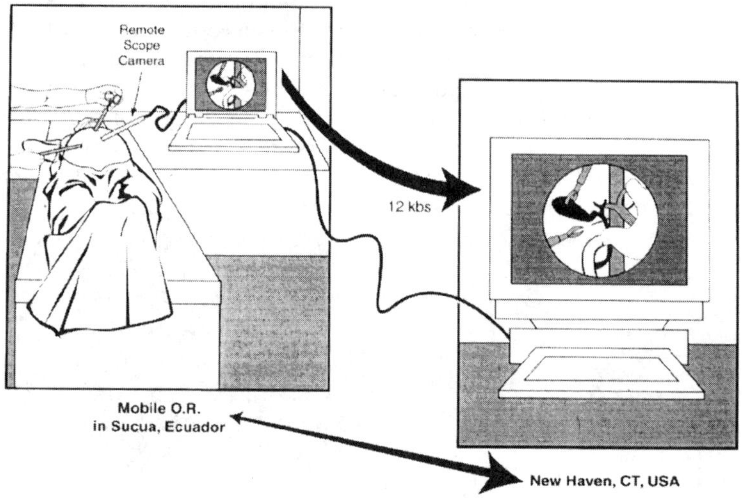

Figure 3. Diagram of connection between operating room in Ecuador and consultant's screen at Yale.

3. Results

To date there have been no injuries or conversions in the early cases involved in all three programs. At the regional hospital, there was no problem at all with the connection for the purpose of consultation or mentoring. The quality of image and ease of connection was completely consistent with clinical need.

Similarly, during the cholecystectomy performed in the mobile unit in Ecuador, the consultant at Yale was able to identify each of the critical anatomical structures and direct the conduct of the operation. Full motion was obviously not possible, but freeze frame capture at the rate determined by the narrow bandwidth was completely adequate to support the visual identification of the critical structures, including the common bile duct. (Figure 4)

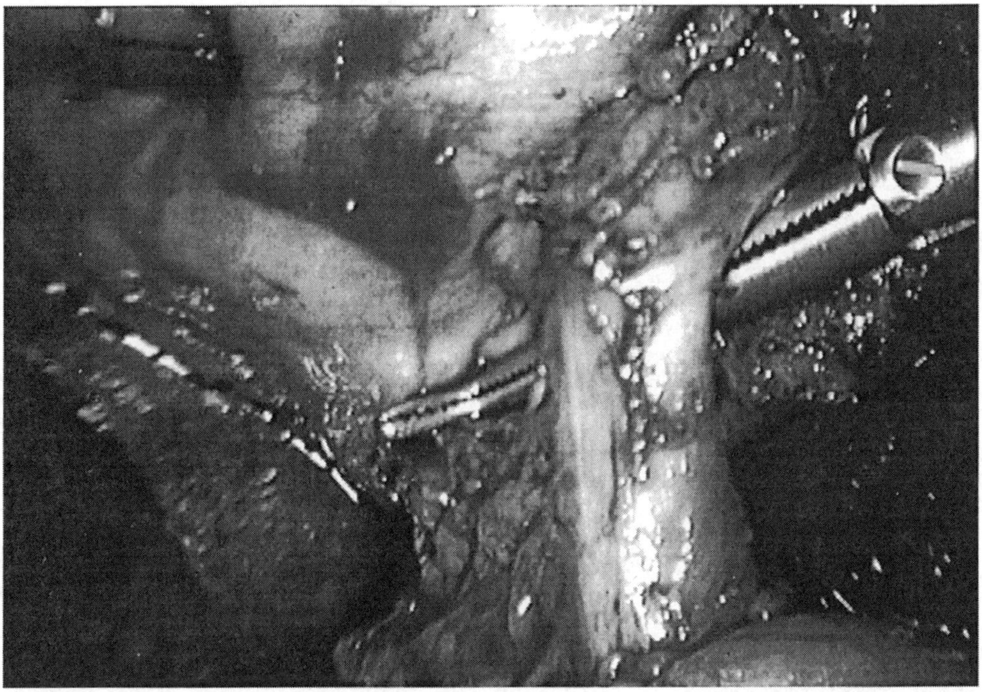

Figure 4. Freeze frame transmission of surgical dissection from Ecuador to Yale. The instrument has identified the cystic duct.

4. Discussion

It is clear that standard telecommunications can overcome the isolation of the operating room. Operations can be directed and mentored in real time. Even remote and primitive technological situations are not incompatible with telecommunications support. The use of telecommunications can allow integration of surgical care standards at widely separated sites. Common standards and a worldwide expectation of excellence should enhance surgical services such that distance will not be a determinate of outcome. Access to expert consultation in real time will change the nature of surgical care by eliminating the isolation of the surgeon in the operating room, and by integrating the surgeon into a world of experience based medicine.

References

[1] Japan Human Relations Association. Kaizen teian 1: developing systems for continuous improvement through employee suggestions. Portland; Productivity Press, 1992.

[2] Warner MA, Shields S, Chute CG. Major morbidity and mortality within 1 month of ambulatory surgery and anesthesia. J of Am Med Assoc, 1993;270(12):1437-1441.

[3] Goonan KJ. The Juran prescription: clinical quality management. San Francisco; Jossey-Bass Publishers, 1995.

[4] Soper NJ, Brunt LM, Kerbl K. Laparoscopic general surgery. New England J of Med 1994;330(6):409-419.

[5] Zucker KA, Bailey RW, Graham SM, et al. Training for laparoscopic surgery. World J. Surg 1993;17(1):3-7.

[6] Kerin MJ, Gorey TF. Biliary injuries in the laparoscopic era. Eur J Surg, 1994;160:195-201.
[7] Lee VS, Chari RS, Cucchiaro G, et al. Complications of laparoscopic cholectystectomy. Am J of Surg 1993;165:527-532.
[8] Orlando R, Russell JC, Lynch J, et al. Laparoscopic cholecystectomy: a statewide experience. Arch Surg 1993; 494-499.
[9] Rosser JC, Rosser LE, Savalgi RS. Skill acquisition and assessment for laparoscopic surgery. Arch Surg 1997; 132:200-204.
[10] Rosser JC. The Yale curriculum for laparoscopic surgery. In: Merrell RC, (ed.). Laparoscopic surgery: A colloquium. Springer-Verlag, New York, 1999; Chap. 20, pp. 235-251.
[11] Merrell RC. Generalist versus specialist in laparoscopic surgery. In: Merrell RC (ed.) Laparoscopic surgery: a colloquium. Springer-Verlag, New York, 1999; Chap. 23, pp. 271-276.
[12] Institute of Medicine. Telemedicine: a guide to assessing telecommunications in health care. Washington DC; National Academy Press, 1996

Address for correspondence

Ronald Merrell, MD
Department of Surgery
Yale University School of Medicine
330 Cedar Street, FMB 102
New Haven, CT 06510
Tel: +1-203 785 2697, Fax: +1-203 737 2116
ronald.merrell@yale.edu

Telemedicine in Neurosurgical Daily Practice

Frank J. SCHULMEYER, Alexander BRAWANSKI
Department of Neurosurgery, University of Regensburg, Regensburg, Germany

Abstract: Telemedicine has been in daily practice at our neurosurgical department for five years. In our experience the standard personal computer-based telemedicine systems Medicom® and especially RADO Look® are reliable, easy to use, and of high quality performance.

Telemedicine makes possible better patient management at regional hospitals and the avoidance of patient transports. Therefore treatment costs in neurosurgical patients can be highly reduced.

1. Introduction

The tradition of telemedicine in neurosurgery started in the late eighties, when numerous neurosurgical departments began to build a network between regional hospitals and their respective clinics. For transmitting cranial computed tomography (CCT) scans by phone, the Photophone®, which was based on analogue telephone technique, was used. In our department the first telemedicine system (Medicom®) was established at the end of 1993. In mid-1998 we installed a new teleradiology system (RADO Look®) in addition.

2. Materials and Methods

The Medicom® system and the RADO Look® system are based on standard personal computers using the ISDN-technology. The RADO Look® system allows the transmission of CCT or MRI data (DICOM 3 standard) without loss of quality. It takes about 7 to 14 minutes (depending upon the extent of the data) to transmit a complete CCT investigation. The scans are received automatically.

We are connected with six regional hospitals-- Cham, Eggenfelden, Mainkofen, Passau, Straubing, Tirschenreuth-- in east Bavaria (Figure 1). The number of teleconsultations is increasing every year: in 1996 there were seventy-two, in 1997 there were eighty-three, and from January to October 1998 seventy-eight scans were transmitted.

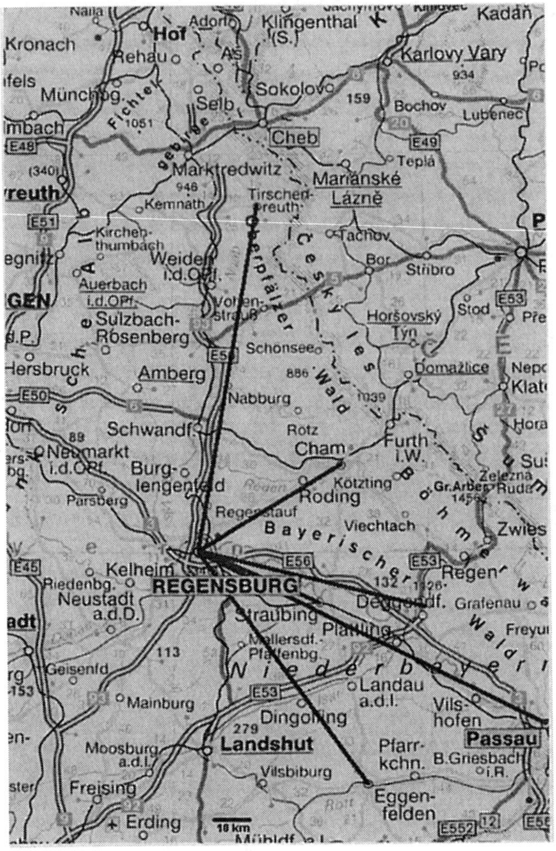

Figure 1:
Regional hospitals connected to our neurosurgical department

3. Results

Both telemedicine systems (Medicom® and RADO Look®) are easy to use, even for someone who is not trained in using a computer. In the last five years we have never had a software or hardware problem which made data transmission impossible.

The usefulness of telemedicine for better patient management and cost-saving becomes clear by analyzing telemedicine consultations. For example, cases discussed by telemedicine from one regional hospital in a single month are summarized in Table 1.

The analysis of these cases shows that in the month of September 1998 alone, two patient transfers were avoided. This was not only to the patients' advantage insofar as it prevented the unnecessary physical strain of transport, but also made possible the reduction of treatment costs in these two cases by at least 12550.- DM (Table 1).

DATE	PATIENT	DIAGNOSIS	TREATMENT	COST SAVING
02.09.1998	A.S.	meningioma	no emergency surgery required, admission of the patient some days later.	no courier transport (taxi) of the CCT scans (220.- DM)
03.09.1998	J. D.	head injury, cerebral contusions	no surgery required, best medical management at the local hospital	no transportation (helicopter) of the patient (7000.- DM) the daily hospital fee at the regional hospital is much cheaper (1500.- DM per day) no return transport (475.- DM)
16.09.1998	J.H.	head injury, epidural hematoma	emergency surgery required, take over of the patient immediately	no cost saving
16.09.1998	H.K.	cerebral hematoma, aneurysmal bleeding suspected	neurosurgical therapy required, but no possibility to take the patient over due to shortage of intensive-care-beds. The patient was referred to another neurosurgical department.	no cost saving
21.09.1998	T.O.	subarachnoid hemorrhage, hydrocephalus	neurosurgical therapy required, but no possibility to take the patient over due to shortage of intensive-care-beds. The patient was referred to another neurosurgical department	no cost saving
24.09.1998	M.W.	intracerebral hematoma	no surgery required, best medical management at the local hospital	no transportation (helicopter or "Intensivmobil") of the patient (7000.- DM or 1600.- DM) the daily hospital fee at the regional hospital is much cheaper (1500.- DM per day) no return transport (475.- DM)
25.09.1998	M.W.	intracerebral hematoma (CCT control)	continue of best medical management at the local hospital	no courier transport (taxi) of the CCT scans (220.- DM)

Table 1: Telemedicine consultations from the hospital of Tirschenreuth (about 100 km. away from Regensburg) in September 1998.

4. Discussion

In our experience PC-based telemedicine systems are reliable, of high quality performance, and easy to use. This is also shown by Anderson *et al.* [1].

In consideration of the data provided in Table 1 and today's prices for software and hardware, the costs of telemedicine systems could be amortized in one or two months (depending on the system used). However, in reality telemedicine systems are financed by the hospitals, whereas the cost reduction is to the benefit of health insurance funds. So it should be in the interest of the health insurance funds to promote telemedicine.

References

[1] E.B. Andersen *et al.*, Image Transmission Between Hospitals: Technical and Clinical Testing of the Equipment for Digital Image Transmission between Hospitals *via* the Ordinary Telephone Network, *Ugeskr-Laeger* **157:15** (1995) 2155-2158.

Address for correspondence

F. J. Schulmeyer
Department of Neurosurgery
University of Regensburg Medical Centre
Franz-Josef-Strauß-Allee 11
93042 Regensburg, Germany
E-mail: frank.schulmeyer@klinik.uni-regensburg.de

The Impact of Telemedicine on Health Care Management
M. Nerlich and R. Kretschmer (Eds.)
IOS Press, 1999

Perfect DiViSy Technology for Video Network in Medicine (Moscow Information Network for Teleoncology)

George VOROZHTCOV, Valery CHISSOV, Andrew DANILOV, Vladimir KAZINOV, Victor SOKOLOV, George FRANK
Moscow, Russia

Abstract: A large telemedicine project is now under development in Moscow. The general task of the project is to link oncology research centres and hospitals meeting the project profile, and to provide on-line (using real-time video conferences) and off-line (*via* distributed database of medical information) information exchange. There was no existing technology available for use at the project's base which was ready to meet all requirements, so we are using specially created technology for video networks (DiViSy V.97). We suppose this technology to be more applicable for use in telemedicine networks than are business video conference technologies and classical Internet/Intranet technologies. We affirm in our conclusion that now is the time for developing special telemedicine standards, recommendations of compatibility, etc., and that we are ready to take part in this process.

1. Introduction

"Teleoncology" is a broad term referring to the various methods of remote diagnosis and advising in the course treating oncology patients which are based on receiving and transmitting video, audio, graphic, and textual medical data through various communications channels.

This term is expressly introduced by the authors, as the major purpose of all and any telemedical consultations is to improve the quality of the medical care to be provided to particular patients, and the authors intentionally concentrate their attention on the programme to build a system of telemedical advising for the diagnosis and treatment of oncology diseases.

Teleoncological advising is like an iceberg, most of which is below the surface and is comprised of organisational, engineering, legal, moral, and other steps which are necessary to make teleoncological advising successful and effective.

In February 1998, the Moscow Government in the person of Mayor Y. M. Louzhkov--jointly with the Ministry of Science and Technology and the Ministry of Public Health RF--passed a resolution to put the programme to create the Moscow Information Network for Teleoncology (hereafter, the MINT) into practice on the basis of the DiViSy technology and facilities developed by the experts at the Research Engineering Centre: DiViSy [Digital Video System]. State Research Centre NIOPIK, RF, was appointed to be the leading organisation in this project.

The main objective for which the MINT has been created is to provide a means of transmitting various medical data, such as high-resolution video in both frame mode and real time, sound data, complicated graphic representations, text, and various official medical information. With this aim in view, provision was made to create a system to transmit the data among users, such as those at Moscow's oncological research centre and oncological hospitals, with the use of optical communication channels with the carrying capacity of 2 MB per second.

The MINT is going to have its own Control and Monitoring Centre, which wil! be connected to the network through a channel of 10 MB per second. To do this, provision has been made to connect remote users from the Russian regions and foreign countries through communication channels of any kind. The IP protocol with its own addressing is going to be used as the basic protocol for data exchange. During the initial stage, Frame Relay technology will be used; a switch to ATM technology will later be made. All operators' stations will be equipped with the DiViSy special purpose units for teleoncology in order to provide advising.

2. Materials and Methods

During its first stage, the MINT will include about 40 telemedicine workplaces in 10 clinics. Most of them will be for telepathology purposes. Other workstations will be experimental variants for telemedicine consultations during endoscopy and ultrasound diagnostics and photodynamic therapy sessions. In every clinic, the entire telemedicine system will be integrated into the telemedicine segment of the clinic's information network (Figure 1).

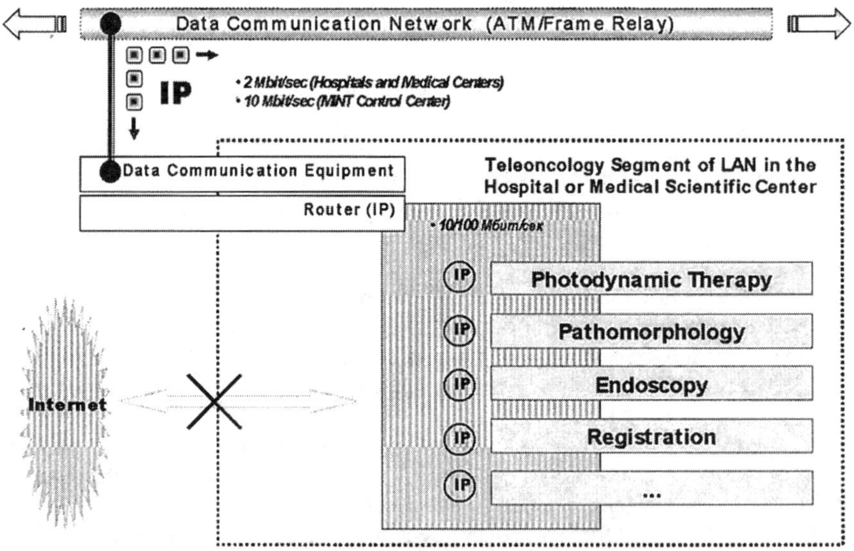

Figure 1: Teleoncology segment

The main software technology being used in this project is DiViSy [Digital Video System] V.97, designed by Research Engineering Centre. This technology was originally created for various types of digital video networks for business and administrative purposes; (the typical the video network structure in a large company (as shown in Figure 2).

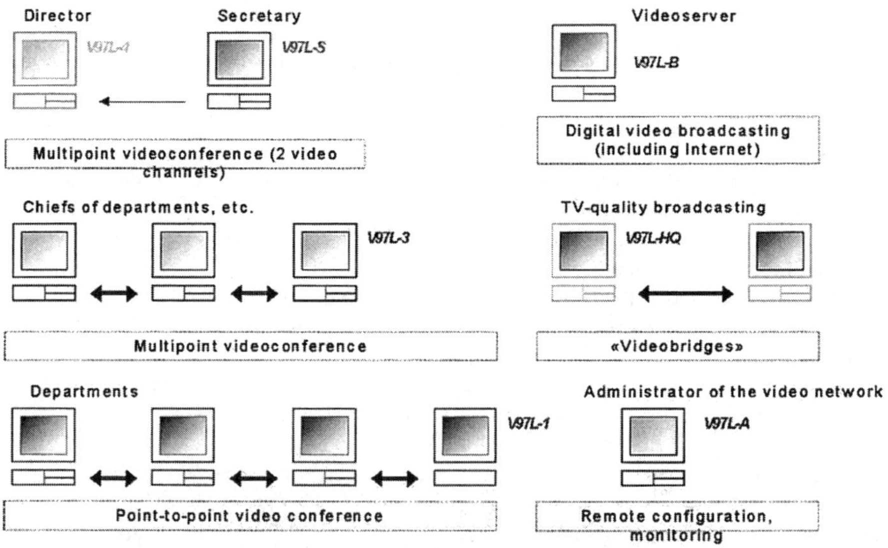

Figure 2: Typical structure of a video network in a large company

DiViSy V.97 is an open software technology. Additional modules for database support, authorization, monitoring, etc., have been created and added to the kernel software. As a result, a universal video conference technology has been introduced into telemedicine technology (Figure 3).

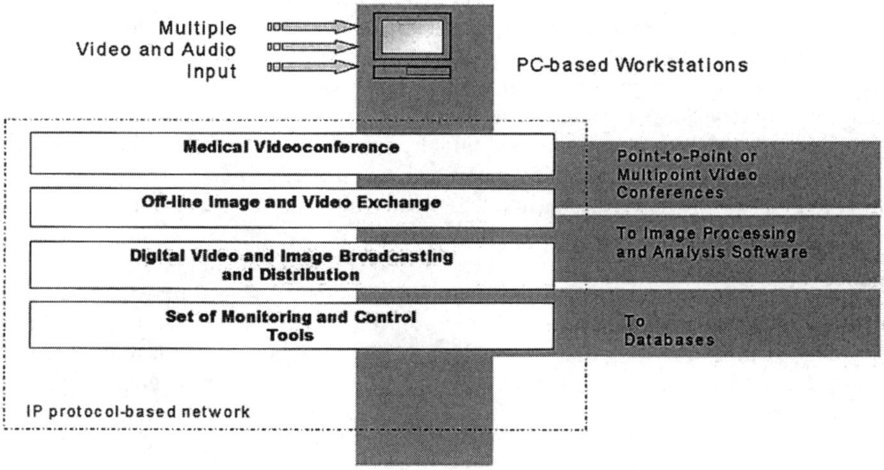

Figure 3: A technology for video networks development in medicine

3. Results

We suppose that there are two ways of engaging in practical telemedicine.

The first way is to provide remote telemedical advising in an offline mode, in which an expert to be advised has acquired the necessary data beforehand and sends it to his partner, an advising physician. The latter, in his turn, provides analysis and study of the materials transmitted and sends back his conclusion. The necessary and sufficient conditions to make such advising efficient are as follows:

a) The level of the skills and education of both advising physician and physician to be advised must be rather high and not differ too widely.

b) The types of medical information and the methods of getting it ready must be, in the best case, standardised-- or must at least be preferred by the physician to be advised and the advising physician.

Should any of the said conditions not be met, the advising services become essentially less effective and at times such advising may give a negative result.

As a rule, during the initial stage of telemedical advising none of these conditions are fulfilled and it becomes necessary to put into practice a rather complicated process of standardising the medical data to be prepared by each participant. Very often in actual practice, physicians of the same trade-- for instance, the pathomorphologists-- use different terms when referring to one and the same oncology diseases. Because of this, it is very important to bridge the gap between their positions to make their mutual advising more effective.

The second way is to provide video conferencing in real time with the use of the conventional equipment for business conferences.

As a rule, this is used mainly to show the potentials of telemedical advising in real time and it is an additional means of discussing medical information transmitted beforehand.

Given the high cost of such video conferencing sessions and the non-availability of the exchange of additional information directly in the course of these sessions, the effectiveness of such advising in real time is not high.

Thus, in developing the technology and equipment for teleoncological advising, the experts of the Russian Research Engineering Centre of Digital Video Systems took the path of creating radically new capabilities, namely:

To conduct teleoncological advising in real time with the availability of simultaneous exchange of any requested information beforehand.

To provide the connection of any additional user whose opinion, relating to a particular part of the medical information being discussed, is directly required-- for instance, if it is required to hear out the opinion of a radiologist when clinicians are discussing the results of a diagnosis.

To conduct training sessions on various methods of diagnosis and treatment of oncology patients. For instance, a famous and highly skilled pathomorphologist may conduct diagnosis sessions of histology specimens in real time, during which he can be seen and heard by several tens of the users in different oncology hospitals. They can follow his methods for analysing the specimen, hear his comments, and ask him questions. It goes without saying that such training sessions will result in improvement of the skills of participating physicians, and that they will be able to get data ready for advising in offline mode within the same standards with which their prospective adviser works.

To conduct video consultations in real time involving physicians of various trades to provide a complete discussion of the results of the different tests of a particular oncology patient.

To derive a conclusion electronically, with its further registration in the electronic case report, in the course of the teleoncological advising.

The major requirements and principles of the MINT structure are shown in Figure 4. This network is to be formed on the basis of the multifunctional potentials to exchange all and any medical information in online and offline modes among any group of users.

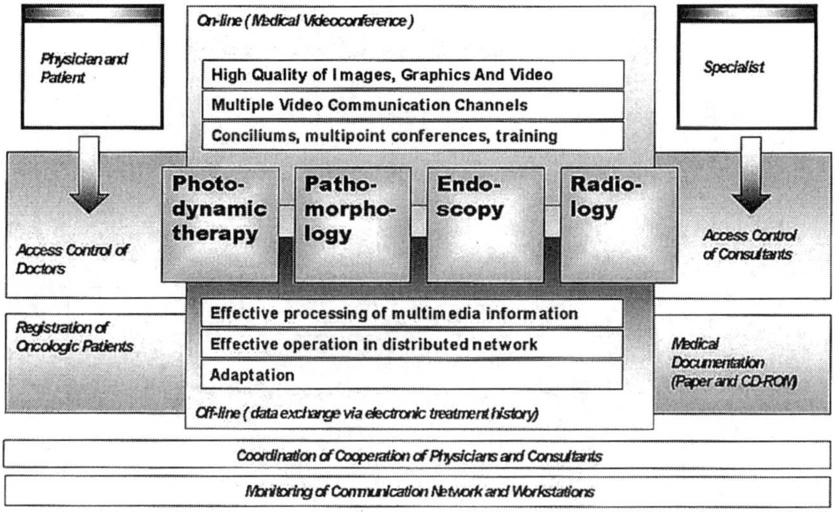

Figure 4: Major requirements and principles of MINT

It is not sufficient to use the conventional equipment to provide capabilities as wide as they are, e.g., for video conferencing. It is then not surprising that the equipment for exchanging medical data has been specially developed to match projected capabilities, in order to meet all requirements of this programme.

The software was developed in the same manner. It comprises not just a set of various software applications, but an entire software complex consisting of interconnected modules which allow connection to various different functions for teleoncological advising. The network has been added with special-purpose capabilities for authorised access, remote diagnosis and monitoring, and a control function to schedule work in the network.

The MINT programme involves the practical introduction of technology and equipment for teleoncological consultations in the course of:

- treatment for oncology diseases by the method of photodynamic therapy in online and offline modes
- pathomorphology examinations in online and offline modes
- endoscopy examinations
- X-ray examinations
- ultrasound examinations

All users of the MINT will be supplied with units for the teleoncology of various modifications and will have equal rights and obligations in the course of advising, notwithstanding whether it is an oncology research institute or a hospital. The first consultations within the network will be performed among the Oncology Clinic Dispensary, the Moscow Research Oncology Institute (named after P. A. Herzen), and the Medical Radiology Research Centre at the Russian Medical Academy.

For diagnosing cases, the automated TNM classification system will be used; this allows diagnosticians and clinicians to be more precise in setting their diagnosis of a case, as well as the form of the disease and its localisation, to make a detailed examination of the zones of close and deep metastasis spread, and to develop an optimal treatment plan. All of this information is registered in the electronic case record of an oncology patient (Figure 5).

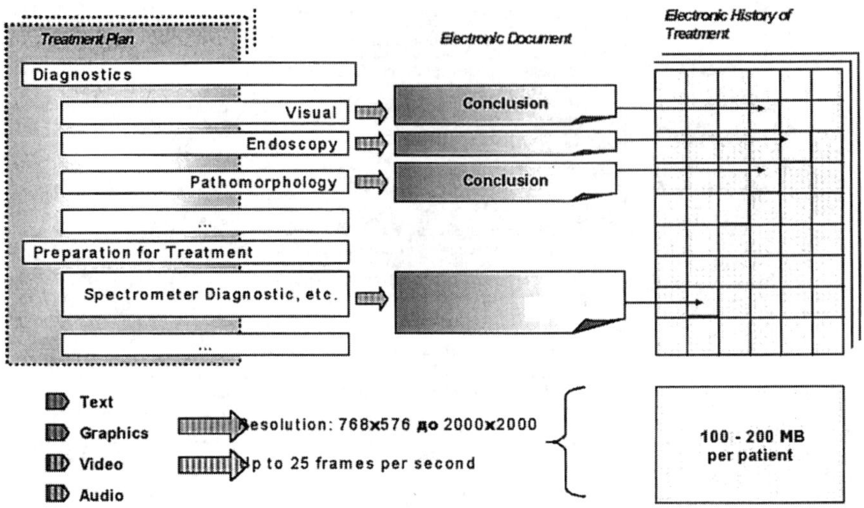

Figure 5: Electronic history of treatment

Within the framework of the programme, the electronic version of the case record of an oncology patient is formed with the use of photodynamic therapy, as well as electronic versions of physicians' reports, in the course of teleoncological advising during pathomorphology examinations on the basis of the main principles of the international standard Dicom 3.0.

Any user of the MINT will be supplied with a special purpose microprocessor card, to be authorised for access to the information resources of the network and participation in teleoncological advising.

Within the information medium of the MINT, not only will point-to-point advising in real time be performed, but also consultations among several users at a time. This will allow involving several experts of both the same and different trades in the discussion of those cases in which a diagnosis is hard to make. Furthermore, within the teleoncological network special-purpose training lectures and seminars for oncologists in various lines of medicine are planned. These lectures and seminars may involve several tens of the registered users of the network at a time.

Upon the completion of treatment each patient will be allowed to obtain a CD-ROM with his/her case record, including all necessary video, sound, graphic, and textual data. The complete information of the case record in all details will be kept in the central database at the Control Centre of the MINT. The said CD-ROM allows a patient to take repeated advice from any expert, and the advisor of such a patient will also be able to receive the complete data of the case record, provided that he is an authorised advising physician of the MINT. Since access to the MINT may be provided through any communication channel, any expert in any country of the world may act as an adviser.

One of the first remote users of the MINT will be the Moscow Radiology Research Centre at the Russian Medical Academy in the city of Obninsk, Kaluga region. This leading institution in treatment of the Chernobyl invalids will be allowed to extend their experience to other medical oncology institutions and to carry out remote monitoring of the health conditions of approximately thousands of Chernobyl invalids in Moscow.

Finally, we feel it necessary to note that the technology and equipment developed for teleoncological advising allows for building similar telemedical video networks for other fields of medicine, as well.

4. Discussion

In the development of this project we have encountered a lot of problems, but two of them are principal:

1. There are no telemedicine standards and recommendations for compatibility; these can be generally useful when a telemedicine system is being developed for practical use and not only for demonstration purposes.
2. It is very difficult (maybe impossible) to create a large telemedicine network using such "bricks" as general purpose business video conference systems, because these systems support necessary video conference interfaces (like H.320/H.323) but have no open interfaces for integration with other hardware and software.

We solve these problems using technology which we can define as a *de facto* "telemedicine standard for us" and which is open enough to make necessary adaptations for practical tasks.

Address for correspondence

Vladimir Kazinov
P.O.Box 113
105122 Moscow, Russia
divisy@iasnet.ru

A Controlled Pilot Study in the Use of Telemedicine in the Community on the Management of Heart Failure
- A report of the first three months -

Simon de LUSIGNAN[1], Karen MEREDITH[2], Sally WELLS[3], Edward LEATHAM[4], Paul JOHNSON[5]
[1]*Honorary Senior Lecturer, St George's Hospital Medical School, London SW17 ORE*
General Practitioner, Woodbridge Hill Surgery Guildford, UK
[2]*Community Nursing Team Leader, Surrey and Hampshire Boarders NHS Trust*
Research Assistant, Woodbridge Hill Surgery Guildford, UK
[3]*Research Assistant and Practice Nurse, Woodbridge Hill Surgery Guildford, UK*
[4]*Consultant Cardiologist, Royal Surrey County Hospital, Guildford, UK*
[5]*Consultant Clinical Physiologist, John Radcliffe Hospital, Oxford, UK*

Abstract: This is a controlled pilot study of twenty patients to see if heart failure management can be optimised in the community using telemedicine. The study seeks to examine the feasibility, acceptability and reliability of using telemedicine in this context. Heart failure is a common condition. It is an important cause of mortality and morbidity and has large cost implications for the NHS. Most patients are managed in the UK in General Practice based on clinical assessment by the practitioner. Twenty patients with a mean age of 75.1 years and mean New York Heart Association grade of 1.75 were randomised in to two equal groups (telemonitoring and control) and observed for a period of three months. All twenty patients had a Cardiologist assessment and quality of life measurement at the beginning and end of the study. Patients in the telemedicine group had their blood pressure, pulse and weight data collected daily and undertook a weekly video conference with the nurse. Control patients had their blood pressure, weight and pulse measured at six weekly intervals. The study has been extended for a further six months beyond its initial three-month observation period to see if the initial short term benefit in the telemedicine group is maintained.

1. Introduction

Telemedicine is defined as medicine at a distance. Although regarded as a new concept, the medical professions have been undertaking remote consultation, "teleconsultation", for years. Telephone diagnosis has been an established part of General Practice as long as this medium has existed. What is happening now is merely exploiting the new media for communications.

In this study we examine the feasibility of using telemedicine to improve the management of heart failure in the community.

Heart failure is a common and increasing problem in General Practice particularly among older patients. It is unclear why it is increasing; in part it is due to the ageing population, but increased survival after myocardial infarction may also be an important factor.

A general practitioner with a list size of 2000 patients will see approximately 20 patients with heart failure each year 10 of who will be new cases. The general practitioner can expect four admissions to hospital in one year with patients with heart failure.

Half of the patients diagnosed with heart failure will die within four years and half of those with severe heart failure will die within one year. It has been estimated that 1% of the NHS budget is devoted to heart failure management, with 60% of this spent on hospital admission [1] Indeed heart failure continues to escalate in importance as a major cause of morbidity and mortality. More hospitalisation may not be the ideal way forward. ACE (Angiotensin Converting Enzyme) inhibitors can reduce mortality and morbidity in heart failure and it is recommended that all patients with symptomatic heart failure should be treated with an angiotensin converting enzyme inhibitor [2]. Yet only 20-30% of patients with heart failure in major studies were prescribed an ACE inhibitor by their general practitioner [3] [4]. However, a local audit suggests these figures may be out of date. Around 40% of patients in West Surrey practices were treated with ACE inhibitors.

Most general practice consultations last eight to ten minutes. In this relatively short period of time it is difficult for GPS to undress and adequately examine patients; particularly the elderly. What measures a GP does make are influenced by the stress of consulting. Without objective measurements at their disposal it is difficult for general practitioners to manage heart failure effectively in the consultation.

"White coat hypertension" is a real phenomenon and other physiological measures such as pulse can easily be influenced at times of stress. Telemonitoring from home has been shown to reduce some of the stress effects and may well lead to improved management of patients with heart failure [5].

Trials of telemedicine were first performed over 20 years ago. These early efforts experienced problems due to financial constraints (building expensive broad band video systems), failure to evaluate the system and recommended proposals for further research to be carried out. Early telemedicine projects failed, after all the initial enthusiasm, because of organisational, technological and communication problems.

Notwithstanding these early failures, home care of some groups of patients with heart failure using of telemedicine has shown to be cost effective. One other important facet of home care to be shown was its positive effect on quality of life in these patients. Telemonitoring can also help to interpret data to determine the effectiveness of therapeutic regimes. Potentially it may effect better symptom control, improve quality of life and improve patient compliance.

When the patient is remote from the health care professional the need for telemedicine is obvious. Useful interaction can still take place in the urban environment. The justification for urban telemedicine will come establishing whether it improves the management of a range of conditions in a cost-effective way. The principal way in which telemedicine can be cost-effective is by reducing hospital admissions. The hardest part of the cost-benefit equation to evaluate is the improvement in quality of life.

Techniques in telemedicine

- *teleconsultation* - Consultation between health professional and patient, separated geographically. In the simplest form this is via telephone but recently full colour two way video and audio links have been used.
- *telemonitoring* - The use of video, electronic or other telecommunication information to monitor patients status at a distance.
- *teledermatolgy* - The use of videoconferencing equipment for dermatology consultation.
- *teleradiology* - the transmission of radiological images for interpretation between health care professionals.
- *telepsychiatry* - the use of video consultation to conduct evaluation and management of psychiatric patients.

Face to face contact has always been fundamental in the delivery of health care. However it has been recognised that it is increasingly expensive to send patients into the secondary care sector rather than managing them in primary care, with the remote support of consultants.

Communication via the written word between the primary and secondary care sectors has been shown to be of varying quality . The NHS recognises that there is a need to improve communication between primary and secondary care and has even prioritised this as an area for research and development. [6]

The subsequent development of an IM&T strategy which included the creation of NHSnet (the NHS own secure computer network) reinforces the importance of communication within the NHS. The most recent white paper has reaffirmed the NHS commitment to NHSnet [7] with the stated intention to connect all General Practices by year 2002. This network provides a secure Intranet across which telemedicine and communications in general can take place. The NHS strategy for implementing its IT objectives are set out in *Information for Health* document (1998.) This not only reinforces the commitment mead above but also sets the objective of creating within the NHS lifelong Electronic Health Records (HER.) A National Health Service with electronic conduits to lifelong electronic records will also be one with the infrastructure over which telemedicine can be practised.

The telephone has long been a medium for communication between specialists both in primary and secondary care but programmes to increase and improve its use have only been partially successful. There is great potential for telemedicine between primary and secondary care to reduce these difficulties. In the UK there are approximately 300 million general practitioner consultations per year which result in approximately 40-50,000 hospital out-patient consultations per day.

There has been a great surge during the Fundholding years in the use of Outreach Clinics. These are clinics where a consultant instead of using their hospital based Outpatient Clinic, consults in a general practice surgery. Outreach has not proved to be cost effective and has done little to develop interactions between general practitioners and specialists . Studies have shown that telemedicine is feasible between general practitioners and hospital specialists and acceptable to all parties involved including patients. It may be that telemedicine could play a better role in improving GP consultant communication than Outreach did.

It has been predicted that telemedicine will play an increasing role in communication in health care in the future. It has been shown that it is potentially cost effective when improving communication between primary and secondary care and may offer a solution to controlling the increasing cost delivery of health care. In addition to delivery of care it can also be used for medical education.

Up to now telemedicine has been used in a way that reproduces current information flows between patients and primary or secondary care or between primary and secondary care. Our approach is to integrate the advantages of more physiological monitoring at home; with supplying objective observations to medical staff. This is intended to be achieved therefore allowing easy communication between patient, primary, secondary and tertiary care consultants, as needed. The web-server storage of patient data allows it to be viewed by any of the involved professionals as required. This is in marked contrast to the conventional flow of information in medical management.

Woodbridge Hill Surgery

This study was carried out using patients registered at Woodbridge Hill Surgery. The surgery is a seven doctor practice in North Guildford. The practice has an age-sex and social class distribution close to the national average. The practice has operated without written records for three years, and makes intensive use of information technology.. Use is made of internal e-mail. External e-mail and web browser access is provided via the Doctors Desk Project and NHSnet [8] The practice has educational links with St George's Medical School where one of the partners leads on the Doctors Desk Project (an NHSnet based information project for GPs).

The latter association and the high level of computerisation at the practice made this an obvious choice for this study.

Project Aim:
To conduct a controlled pilot study to see whether patients with heart failure can have their management improved using telemedicine.

Project objectives:
- To discover if the technique is acceptable to patients
- Are the recording devices reliable
- Are patients in the telemedicine group more likely to be managed according to guidelines.
- Is compliance with drug therapy greater in the telemedicine group
- Measure and compare the level of hospital admissions and outpatient attendances in both groups.
- Record quality of life change
- Manage the secure passage of data into NHSnet based database
- Allow interrogation of that data by community nurses, GPs and Consultants.

We wish to discover whether telemedicine can assist in optimising the management of heart failure. We also wish to test if there is a greater improvement in patient's quality of life in the telemedicine group, as compared with the control group. It is widely recognised that ACE inhibitors improve survival and reduce morbidity.

Studies have also shown that exercise tolerance of patients with heart failure prescribed an ACE (Angiotensin Converting Enzyme) inhibitor improved but that it was less clear whether there was overall improvement in terms of general wellbeing.

Quality of Life in heart failure

Quality of life is an important outcome for measuring health care benefits. Quality of life refers to many subjective and objective experiences among which, health, wellbeing and the ability to function in day-to-day activities are important [9]. Heart failure not only exerts its toll on the patient by shortening the duration of life but also by worsening the quality of life with chronic symptoms such as dyspnea and fatigue as well as significant impairment of psychological functioning.

Acceptability of telemedicine to patients

We aim to test if telemedicine as set out in our methodology, is feasible, reliable and acceptable to patients as a method for managing heart failure

Compliance

Studies have examined patient's response to teleconsulting in other disease areas, but we wish to examine this in the context of heart failure. We wish to examine the influence of telemedicine on compliance. Sharman [10] found that home monitoring of patients with heart failure increased compliance but studies of telemedicine have yet to show this. Will telemedicine foster dependency and high levels of use of medical services?

NHSnet – Working in a Secure Intranet

We intend to test the effectiveness use of NHSnet for the transmission of clinical data. This secure network is currently very little used. We wish to establish whether it is a reliable medium within which direct patient data can be collected and forwarded to different specialists. We plan to record the impact of these interventions on the interface between primary and secondary care and on the use of care services.

2. Method

Approval for this research was obtained from a Local Ethics Committee. The local Data Protection Registrar was also consulted. His view was that what was of importance to him was the purpose to which the data was being put, not the form in which it was being stored. Application was also made to our Regional Branch of NHS Telecommunications, and their Security Board has approved this project, on the basis of the security information supplied . It was noted that the Data Protection registrar made mention of the desirability of taking advantage of the security provided by NHSnet.

Identifying patients with heart failure

A search was carried out on the practice's computer system EMIS (Egton Medical Information System), the most widely used GP database software in England, to identify all current patients with a diagnosis of heart failure. We used the Read Codes set out below in the search:

G580	Congestive Heart Failure
C58z	Heart Failure NOS (Not otherwise specified, a Read coding classification)
G58	Heart Failure
14A6	H/O Heart Failure (History of)
C581	Left Ventricular Failure
G2111	Benign Hypertensive Disease + CCF (Congestive Cardiac Failure)
G2101	Malignant Hypertensive Heart Disease+CCF

This search identified a total of 152 patients.

Exclusions:

Exclusion Criteria
• Dementia • Terminal illness • Nursing Home • Severe respiratory disease • Physical impairment • No home telephone

The patients unable to co-operate with the study either due to dementia or severe physical impairment were excluded. We didn't want to impose the stress of participating in a study on a patient with a terminal diagnosis and these patients were also excluded. We also excluded patients resident in Nursing homes as they have a large amount of supervision already.

Patients with severe respiratory disease were excluded because it is diagnostically difficult to differentiate between cardiac and respiratory symptoms in this group.

Our working definition of a severe respiratory disease was patients requiring home nebulisers. At a later stage it became necessary to exclude patients who had no home phone. While many of these diagnoses were recorded on the patients electronic records, it was necessary to go through their written notes manually to check for exclusion criteria.

The exclusions reduced the sample from 152 to 137 patients.

ACE Inhibitor Use

A search was carried out to identify all current patients prescribed an ACE inhibitor. There were 324 patients using ACE inhibitors. This number is not surprising as this drug is also used to treat hypertension.

For the purposes of this pilot study (for which we could only investigate 20 patients), we decided only to include patients with a diagnosis of heart failure who were taking an ACE inhibitor. This reduced our heart failure population from 137 to 54 patients. We also excluded those patients who were not on the telephone.

Looking for patients with heart failure taking ACE inhibitors, on the phone, produced a sample of 51.

Heart failure diagnosis confirmed by specialist

At this stage we again examined through the patients notes for a specialist confirmation of the diagnosis of heart failure. This was done to ensure patients in this small pilot study genuinely had heart failure. This gave a final number of 29 patients for the project.

Randomisation

The remaining 29 patients were given an individual number of 1 -29 and the first twenty were allocated to the study using a random number generator.

Consent

The 20 patients identified were then contacted by telephone to determine whether they would be interested in taking part in the project. At this stage 4 patients declined to take part due to differing reasons (See table below). The remaining 25 patients were again allocated using the same random number generator and the 4 new patients contacted to see if they would be interested in taking part in the project. These patients agreed to the initial proposal.

Reasons for declining to take part
• Depression - 2 patients
• Husband seriously ill
• "Seeing too many doctors"

An appointment with each patient was made, at their convenience, in their home or at the surgery. At this consultation the project was fully explained and consent to take part requested. After these interviews all the patients gave their consent to take part in the project.

No of patients	*Group of Patients*
11169	Total Practice List
324	Patients prescribed ACE Inhibitor
152	Patients with a Read code for heart failure
137	Patients read coded for heart failure without any exclusion criteria *"Eligible patients"*
54	*Eligible patients* taking an ACE Inhibitor
51	*Eligible patients* taking ACE Inhibitors and on the phone
29	*Eligible patients* on ACE Inhibitors, on the phone with written specialist confirmation of diagnosis
25	The number of patients from the above group willing to give consent
20	The first 20 patients identified by random table allocation 10 to Telemedicine, and 10 to the Control Group. *"The Study Patients"*

Cardiologist's Assessment

The 20 patients included in the study were given an appointment to see a Consultant Cardiologist at the local hospital to confirm their diagnosis of heart failure.

Key information about their medical history and therapy was recorded on a proforma, on which the consultant would add his findings and guidelines for management. The consultant at this stage did not know which group the patient had been allocated into (telemedicine or control). A clinical examination was carried out. An echocardiogram was done unless performed already in the last year. A programme of care was determined for each patient to be managed in primary care, with reference back to the consultant as requested. These were the findings of the initial assessment:

- All the patients had their diagnosis of heart failure confirmed by echocardiogram.
- On the NYHA grading of heart failure
  10 patients = Grade 1
  6 patients = Grade 2
  3 patients = Grade 3
  1 patient = Grade 4
- 12 patients had their ACE inhibitor changed to a once a day preparation.
- 13 patients were not on optimal ACE inhibitor therapy.
- 4 patients had their diuretic therapy increased.

- One patient was commenced on anticoagulant therapy
- One patient had their anticoagulant therapy discontinued.
- 5 patients were commenced on antihypertensive therapy.
- One patient required a coronary angiogram.

Installation of Telemedicine Equipment

Telemedicine equipment in patient's home

- Wrist blood pressure monitoring device
  - Teleconsulting equipment
- 8 x 8 ViaTV system
- Telemonitoring equipment
  - HP Heart Link home hub
  - HP Heart Link scales

The 10 patients who were allocated into the telemedicine group were then visited and the equipment installed and installation checklist and questionnaire completed

Wrist blood pressure-monitoring device

This was chosen as a convenient way for patients to monitor their own blood pressure. A small questionnaire based trial was carried out in the surgery and community to determine the patients' preference to arm or wrist blood pressure devices [11]. Overall, patients preferred the wrist device, which was selected for the study. In order to achieve accurate and consistent readings, the patients were supplied with a foam wedge. The patients placed their left arm on it each time a blood pressure was recorded. This meant their wrist was kept at a consistent height during blood pressure measurement. Our experience was that the device appeared very sensitive to wrist height.

Patients were able to store each recording in the memory and this information was down loaded weekly by the community nurse and recorded with their other computer data. The blood pressure and pulse device we chose to use in this project was CE marked. This is a Europe wide quality standard.

CE Marking

- Background – The main purpose of the marking is to bring about the completion of the Single Market by introducing harmonised and statutorily based controls to regulate safety and marketing of products throughout the European Community (EC).
- What the marking means – CE marking means that a manufacturer claims his product satisfies the requirements essential for it to be considered safe and fit for its intended purpose
- Is the device safe? – The CE marking ought to indicate that a device is safe, but should not be viewed as a guarantee of safety. Rather users should see CE marking as a declaration by the manufacturer that his product meets all the relevant provisions and has been assessed accordingly. The CE marking means that the product can be freely marketed anywhere in the community without further control.

Teleconsulting equipment

This consisted of videoconferencing equipment. A ViaTV 8 x 8 (™) system was connected to the patients television and home phone. The system allowed the patient and the community nurse to see each other whilst they talked on the phone. A link was made from the patient's home to the general practitioners surgery. Both parties were equipped with the system which was connected via the television and compatible telephone.

Telemonitoring equipment

This consisted of HP (Hewlett Packard) Heart Link Home Hub and HP Heart Link scales. The hub sits by the telephone and collects the data from the scales via radio transmission. It stores the data and sends it by telephone to the telemedicine server daily. This set up meets NHS Telecommunications Department Security Board requirements.

The baseline visit

The 20 patients who had been confirmed to take part in the study had a management plan completed.

The 10 patients in the telemedicine group had all the equipment installed and running. A baseline visit was made to each patient. An initial blood pressure and weight was taken on all the patients and a quality of life questionnaire completed [12]. After a baseline period of observation the patients attended the consultant cardiologist for assessment.

Monitoring during the Study

The study will run for a three-month observation period. During this period the following observations were planned:

Telemedicine Group: The telemedicine group will carry out the observations set out in the grid below:

Observation	*Timing*	*Special Instruction*
Body weight	First thing in the morning	Measured in night attire.
Pulse & BP	Twice a day mid morning and evening (2hrs after morning medication and12 hrs after that depending on patients lifestyle)	This will be stored in blood pressure machine's memory.
Teleconsultation	Once per week	Scheduled interview to cover items set out in the Teleconference prompt sheet

Control Group

The intention with the Control Group is that they should have best practice. However it is possible for members of the control group to have consultations with medical practitioners that might not get recorded in their notes and therefore be missed in the study.

Members of the control group will have a baseline visit, as described above, to measure weight, blood pressure and assess quality of life.

This group will then have further regular assessment visits from the nurse (this will be a departure from normal best practice for this group of patients).

However it is possible at the end of the study that they will not be able to remember all the medical interventions they have had over the three-month period. It is also important to know whether this group of patients has a substantial number of untreated problems that this visit might identify.

Final Visit

At the end of the study, all patients will complete a final Quality of Life Questionnaire. Any medical inputs or changes will be noted.

Both groups of patients, will, on a monthly basis, have their medical records examined by the Research Nurse for the changes, or medical input not identified from the telemedicine or the Intermediate assessment visit. Compliance with medication will be particularly carefully checked at this time.

3. Results

The concept of Telemedicine was accepted readily by our Pilot Telemedicine Group. Although the average age of the group was 73.5 years and the group were not used to this technology they were keen to start and to be involved in the project. Qualitatively, our patients associated telemedicine with their General Practice as being up-to-date and innovative. They did not necessarily associate the study as being beneficial to there own clinical care but saw it as furthering the progress of medicine for future generations.

Of the patients invited, only four declined. One patient (in the telemedicine group) transiently dropped out of the study, telephoning the surgery asking for telemonitoring equipment to be removed. On visiting the patient they explained that they only wished to have the equipment removed whilst they were on holiday but wished that the equipment be replaced on return! Two patients died in the control group, one of an unrelated cancer, the other of myocardial infarction.

The biggest subjective problems presenting were the technical difficulties to allow the teleconsulting to take place. There was no uniform standard of television connection. One patient did not have a television and another patient's television was unable to be connected. Therefore two new televisions had to be purchased to allow teleconsulting to begin. A secondary problem was the amount of wiring involved in the connection of the system from phone to television. In some cases this involved wires stretching across the length of a room, or between rooms This was considered it to be a physical hazard to the patients and they were most anxious that it be placed well out of the way. This meant with some patients the wiring being fixed above floor level. Patients were also concerned that the system did not interfere with other electronic equipment, and in particular their own regular television viewing. Patients also were required to have a touch–tone phone as part of the dialling system. Two patients required new phones to be purchased, as they did not have the correct dialling system

9 out of 10 patients showed a reduction in their systolic blood pressure and 7 out of 10 a decrease in weight over the first 60 days of telemonitoring. There is a significant correlation between reduction in weight and systolic blood pressure.

Results – Telemedicine Group		
	Weight Increase	*Weight decrease*
Systolic B/P Increase	1	
Systolic B/P Decrease	2	7

Results – Control Group		
Mean (+range)	*Day 1*	*Day 60*
Systolic	190 (120-200)	146 (130-160)
Diastolic	78 (60-100)	81 (70-90)
Pulse	84 (66-110)	81 (70-90)
Wt in Kg	86 (63-106)	85 (64-99)

Average systolic blood pressure appeared to fall among the controls, although these observations are suspect as they are only based on two readings. There was no significant change in diastolic blood pressure, or weight in kilograms. The entire reduction in weight in the control group can be attributed to a single patient who went from 106 to 99 kgs during the first 60 days.

Results – QoL (GHQ – General Health Questionnaire)		
	Telemedicine Group	*Control Group*
Day1	22	25
Day 90	17	31
No relationship between QoL score and rise in BP and/or weight was found		

On Day 1 there was no significant difference in quality of life scores between the telemedicine and control group. A low GHQ score is associated with high quality of life, and visa versa.

Over the study period, the quality of life of the Telemedicine group appeared to improve significantly whilst the control group deteriorated. There was no correlation between the individuals in the Telemedicine group or control group who gained weight or increased their systolic blood pressure, and those who had a decline in their quality of life.

4. Discussion

The Telemonitoring and observation of patients was surprisingly acceptable to patients. No one has dropped out of the study other than the two deaths in the control group. The technique appears to be robust and reliable. Clinical benefit (in terms of improved systolic blood pressure) appears to be measurable in 70% of the telemonitoring group and 90% reduced their weight. It might be assumed that this was associated with better compliance with ACE inhibitors and diuretics.

Modular units are needed to overcome the technical difficulties and to ease patient anxieties for teleconsulting to take place. They would reduce the amount of technical knowledge and support required from the medical professionals involved.

Further research is needed to see if these initial benefits are maintained, and if this intervention is cost effective. We are continuing this study for a further six months to see whether the improvements in clinical condition and quality of life continue. We are looking as to whether trend lines that monitor change in systolic blood pressure and body weight can be used as markers as to the improvement or worsening of a patient's clinical condition.

A larger study is needs to be conducted to separately evaluate the contribution made by the videophone consulting and the telemonitoring equipment. We also need to compare this equipment with that capable of recording continuous ECG and possibly other modalities to see if more information can be gleaned from about a patients clinical condition from more sophisticated equipment.

References

[1] McMurray, W Hart, G Rhodes. An evaluation of the cost of heart failure to the National Health Service in the UK. *Br J of Med Econ* 1993;6:99-110.

[2] The treatment of heart failure. Task Force of the Working Group on Heart Failure of the European Society of Cardiology. *Eur Heart J* 1997 May;18(5):736-753.

[3] Mair FS, Carowley TS, Bundred PK. Prevalence, aetiology and management of heart failure in general practice. *Br J Gen Pract* 1996;46:77-79.

[4] Clark KW, Gray D, Hampton JR. Evidence of inadequate investigation and treatment of patients with heart failure. *Br Heart J* 1994;71:584-587.

[5] Johnson P, Andrews DC. Remote continuous physiological monitoring in the home. *Journal Telemedicine and* Telecare1996;2(2):107-113.

[6] Department of Health. *Research for health: a research and development strategy for the NHS.*London: DoH, 1991.

[7] Secretary of State for Health. The New NHS - Modern, Dependable - HMSO 1998

[8] de Lusignan S. The Doctors Desk. One vision of the future information and communication needs of General Practice. Journal of Informatics in Primary Care. May 1998; 19-22.
de Lusignan S, Whitelaw R, Scanning for Networked EMIS, Part 1, EMIS user Sept(3) 1997.
de Lusignan S, Whitelaw R, Scanning for Networked EMIS, Part 2. EMIS user Jan(1) 1998.

[9] Palmore , Luikhardt C. Health and social factors related to life satisfaction. *J Health Soc Behav* 1972;13:68-80.

[10] Sharman A. Critical care management of the heart failure patient in the home.*Crit Care Nurs Q* 1995 :18(1);77-87

[11] de Lusignan S et al, Measuring blood pressure at the wrist: more comfortable for patients and more convenient for doctors. *Submitted for publication*

[12] Goldberg and Hiller. General Health Questionnaire 28: A scaled Version of the General Health Quest ionnaire. *Psychol Med* 1979;9:139-145.

Address for correspondence

Simon de Lusignan
Honorary Senior Lecturer
St George's Hospital Medical School
London SW17 ORE, UK

Telematic-Based Model of Early Diagnosis and Treatment of Acute Coronary Syndromes

R. GRIEBENOW[1], Ch. DANG[2]
[1]Med. Klinik Merheim (Kardiologie), Med. Universitätsklinik II, Köln, Germany
[2]Telemedizinisches Konsultationszentrum, Johanniter-Unfall-Hilfe e.V. Regionalverband Köln, Germany

1. Introduction

In Germany, diseases of the heart and circulatory system continue to be the leading cause of death, most often in the form of acute myocardial infarction and its subsequent sequels.

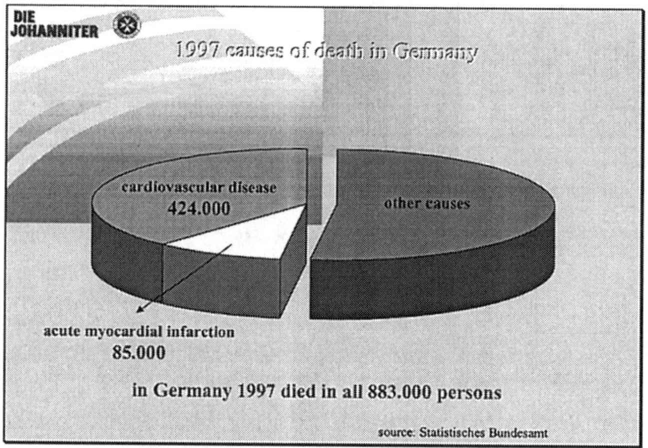

Fig. 1 Causes of Death in Germany 1997

The aim of therapeutic efforts of the past ten years has been to limit the magnitude of infarcts. A keystone of this concept has been the rapid re-opening of the infarct related artery, which is obstructed in the majority of patients. The most common method is that of intravenous thrombolysic therapy, which has been shown to significantly reduce acute and delayed mortality [6]. The greatest therapeutic effectiveness is consistently achieved when the time between the onset of the infarct and the reopening of the artery by means of thrombolysis is as short as possible [3].

Germany provides excellent conditions for delivering emergency care to patients suffering from an acute coronary syndrome, thanks to: a) the high density of physicians, b) an emergency system which ensures that physicians in private practice are on call 24 hours a day and c) a well-developed emergency-medicine system equipped with a veritable arsenal of therapies for acute treatment of life-threatening situations. The syndrome of acute thoracic pain continues to be observed frequently within the context of emergency medical care [1], but cannot always be adequately interpreted, as it is not always possible to examine the patient using a 12-channel ECG, or to have the record evaluated by a physician with experience in ECG interpretation. Thus, although early diagnosis of myocardial infarction is highly desirable, it is often not possible as the physician providing initial care does not possess the requisite experience in such diagnosis. On the other hand, the high rates of admission to stationary care facilities which this situation engenders is economically undesirable. In such situations, the ECG is decisive, because of all diagnostic methods this is the one which becomes positive early, which permits recordings in an easy and standardizable manner, and which enables early diagnosis of a myocardial infarct with a high level of diagnostic sensitivity and specificity [5].

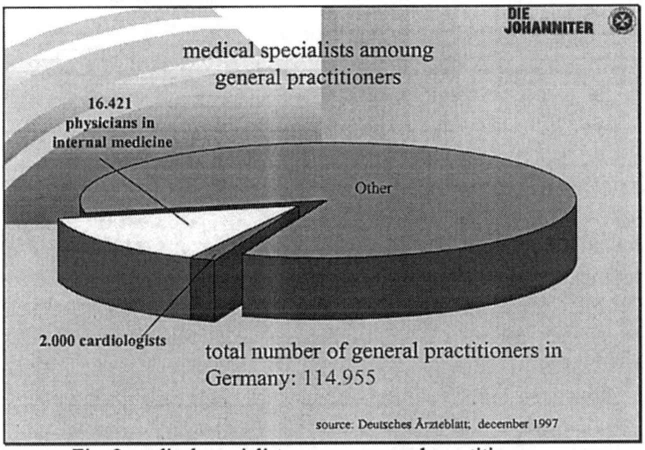

Fig. 2 medical specialists among general practitioners

For these reasons, a plan has been conceived to create a telematics-based ECG diagnosis service in order to provide prompt, competent analysis of the ECG 24 hours a day in the event of suspected acute coronary syndrome.

2. The Model

Technically, this concept requires a miniaturized ECG-measuring apparatus capable of recording and transmitting the ECG in digital form. The unit must be as small as possible, so as not to make providing emergency care even more difficult. This device must also be equipped with an integrated display, in order to allow experienced physicians to diagnose the condition immediately without having to transmit data, and to permit continuous monitoring of both the ST segments and the heart rhythm. A chip card reader would be an additional desirable feature to facilitate billing. A further important requirement is a mains-independent power supply. Data is transmitted in digital form, *via* a fax modem (integrated into the ECG recorder) and analog telephone lines where possible. The device must also supply a simultaneous voice link to permit contact with the physician at the scene. The requirements which the ECG recorder must fulfill are summarized in Table 1.

Requirements for an Innovative ECG Recorder

Small enough to be held in one hand

Easy to handle, with at most **3 buttons**

- *one to switch between speech and modem connection*
- *one to start the registration*
- *one to send the ecg-file*

Display to control

- *a screen to define a clear ECG-wave*
- *preferably all 12 leads to click through*
- *with a warning signal to control the leads attachment*

Integrated **chip card reader**

- *personal data and ID number from this card should be taken into the ECG-file*

Power supply should be guaranteed over an **accumulator**, alternatively over an external cable

Table 1

A high-performance server is required at the receiving end to ensure minimum time delay in receipt of the ECGs. The analysis software must enable the user to interactively access the recording, e.g., for precise evaluation of the time intervals. In this regard, further desirable features include the simultaneous display of multiple leads (e.g., thoracic wall leads), or the high-resolution "zoomed" display of individual sections of a lead. The written diagnosis is electronically transmitted to the physician on site, as well as to the patient's primary care provider.

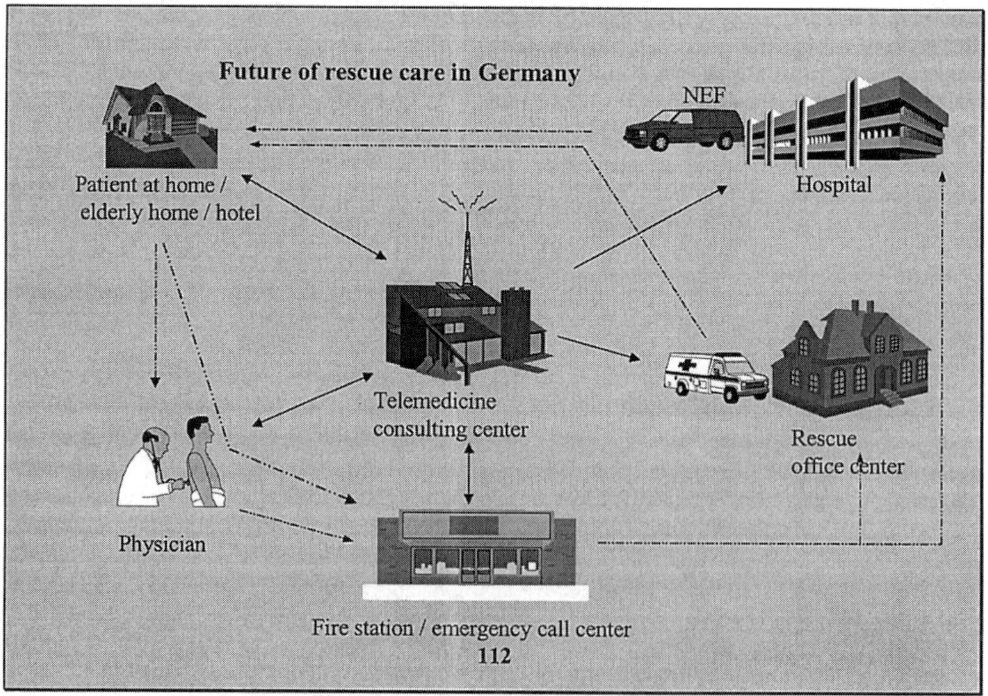

Fig. 3 Future of rescue care in Germany

As the ECG diagnosis is accomplished outside of existing medical facilities (such as a hospital) and their hierarchically structured chains of responsibility, it is especially important to ensure that the diagnosing physicians receive the best possible training and supervision. To this end, a structured training program with final certification is being developed. In addition, regular supervision will examine randomly selected ECG diagnoses and organize discussions between diagnosing physicians and experienced cardiologists to deal with special problems. Diagnosing physicians will also be required to renew their certifications at regular intervals.

3. Discussion

The development of new, miniaturized ECG recorders makes it possible to record a 12-channel ECG on site without impeding emergency care provision. The display to be integrated into the device to be developed for this application will permit rapid diagnosis by an experienced physician without prior data transmission, and also ensure continuous monitoring of both the ST segments and possible arrhythmia. The possibility of simultaneous voice communication allows an exchange of clinical-anamnestic information, which is absolutely vital for interpreting the ECG.

The ability to transmit ECG diagnoses *via* fax additionally involves subsequent treatment facilities (e.g., clinics) at the earliest possible stage, helping to save even more time. Studies have repeatedly shown that an ECG analysis under emergency-care conditions can help to further shorten the time between the onset of symptoms and the start of therapy, and thus improve the patients' prognosis [4, 2]. The model described here makes possible for the first time a broadly available capability for early diagnosis of acute myocardial infarct under emergency-care conditions, enabling definitive therapy to commence at the earliest possible moment. At the same time, it will also help to improve patient selection and thus more effectively use precious health care resources.

References

[1] H.R. Arntz, R. Stern, Th. Linderer, and R. Schröder, Efficiency of a Physician-Operated Mobile: Intensive Care Unit for Prehospital Thrombolysis in Akute Myocardial Infarction, *Amer. J. Cardiol.* **70** (1992) 417-420.

[2] The EMIP Study Group, Prehospital Thrmbolytic Therapy in Patients with Suspected Myocardial Infarction, *M. Engl. J. Med.* **329** (1993) 383-389.

[3] GISSI 2, A Factorial Randomized Trial of Alteplase versus Streptokinase and Heparin versus No Heparin among 12.490 Patients with Acute Myocardial Infarction, *Lancet* **336** (1990) 65-71.

[4] GREAT Group, Feasibility, Safety and Efficacy of Domiciliary Thrombolysis by General Practitioners: Grampian Region Early Anistreplase Trial, *BMJ* **305** (1992) 548-553.

[5] R. Stern, H.R. Arntz, S. Klatt, Th. Linderer, J. Beneker, B. Levenson, H. Cöller, W.H. Storch, H. Schäfer, and R. Schröder, Ist die prästationäre Thrombolyse bei akutem Myokardinfarkt als Routinemaßnahme sinnvoll? *Z. Kardiol.* **81** (1992) 199-204.

[6] A.C. Weis and D.C. Gulba, Thrombolysetherapie des akuten Myokardinfarktes und angewandte Therapien. In: R. Griebenow, P. Dominiak, and H.M. Piper (eds.), Autonomes Nervensystem und Koronare Herzkrankheit (i.Druck).

Address for correspondence

R. Griebenow
Med. Klinik Merheim (Kardiologie)
Med. Universitätsklinik II
51109 Köln, Germany
E-mail: tele-ekg@juh-cologne.de

The Impact of Telemedicine on Health Care Management
M. Nerlich and R. Kretschmer (Eds.)
IOS Press, 1999

Telemedicine and Diabetes

Rolf ENGELBRECHT, Claudia HILDEBRAND
GSF-MEDIS Institute, Neuherberg, Germany

Abstract: Telecommunication technology has reached a maturity which can effectively support the promotion of health, prevention and management of diseases and rehabilitation. To achieve effective support harmonisation and interoperability of technologies are main requirements. This article tries to point out how interoperability is being met and how the requirements are being applied using DIABCARD as an example. DIABCARD has developed a chip card based medical information system for the care of persons with diabetes.

1. Introduction

Telemedicine is the application of telecommunications technology to healthcare using methods of informatics It has, over the past decades of implementation, proven to be clinically effective in an increasing number of medical specialities. Improvements in information technologies have made technologies available to the health care professional, as for example, high definition video teleconferencing. Applications in diabetes care include decision support on the management of diabetes, telecommunication for managing patients at home, internet technologies to support professional and patient educational processes, diabetic retinopathy screening and a chip card for improving the quality of care. Nevertheless, information processing in health care is still primarily being used for administration, statistics, and economy. What is hampering the wide-spread use of telemedicine?

There are, of course, the (initial) costs. Additionally, effective use of telemedicine requires effective telemedicine software which must be long-living, adaptable, easy to update (without requiring new hardware) and can be implemented with mature, off-the-shelf technologies, such as personal computers networks using internet access. On top of that, they must be accessible by various people of the healthcare team thus supporting shared care. This, on the other hand, asks for an electronic patient record, interoperability, harmonisation and standardisation. Different activities on European (TAP, CEN) and on international (G7) level are dealing with these topics. First results have been presented.

2. Electronic Medical Record

The medical record is in most Western health care systems not held centrally but distributed. This poses many problems especially for a patient with a chronic illness who is being treated by a multidisciplinary and decentralised team. Double examinations cause discomfort to the patient and increase the costs for healthcare, ignorance on the overall medication or allergies may even put the patient at risk.

A patient record is best characterised by the need to support the care of individual patients based on a detailed representation of the individual's record thus improving its quality of care

[1]. At the same time it should enhance the productivity of health care professionals and reduce costs associated with health care delivery and financing. It also could support clinical and health services research. This requires a patient record that is up-to-date, complete and available.

Telecommunication facilitates the access to medical data and knowledge and it enables computer systems to solve problems that without it could hardly be solved, e.g. retrieving some important information from a patient's record that otherwise would go unseen [2]. It meets the growing demands of our society like continuous mobility, optimal support of an ageing population with multiple diseases and the increased use of information technology.

In 1991 the Institute of Medicine, National Academy of Sciences/USA, published a study on the state of the Electronic Patient Record (EPR) and gave recommendations on the requirements of a future EPR system [2]. It stated that an EPR is more than a paper record put onto a computer: it has to enhance patient management, link to other systems, improve communication between the different health services and health care levels, allow for further developments and provide confidentiality and security.

Among different storage technologies an intelligent chip card seems to be an ideal carrier for an EPR. The patient health card contains essential data, it is patient based, can be taken everywhere at the same time providing privacy and security to patient and health professional in a balanced patient-doctor relationship. Each health professional is able to assess the patient's actual state-of-health at any time. She/he can take into consideration the results from the patient‘s contact with another health care professional.

The DIABCARD project team has developed an information system for the treatment of persons with diabetes based on an electronic medical record held on a smart card -a portable patient record.

3. Chip Card and Smart Card

Since the middle of the 80s chip card applications are booming world-wide. More than 50 countries have introduced telephone cards equipped with a chip, all French banking cards are chip cards and the mandatory German Health Insurance card also carries a microchip [3].

Most applications in the health care sector concern the administrative sector. In Germany most insured people have been equipped with a health insurance card. Even though the health insurance card is a read-only memory card by definition and contains administrative data only (name, address of the insured, date of birth, insurance company, insurance number and date of expiration of the card, 238 bytes in total), it helped reduce the administrative workload, proved to be cost saving and has prompted the use of doctor office computer systems [4].

A smart card is a chip card which has one or more processors and memory and whose access is protected [5]. Applications that need a high degree of confidentiality and ensure data integrity to the user can be realised in smart card technologies, e.g. encryption, digital signature, access matrixes or on-going developments in biometrical identification methods like finger print on a chip card, voice recognition or eye movement interpretation [6]. A typical smart card architecture is presented in fig. 1.

The introduction of the patient data cards does not require vital modifications of existing structures and practices. Not even the reading device poses a problem: Bill Gates -the chairman of the leading institution for PC system software- announced at the Harrogate 98 conference in March 1998 that he expects within short time to have each desk top computer equipped with a smart card reader. Smart cards can be used as part of a network or as stand-alone system. Their integration into a workstation offers the possibility to aggregate the data of individual patients and to analyse the state of care. In any case they are part of a medical information system (MIS).

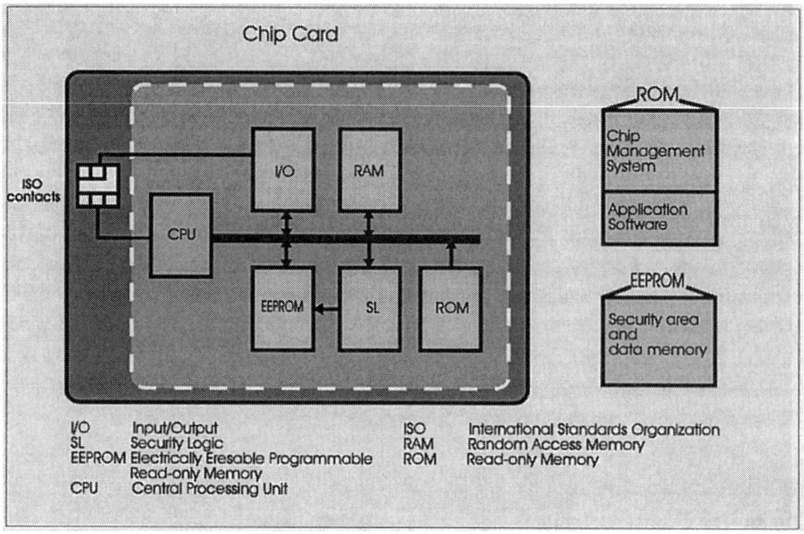

Fig.1: Smart card architecture

There are a number of interesting limited trials based on clinical cards that have been, or are on the point of being implemented [7]. These applications are highly specific and dependent on the issuer system. If we do not prepare for interoperability now, the extension of these clinical card applications will lead to a situation in which health professionals who have patients of different origins and with different portable medical devices will have to handle a multitude of specific elements to access the data.

It is unlikely that healthcare facilities will be equipped with all the specific card terminals, interfaces, protocols, software, necessary to access the full range of clinical cards because this would mean that each time a new application is developed, all the participating healthcare structures would have to invest in the specific card and new hard- and software

At this stage, only few clinical card applications are actually in use and none is ready yet for European-wide diffusion. It is necessary to establish interoperability guidelines now to prepare the future.

4. Interoperability

The target for interoperability is to offer a clinical card that can be considered as a transparent device for all healthcare users regardless of card technology or contents and can be used across borders. The information necessary to treat the patient as well as security functions will have to be available in the preferred language of the health professional. Under strict security conditions, authorised healthcare personnel will be able to read and write information.

The interoperability of healthcare cards therefore defines as follows: Interoperability of computer readable health care cards is the ability to access, use and update computer readable data held on cards issued by any healthcare organisation, any healthcare facilities to the extent that accessing, managing and processing these data is possible for those healthcare facilities and healthcare professionals that are legally authorised.

The card needs an information processing environment to communicate. Therefore interoperability must not only be considered at the level of the card and card terminal but also in terms of solutions integrating the communication devices. Four levels can be distinguished:

- Technical, enabling the use of cards and readers from different producers;
- Data, a common definition of the content;
- Data presentation, in order to integrate the different applications;
- Security, to ensure a trustful environment.

To show interoperability a smart card designed for the care of people with diabetes seems a good starting point. Diabetes can be seen as a paradigm of a chronic disease including its need to be treated by a multidisciplinary team. The rising figures of persons concerned are another indicator for the necessity to provide effective diabetes health care systems. Quality assurance is part of this provision. It will reduce acute and long-term complications, support preventive care and improve the patient's well-being. This will save costs, direct costs, and indirect costs, for example, by increased employment of the persons with diabetes.

5. Interoperability on the technical level

5.1. EU/G7 interoperability architecture

In the 4th framework of the EU research programme "Health Telematics" (then called "Advanced Informatics in Medicine") the concerted action EUROCARDS was initiated with 6 working groups and additional activities. One was the "European Healthcard Interoperability Feasibility Study". The EU-sponsored projects DIABCARD and Cardlink [8] –another EU-funded project on healthcards- participated actively. It resulted in an architecture for medical cards which should be applied in the EU and G7 countries and piloted by DIABCARD and Cardlink.

The priority of the EU Interoperability Feasibility Study was on interoperable access to the patient's administrative and emergency data. It was thought that the technical architecture for interoperability should allow the card issuers to meet their own priorities [9]. Therefore the interoperable elements of the system are divided into the „Local System Components" -which are the responsibility of the supplier of the local healthcard system- and into the „Card Dependent Components", which are the responsibility of the card issuer. Fig. 2 shows the interoperability architecture as proposed by the EU feasibility study. It includes the following interfaces

- the card interface for the communication between the card and the card terminal
- the card terminal interface to allow healthcard servers to access different card readers
- the healthcard server interface to request the interoperability data sets from the healthcard server.

The physical characteristics, the dimension and location of contacts, the electronic transmission and signal protocols and the location of contacts have been standardised in ISO 7618. Standards have also been drafted for "inter-industrial commands for interchange" and the "registration system for application in IC cards", standards for security and on the application level are on the way.

More information on the EU Feasibility Study and the proposed architecture is to be found on the internet [10,11] and in [9]. The actual DIABCARD architecture described below is based on the EU/G7 architecture but has taken recent developments into account.

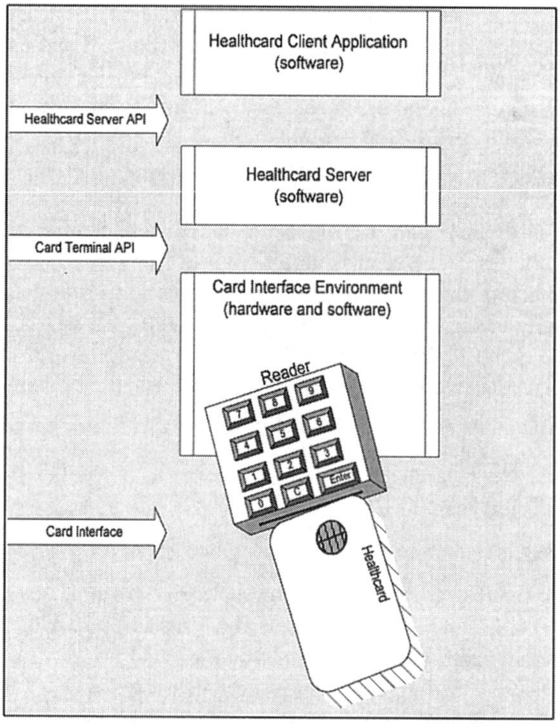

Fig. 2 Interoperability architecture as proposed by the EU feasibility study.

5.2. Joint Panel on Health Cards

In 1995 working groups were found in Germany to harmonise the German on-going health card projects and to prepare the input for national and European standardisation committees [12]. At the same time it enforces the use of standards and recommendations, for example, the use of the EU/G7 interoperabilty data set and ASN.1-structure for data storage. This Joint Panel on Health Cards is split up into six working groups which deal with the following topics

- Health Professional Card
- Checklist
- Data Structures
- Security Infrastructure
- Multifunctional Card Terminal
- Further Development of the Health Insurance Card.

5.3. PC/SC (Personal Computer/Smart Card) specification and the OpenCard Framework

PC/SC standard (Personal Computer/SmartCard) [13] was developed to ensure compatibility between smart cards, card reader/writer and computers produced by different manufacturers. The technology integrating smart cards and PCs was built on the current ISO 7816 standard, and supports business-specific application standards such as EMV (Europay, MasterCard, Visa) and GSM (Global Standard for Mobile Communication). It allows application developers to take advantage of the smart cards portability and hardware-based security, both critical factors for the development of secure applications.

PC/SC includes

Different layers for describing the cards and card terminals:

- Programming interface for communication with smart card and reader device connected to a PC;
- High-level application interface - to make it easier to build smart card applications.

Specifications for cryptographic functionality and secure storage.

PC/SC is an emerging industrial standard which has not yet been not finally defined on all layers. So, for an intermediate time, OpenCard Framework [14] as a smart card standard enabling access to personalised data and services from any network computer is being used additionally. It provides a high-level interface which can support multiple smart card types independent from the supplier. It enables interaction with existing PC/SC standard. The OpenCard Framework supports digital signatures and uses cryptographic keys for security.

This PC/SC specification, and the OpenCard Framework were both incorporated into the DIABCARD architecture (see fig.3).

5.4. DIABCARD architecture

The DIABCARD architecture (fig.3) defines the required functionality that should be provided by a high level DIABCARD application interface (the DIABCARD Server), easily to be integrated into existing medical information systems and other applications. Apart from the EU/G7 Interoperability Specification it incorporated the PC/SC (Personal Computer/Smart Card) specification and the OpenCard Framework.

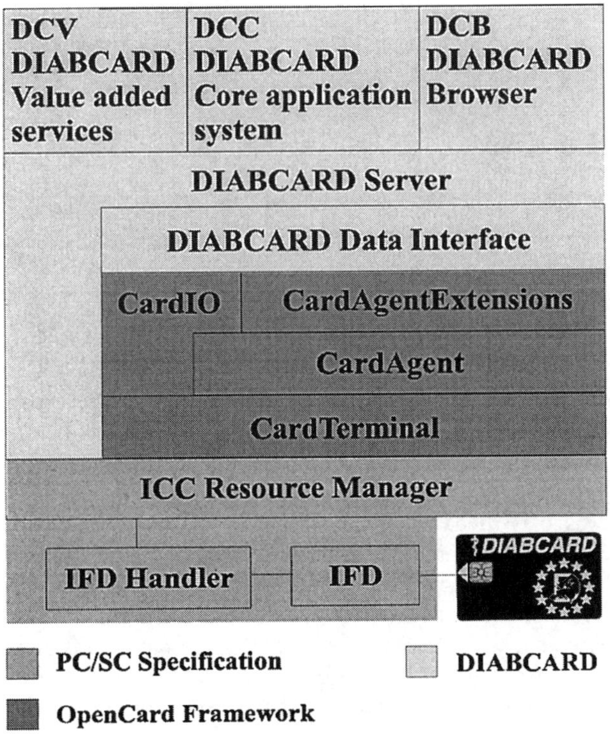

Fig.3 DIABCARD architecture

The interface allows access to the EU/G7 interoperable data and to DIABCARD patient data (see 7). The server ensures that application programmes gain independence of the used chip card reader, chip card respectively chip card operating system, security algorithms and of details concerning data location and file structures on the card. It supplies functions to access both the structure of the DIABCARD data set (DCDS) (e.g. data item types, allowed values) and the data itself (single item values, item value groups).

Part of the architecture is the DIABCARD Browser which is integrated. This is available to all applications and gives comfortable access to EU/G7 and DIABCARD data without any programming effort.

6. Interoperability on data

6.1. EU/G7 Interoperability Data Sets

Within the EU/G7 Interoperability Feasibility Study three data sets were defined for the interoperability of heath cards [11]. These are

- Card Application Data for identifying the card issuer and the method to read interoperable healthcard data from the card and which contains the minimum set of essential information about the healthcard
- Administrative Data
- Clinical Data which provides minimum data for emergency.

All these data sets have been incorporated into the DIABCARD data set (DCDS).

6.2. Diabetes Data Sets

In the field of Diabetes activities have been on-going in the standardisation of data. For the medical data these are

- the approved EURODIABETA Diabetes Data Set [15];
- the DiabCare Basic Information Sheet (BIS) as part of the implementation of the St. Vincent Declaration) [16];
- the Diabetes a Care Card as a passport and tool for monitoring the state of the diabetes patient.

6.3. DIABCARD Diabetes Data Set

DIABCARD developments are based on the above mentioned data sets. The DCDS does, in fact, completely cover the EU/G7 Interoperability data sets and the BIS. This provides the basis for interoperability. The DCDS was then supplemented with the necessary medical data items which had been found by medical scenarios, designed by the medical partners of the project. The scenarios describe in detail the different medical situations of a diabetic patient's treatment.

The diabetes data was classified and constitutes the following data categories/groups: administrative, emergency, general medical, education, laboratory, self-monitoring, kidney, heart, foot, eye, complications, pregnancy, anti-diabetic treatment, additional medication and diet. Groups are logical collections of data items.

A hierarchical tree structure was chosen for structuring the data items. This provides the basis for the application software and at the same time the data structure for the terminology glossary, which will at a later stage be added to the DIABCARD system.

There will be a minimal data set in each DIABCARD implementation. Beside the site specific data this will be the

- EU/G7 administrative data set;
- EU/G7 clinical data set for interoperability;
- Diabetes passport as a basic monitoring tool;
- Basic Information Sheet (BIS) for DIABCARE quality improvement.

Version 2.2 of the DCDS is at this stage available [17] and fully implemented. Data items necessary to allow cards from DIABCARD to interoperate with cards from Cardlink [8] have been defined. The DCDS has been implemented as a meta-database using a standard SQL-database tool. Interoperability will be shown between DIABCARD and Cardlink [9] in a first step on the emergency data and in a second step on BIS-data of both projects.

7. Interoperability on data presentation

7.1. EU/G7 data presentation

In order to reach interoperability the server of any system must be able to read and represent the data on the card. The EU/G7 Interoperability Feasibility group therefore also made a recommendation on the structure and on the representation of the data at the Server Application Interface. Some of the main points are

- Each of the interoperable data group must be accessible by itself
- The format used at the Server (Interface) complies with ASN.1 Basic Encoding Rules
- Each element is represented by a Tag-Length-Value (TLV) combination.

7.2. DIABCARD data presentation

DIABCARD complies to these rules. Tab. 1 provides some data item groups of the DCDS that can be read from and written on the chip card via DIABCARD Data Interface functions. The format is ASN.1 (TLV format). Most of these groups are low level groups within the DCDS hierarchy, e.g. the group diet in tab.2.

ID	name	tag	content	size
1020	General:Symptoms	A0A0	80-83	4
1070	General:Complications	A0A1	80-84	5
1130	General:Problems	A0A2	80-84	5
2250	General:BIS	A0A3	80-89	10
3150	Foot:Symptoms	A1A0	80-93	20
4200	Foot:Symptoms:BIS	A1A0B4	80-88	9
4700	Foot:Examination	A1A1	80-92	19
5700	Foot:Examination:BIS	A1A1B3	80	1
5850	Foot:Amputation	A1A2	80	1
5940	Foot:Amputation:Amputation Details	A1A2A1	80-87	8
7750	Foot:Amputation:BIS	A1A2A2	80-83	4
8000	Foot:Bones	A1A3	80-91	18
8950	Foot:Outcome	A1A4	80-98	25

Table 1: Groups provided by the DIABCARD Data Interface

The file structures on the DIABCARD chip card implements an ISO 7816 file system. EU/G7 interoperable data, ensuring interoperability with Cardlink, will be stored in three distinct elementary files (EFs). DIABCARD medical data (DCDS), not contained within the three interoperability data sets, will be stored in one single EF. This is also where specific European defined data like the BIS will be exchanged between different projects and applications.

id	name	dctag	dctype	dcvalue	dccodes	dcoccur
31200	Kind of Diet	A9	GROUP [1]			0,1
31250	>diet formulation: calories	80	NUM [4,0]			0,1
31300	>diet formulation:	81	NUM [3,0]			0,1
31350	>diet formulation: fat	82	NUM [3,0]			0,1
31400	>diet formulation: protein	83	NUM [3,0]			0,1
31450	>base: calories	84	NUM [4,0]			0,1
31500	>base: carbohydrates	85	NUM [2,0]			0,1
31550	>base: cholesterol	86	CODED	Y, N, U	0,1,2	0,1
31600	>base: salt	87	CODED	Y, N, U	0,1,2	0,1
31650	>base: fiber	88	CODED	Y, N, U	0,1,2	0,1
31700	>breakfast: time	89	NUM [2,2]			0,1
31750	>mid a.m.: time	8A	NUM [2,2]			0,1
31800	>lunch: time	8B	NUM [2,2]			0,1
31850	>mid p.m.: time	8C	NUM [2,2]			0,1
31900	>dinner: time	8D	NUM [2,2]			0,1
31950	>bedtime: time	8E	NUM [2,2]			0,1

Table 2: The patient's kind of diet is an example of an item group

Views are used to display data for a certain purpose. They can consist of a set of single data items and/or groups and they are application defined. At the moment there are two views relevant to all applications: the Diabetes passport and the BIS. For interoperability of different sites a cross table has been established between the German and the English language (tab. 3), the other languages are in preparation. Fig. 4 shows the multi-lingual application of the BIS as realised in DIABCARD.

id	germanName	name
1010	Allgemeindaten	General
1020	Symptome	>Symptoms
1070	Komplikationen	>Complications
1130	Probleme	>Problems
2000	Probleme DP	>>Problems DP
29000	Kontrolle	>>Follow up

Table 3: Examples for English and German group names of the DIABCARD Data Interface

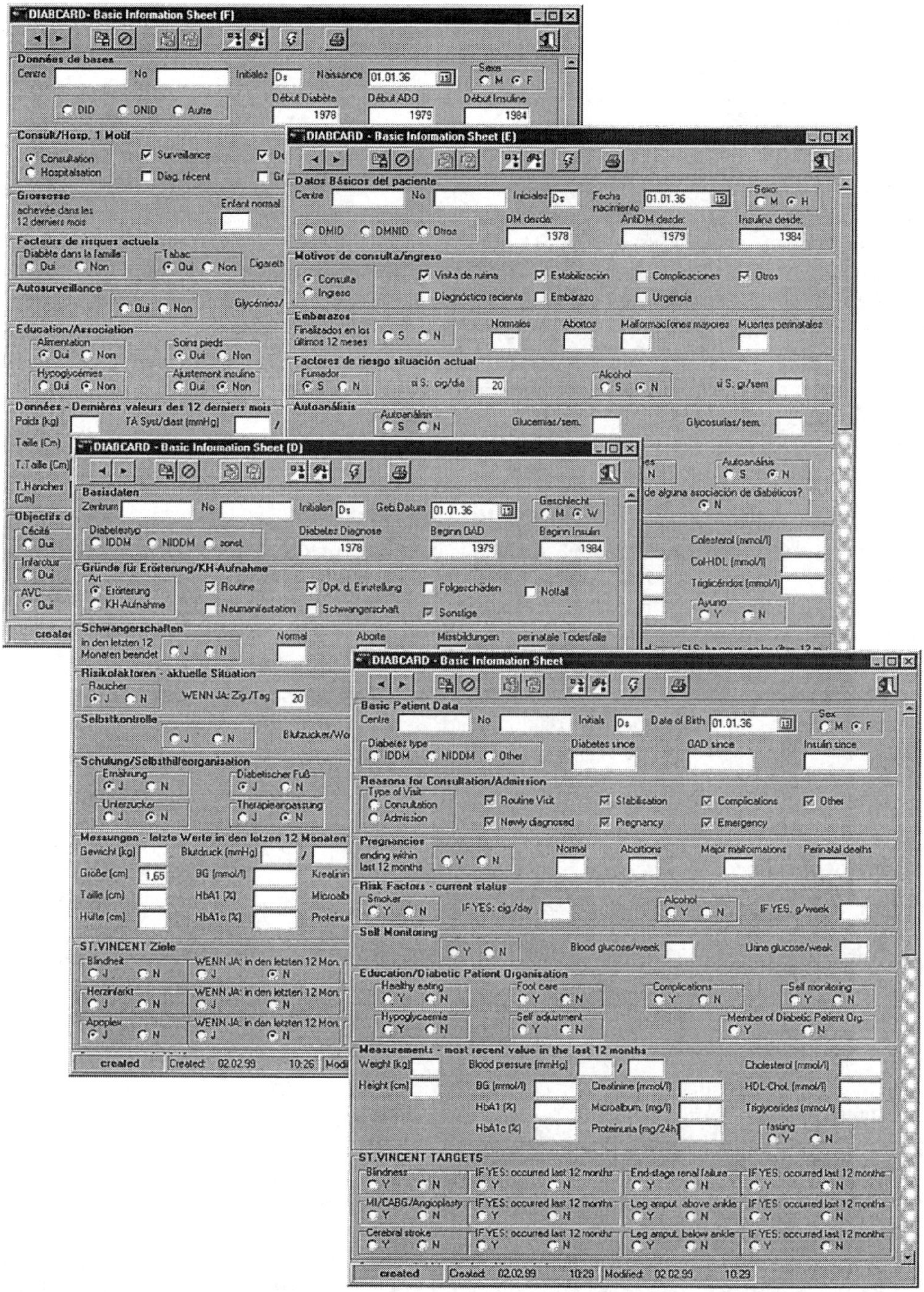

Fig. 4 Excerpts from the DIABCARD-BIS in English, German, Spanish and French.

8. Interoperability on Security

8.1. European Initiatives

Security in healthcare systems concerns various areas such as data access, data protection, data integrity, privacy or confidentiality.

The basic legal issues about security for personal and medical information are ruled in the „European Directive on the Protection of Individuals with Regard to the Processing of Personal Data and on the Free Movement of such Data" [18] and in the „European Recommendation No. R(96) of the Committee of Ministers to Member States on the Protection of Medical Data (and Genetic Data)" [19]. In order to enforce security in healthcare the European Commission has been funding several projects, for example ISHTAR [20], Seismed [21], Trusthealth [22], EUROMED-ETS [23], and also founded the working group CEN/TC 251/WG 6: Healthcare security, privacy, quality and safety [24]. In Germany one of the working groups within the Joint Panel on Health Cards (see 6.2) deals with the security infrastructure.

8.2. DIABCARD Security

High security standards are part of the DIABCARD design. The patient will be the owner of his card and its data. The use of the card will be voluntary. The final development DIABCARD will consist of a "Patient Card" for the person with diabetes and an "Access-Card" for the Health Care Professional which will authenticate the health care professional to the Patient Card.

For the current version of the DIABCARD Server, the DIABCARD medical data is protected by the patient's PIN which has to be provided by the patient before data within the EF can be accessed. Authentication of the health care professional is done by insertion of a DIABCARD Access Card [25]. This is included in the open DIABCARD architecture and realised as a software security access module which later can be exchanged by any standard easily.

Health care professionals can access data within the EU/G7 Emergency data set at the moment without special security measures or by providing their DIABCARD Access Card. PIN entry of the patient is in emergency case also not required. More detailed security measures (e.g. digital signature) will be integrated in a later stage in close co-operation with the Trusthealth project [22]. This includes concepts and implementations on the patient card and on the network level.

9. Conclusion

The long-term vision of a physician's office is one where telemedicine is prevalent and the electronic portable patient record is one that provides routine access across a range of clinical users and settings. The medical smart card is just one of the tools used to apply better service, get faster information and to improve communication. Interoperability is the key problem, standardisation a vital issue.

Smart cards are just one part of a healthcare information system and the problems met for the healthcard also apply to other telecommunication systems. Problems, like missing legal statements on an electronic patient record or missing European and international standards, remain to be solved and have to be overcome in a common effort by all parties involved including health authorities and governmental and European bodies.

Innovative telemedicine programs should gain the necessary governmental and industrial support which should consider that telemedicine is not only a technology for solving health care delivery problems and saving costs, but also a technology to promote the export of medical technology, expertise and economic development.

References

[1] W. A. Nowlan, Synopsis, Patient Record Systems. In: Yearbook of Medical Informatics `93. Schattauer Verlag, Stuttgart, 1993, pp. 173 – 175.
[2] R.S. Dick, E.B. Steen (eds), The computer based patient record. National Academy Press, Washington D.C., 1991
[3] W. Rank, W. Effing, Handbuch der Chipkarten. Carl Hanser Verlag, München, 1995.
[4] E. Fiedler, The Introduction of the German Health Insurance Card and its Effects on Data Communication on the System of Statutory Health Insurance in Germany. In: Health Cards 95 - Proceedings of the Health Cards `95 Conference (Köhler C.O., Rienhoff O., Schaefer O.P. eds.). IOS Press, Amsterdam, 1995.
[5] Intercai Telematics Consultants (eds.), Chipcards - Applications and Opportunities. Telematics Research Centre, Enschede, 1993.
[6] Glade A., Reimer H., Struif B. (Eds.) Digitale Signatur & Sicherheitssensitive Anwendungen. Vieweg. Wiesbaden. 1995.
[7] L.van der Broek and A.J. Sikkel (eds.), Health Cards'97.ISBN 90 5199 379 X. IOS Press, Amsterdam, 1997.
[8] The Cardlink Project. http://www.ehto.be/projects/cardlink
[9] D.C. Markwell, Healthcard Interoperability. In: L.van der Broek and A.J. Sikkel (eds.), Health Cards'97.ISBN 90 5199 379 X. IOS Press, Amsterdam, 1997, pp. 197-205.
[10] EU-projects: http://www.ehto.be
[11] EU/G7 references: http://www.clinical-info.co.uk/euhci.htm.
[12] J. Sembritzki, German Patient Cards. In: L.van der Broek and A.J. Sikkel (eds.), Health Cards'97. IOS Press, Amsterdam, 1997, 31-39.
[13] The PC/SC Workgroup[1], Interoperability Specification for ICCs and Personal Computer Systems. Draft Revision 0.9 (1996). Available at: http://www.smartcardsys.com.
[14] The OpenCard Workgroup[2], The OpenCardTM Framework (1997). White paper available at http://www.nc.com/opencard.
[15] EURODIABETA (1990) Information Technology for Diabetes Care. In: Europe: The EURODIABETA Initiative. Diabetic Medicine, 7, 536-560.
[16] DiabCare homepage: http://www.diabcare.de.
[17] DIABCARD homepage: http://www-mi.gsf.de/diabcard.
[18] Council of Europe (1995) Directive 95/46/EC on the Protection of Individuals with Regard to the Processing of Personal Data and on the Free Movement of such Data. Strasbourg.
[19] Committee of Ministers (1997) European Recommendation (Draft) No. R(96) of the Committee of Ministers to Member States on the Protection of Medical Data (and Genetic Data). CJ-PD (96). Strasbourg.
[20] ISHTAR Consortium. Implementation of Secure Health Telematics Applications in Europe. Project of the Fourth EU Health Telematics Applications Programme. http://www.ehto.be/projects/ishtar.
[21] The SEISMED Consortium, eds. (1996) Data Security for Health Care. Volume I-III. Studies in Health Technology and Informatics, Vol. 31-33. IOS Press, Amsterdam.
[22] Klein G. (1995) Creating an Infrastructure of Trusted Third Parties for Issuing of Cryptographic Cards for Signatures and User Identification. In: Health Cards 95 (Amsterdam: IOS Press), 100-103.
[23] ETS Consortium. EUROMED - European Trust Structure. Information Society Standardisation Programme. http://euromed.iccs.ntua.gr
[24] CEN/TC 251/WG 6: Healthcare security, privacy, quality and safety. http://www.ehto.be/ikb/standards/centc251/booklet/wg6.html

---

[1] Bull, Hewlett Packard, GemPlus, IBM, Microsoft, Siemens-Nixdorf, Schlumberger, Sun Microsystems, Toshiba, Verifone
[2] Apple, IBM. Netscape, Oracle, Sun Microsystems

[25] Engelbrecht et al. (1994) A chip card for patients with diabetes. Computer Methods and Programs in Biomedicine, 45, 33-35.

Address for correspondence

Rolf Engelbrecht
GSF-MEDIS Institute
Ingolstädter Landstraße 1
85764 Neuherberg, Germany
E-mail: engel@gsf.de

The Impact of Telemedicine on Health Care Management
M. Nerlich and R. Kretschmer (Eds.)
IOS Press, 1999

Telemedicine Based Screening of Infants at Risk for Retinopathy of Prematurity

Birgit LORENZ[1], Markus BOCK[1], H. Michael MÜLLER[1], N.A.(Bert) MASSIE[2]

[1]*Department of Pediatric Ophthalmology, Strabismology and Ophthalmogenetics, University of Regensburg, Regensburg, Germany*
[2]*Chairman and CEO, Massie Research Laboratories, Inc. Dublin, CA 94568*

Abstract: Retinopathy of Prematurity (ROP) is a major risk for permanent visual loss in extreme prematures. In stage 3+ (zone I and II), defined as threshold disease, the risk for retinal detachment with subsequent blindness is about 50% without treatment, compared to only a few percent with laser photoablation. Visualisation and interpretation of the critical retinal changes requires a high degree of expertise. Therefore, screening by general ophthalmologists will not identify all cases at threshold necessary to prevent blindness in as many infants as possible. The development of a new digital wide-field camera system (RetCam 120) allows documentation of nearly the entire retina within minutes. Recently, sensitivity, specificity, positive predictive power and negative predictive power have been evaluated to be high. Data collection is also possible by trained staff of the neonatal care units. Data can be transferred electronically, even though it could be transferred through physical transport. Analyzing the data in a central reading center specialized in the treatment of ROP will allow optimal timing of treatment and thus salvage vision in more infants. In additon, unnecessary referrals that are not only expensive but put also stress on the very vulnerable prematures can be avoided.

At present, efforts are made to realize a pilot project in Eastern Bavaria that will test the potentials of telemedicine based screening for ROP. In addition, the potential of the system will be evaluated in other neuroophthalmological diseases

1. Introduction and summary of the problem

Advanced technology and improved clinical protocols have been developed to salvage premature infants at ever lower birth weights. Accompanying this achievement has been a host of clinical problems with caring for the yet-developing infant. One such problem of great consequence is related to the eye, i.e. the development of retinopathy of prematurity (ROP). ROP is a potentially blinding disease in prematures that is characterized by defective maturation of the retinal vasculature that physiologically reaches the retinal periphery only at the end of the third trimestor of pregnancy. There are different degrees of severity, the milder stages usually resolve spontaneously but can be detected by expert screening in a large percentage of prematures with a birth weight below 1500 g. Classification of acute ROP is in terms of radial extent (zones I to III) and circumferential extent (clock hours), severity of vascular changes at the border of the vascularisation (ridge) i.e. where the retinal vessels end in the periphery (stages 1 to 3), presence of a tractional retinal detachment (stages 4 and 5), and the presence of vascular dilatation in the posterior pole (plus disease). Stage 3+ disease in zone I or II is known to end in retinal detachment with blindness in 50% of the cases if untreated [1].

A multicenter study conducted in the eighties showed the beneficial effect of cryoablation of the avascular retina peripheral to the ridge in stage 3+ disease zone I and II, thereafter defined as threshold disease. With treatment, the risk for retinal detachment was reduced by 50% [1]. Since then, diode (and Argon) laser photocoagulation has been used instead of cryo with even more favorable results which may be related not only to the different treatment modality but also to a slightly modified timing of treatment. With laser, resolution of the disease can be achieved in up to 100% of the eyes with ROP3+ zone I and II [2-6]. In other words, only few children will have an unfavorable outcome if treated in time. This unfavorable outcome is not only related to cicatricial stages of ROP but to optic nerve atrophy and other central visual pathway problems as sequelae of intracranial hemorrhages related to the extreme immaturity of the infants.

As ROP is a progressive disorder, monitoring the progress of the retinal development is key to determining the requirement for treatment. Thus, the first task in preventing blindness is accurate screening. Screening programs have been established in many countries [7-9]. Screening is not an easy task given the tiny and fragile nature of the patient. The exam is stressful for infant and physician alike.

1.1 Current practice

Currently, a binocular indirect ophthalmoscope (BIO) is used to visualize the retina. The BIO is comprised of a pair of lens mounted on head-band which the physician looks through, a centrally mounted light source, and a third lens which the physician holds close to the infant´s eye. Proper use of the BIO in infants requires considerable skill and training. Ideally, screening is performed by a pediatric ophthalmologist (PO).

Unfortunately, the BIO only gives the physician an image of a small portion of the retina at a time (figure 2), about 15 degrees (with a 20 diopter lens), and the physician must integrate the wider picture of the state of the retina and the location of various features mentally. By manipulating the eye and the lens a skilled practitioner can scan the eye and conduct an exam, forming a mental picture of the disease which manifests itself over a good portion of the back surface of the eye. At the end of the exam, notes are made on the chart and part of the assessment is to estimate the radial location of the margin of the retina. Clearly communicating between different physicians who may see the child is difficult based solely on the notes. Further, the patients are fragile and in some instances, because of the particular state of the patient, the exam may not be completed. The eye must be moved about (after topical anesthetics are applied) to examine various peripheral portions of the retina and this places forces on the muscles controlling the eye. Through the vasal vagal response, the infant's heart rate may be substantially decreased, placing stress on the already fragile infant.

Complicating this process is that the infant being cared for is in a neonatal intensive care unit (NICU), and the physician must travel to the child. Immediately one can understand the high cost and low financial efficiency of ROP screening.

In the USA, birth centers and therefore NICUs tend to be located in diverse community based centers. Thus, the PO is faced with spending substantial time in driving from center to center. In fact, the PO will actually spend more time commuting than in caring for the patient. Consider also that the PO must, after arriving at the hospital, park, go to the NICU, scrub, gown, and then perform the exam and document the results. It is easy for the PO to spend a total of four hours to examine one patient. During winter months in many locations travel to the patients is problematical.

In Germany, the situation is different. Travelling long distances is less common. POs will do the screening only in the NICUs attached to the Universities. In community based centers, screening will usually be performed by local general ophthalmologists who due to much smaller numbers of infants at threshold than in a referral center will inevitably have less expertise.

1.2 Efficiency and problems of current screening programs in Eastern Bavaria

The Department of Pediatric Ophthalmology of the University of Regensburg (DPOR) is in charge of the screening program of the NICU of the Department of Pediatrics, St. Hedwig Hospital Regensburg located at some distance from the University Hospital. In addition, it is the referral center for 4 NICUs in Eastern Bavaria where the local general ophthalmologist is in charge of the screening. The infants will be referred only in case of query of treatment. There are additional smaller NICUs who also occasionally refer infants.

In the 5 centers, about 250 to 300 babies at risk are seen per year requiring up to 900 examinations. During the last 5 years (from 1992 to 1997), 35 children were treated with ROP stage 3+ zone I and II or above at the DPOR . During the same time period, about 30 children were sent to the DPOR for treatment but did not require treatment. On average, 2 control examinations were needed. This means that about 30 transports per year were necessary from the peripheral NICUs to the DPOR. At the time of transportation the children were still extremely fragile, usually they were at the 32nd to 38th week postmenstrual age i.e. still preterm. Those transports therefore put considerable physical stress on the infants.

Thirteen of the 35 treated children were above threshold. 62% of the 13 children subsequently became bilaterally blind, and 38% in one eye due to progression of the disease to ROP stage 5. In the 22 children who received treatment at threshold, the acute disease was successfully treated in all but one case. Yet, 23% became legally blind, the bad functional results being related to pathologies other than ROP of the visual pathways. Treatment at threshold is most critical for a favorable outcome in ROP stage 3+ zone I and II. Therefore, all efforts must be concentrated on improved screening methods. The problem with conventional screening is that examination of these extremely small and optically non-optimal eyes is difficult, and therefore requires a high degree of expertise. This expertise is difficult to get outside specialised eye centers as stage 3+ disease is relatively rare i.e. present only in about 4% of the children at risk. The difficulties are mirrored in the unacceptable high percentage of late referrals from external NICUs.

1.3 Actual screening strategies and additional aspects

As a further expensive and problematical difficulty, the child in many cases may not be immediately dismissed when stable in the general medical sense until a final eye exam is conducted. Thus, the infant may be retained in a very expensive intensive care unit awaiting the arrival of the PO, or, dismissed with instructions for bringing the child back for the exam and the infant faces the risk of the parent not complying.

It is certainly true that a highly skilled physician must perform the delicate treatment but at most only one in fifty exams leads to a treatment event. Clearly, if there were a way in which a screening exam could be conducted by a technician who could report the exam to the physician a substantial cost savings would be achieved and likely with better outcomes as well. This problem is ideally solved by Telemedicine based on the availability of the appropriate imaging device.

What is required is an instrument which can obtain wide-field images of the retina ideally not only in the hands of a physician but also in the hands of a skilled nurse or technician. It should be digital for transference by electronic means. A further benefit will be documentation and communication between physicians who may sequentially see the patient. In summary, this clinical dilemma is as ideal for Telemedicine as any clinical application can be as it is the promise of bringing expert care to remote sites electronically.

2. A Telemedicine based solution

The problems of using the BIO were discussed above but in summary they are the difficulty of use, the small field of view (FOV) as compared to the need for a global assessment, and the lack of quantitative documentation. Retinal cameras may be considered but do not meet the needs for ROP imaging. The classical retinal camera is a table-top device and requires a good deal of skill to use. When converted from film to digital, the cameras have grown in size and cost. A hand held narrow field camera was brought to market some years ago with a FOV of 30 degrees. The problem of the narrow field can be reduced by using it as an indirect ophthalmoscope together with a 30 diopter lens, however this method is hardly applicable in the awake infant.

Recently, a wide-field palm sized camera was developed. The camera is called RetCam 120 where the 120 refers to the image angular width as measured from the center of the eye (For reference, the retina measures 225 degrees in total.). The camera is hand-held and produces a real-time image on its computer screen to assist the clinician in obtaining the best image. The images are stored on command on an optical disk and can be readily emailed to a central review center.

The system is comprised of the imager which is a palm-sized cylinder about 4 cm in diameter and 15 cm long which has a contact lens at one end and a three-chip CCD at the other. An umbilical connects the imaging unit to a cart containing a control box, a computer system, and supporting items such as a printer. The contact lens is used to achieve wide-field imaging (figure 1) and is touched against the cornea after using anesthetizing drops. The umbilical connects to a control box which provides light to the camera via a fiber optic cable, electrical control signals to the camera to control the focus motor, and bi-directional signals

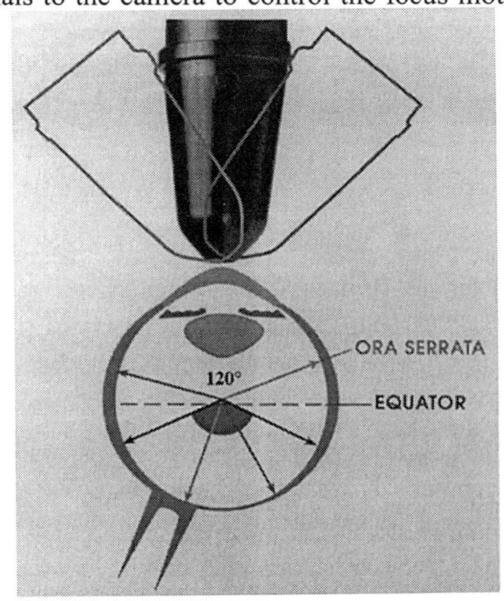

Figure 1: Wide field imaging system RetCam 120: key concept

to the CCD camera and its controller. The control box then communicates to the "frame grabber" or image digitization board in the computer. The camera is a three-chip CCD where there is a CCD chip for each color providing high resolution in all colors. Being of the latest generation of chips and controls, the camera has a very good sensitivity, which means that the light level on the retina is minimized. The images are stored uncompressed on optical disks which can store 600 images for permanent archival.

A modem and standard Internet software allows the images to be transferred. As provided, the system does not transmit the images with any labeling. That is, patient identification is not included with the images, avoiding issues of confidentiality. In more advanced software, the images could be sent with identifying information with encryption or perhaps by a direct dial-up line.

With the real-time image visualized on the CRT, the examiner can see the image and obtain the best focus and aiming point. Each digitized image is 120 degrees in width (figure 3). By tilting the camera, several overlapping images can be stored and the retina can be documented to the equator and beyond. Thus, the camera is functional in even the hands of a nurse or technician for documenting the posterior half of the eye and therefore the existence of plus disease. In the hands of an experienced physician and using the traditional technique of scleral depression similar to the used for the BIO exam, the retina can be imaged to the periphery.

Several centers in Europe and the US are currently using the camera for ROP screening. In a recent study in 35 premature infants in whom the camera was used to diagnose ROP against the „Gold Standard-“ ophthalmological screening exam, a sensitivity of 0.94, specificity of 0.88, plus predictive power of 0.89 and minus predictive power of 0.93 have been evaluated (J.Flynn, personal communication). The images were read in masked fashion by two independent observers.

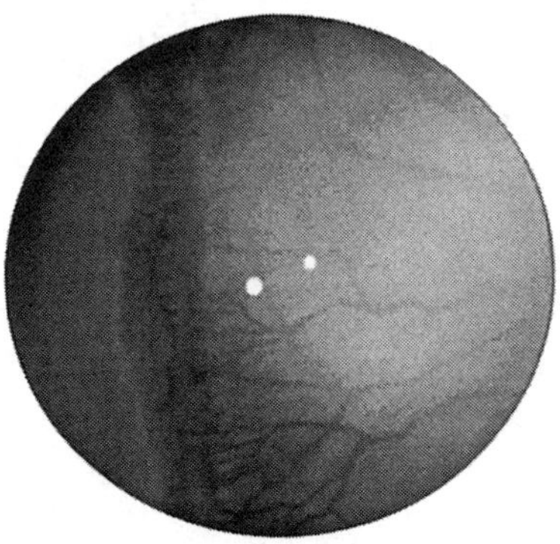

Figure 2: Fundus photograph with a hand-held Kowa fundus camera and a 30 dpt lens of a stage 3+ disease in zone II

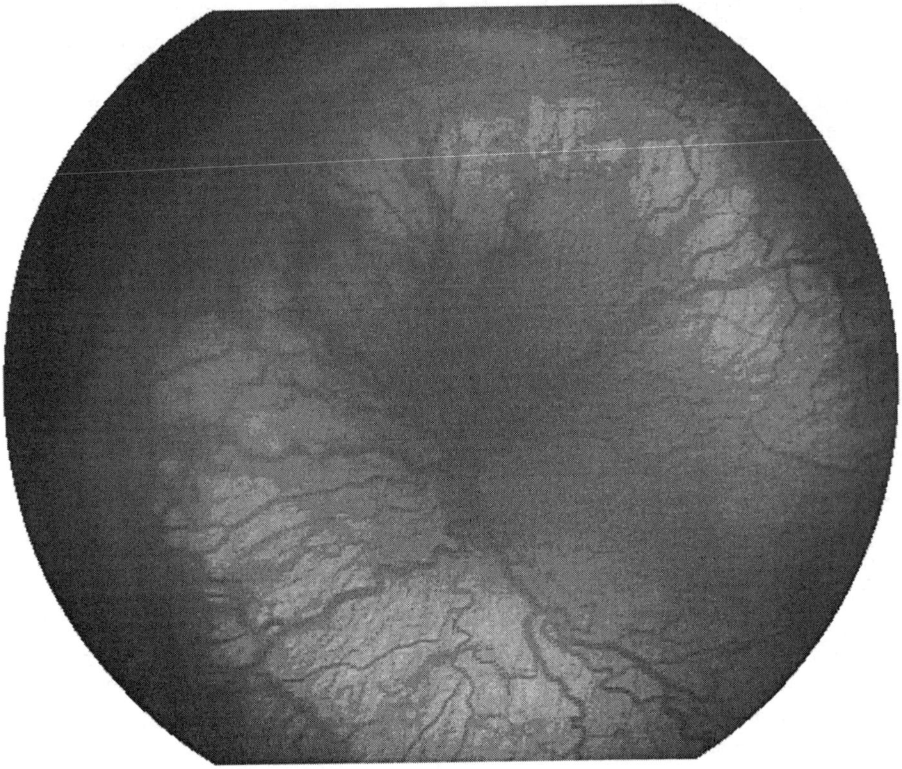

Figure 3: Digital image with a RetCam120 system of severe stage 3+ disease zone I (rush disease, Image courtesy of Steven Schwartz, M.D., Jules Stein Eye Institute, UCLA Medical Center, Los Angeles)

3. Potentials of telemedicine based screening for ROP

3.1 Overview of advantages

In addition to objective documentation of the disease, a number of further potential advantages are evident (table 1).

Table 1.

Potential advantages of telemedicine based screening in ROP

- objective documentation of stage of ROP
- online-control of image quality
- uniform data evaluation by experts in the field
- less stress to the patients
- improved control of time course of disease process
- optimized timing of treatment
- improved outcome
- permanent availability of stored images

- comparative studies
- medicolegal aspect

- improved parents′ information
- improved training of students and medical staff

3.2 Socioeconomical aspects

(a) In the USA

The cost of a lifetime of blindness is USD $1 to $5 M. The cost of screening a given child for three visits for a PO is about $1,000. The cost of screening via Telemedicine is about $100. Thus, the savings for each child is about $900. Based on a five year amortization of the camera the monthly cost of a RetCam is $ 1200 USD per month. Thus, if more than one child is screened per month the camera more than pays for itself irrespective of improve outcomes and less unnecessary costs for transferal of infants.

(b) In Germany

The cost of a 50 year blindness is about 400 000 US$ based on actual German rates. The cost of conventional screening is much lower than in the USA, therefore the telemedicine based screening will be more expensive. The costs of the infants´ transport from the NICUs to the PO at the referral center must be taken into account. Those costs however will not cover the price of the camera. The main saving therefore comes from saving children from blindness. The medical aspect of preventable blindness is most important.

3.3 Medicolegal aspects

Objective documentation of the disease will protect both pediatrician and PO (eventually also nursery staff skilled with the examination technique) from unjustified reproaches. On the other hand it will provide optimal judgement of the disease status thus optimizing the infant´s chances for the best visual outcome possible.

4. The Eastern Bavarian Project

Now that the technology is available for ROP imaging, there are several key steps for widespread use. First, additional studies at key sites will assist the community in establishing this as standard of care. Second, the economic case needs to be documented, both in terms of lower cost of care but also in terms of better outcomes. Thirdly, the community of those caring for the premature infants needs to bring this dilemma and its solution to the attention of those who determine care patterns.

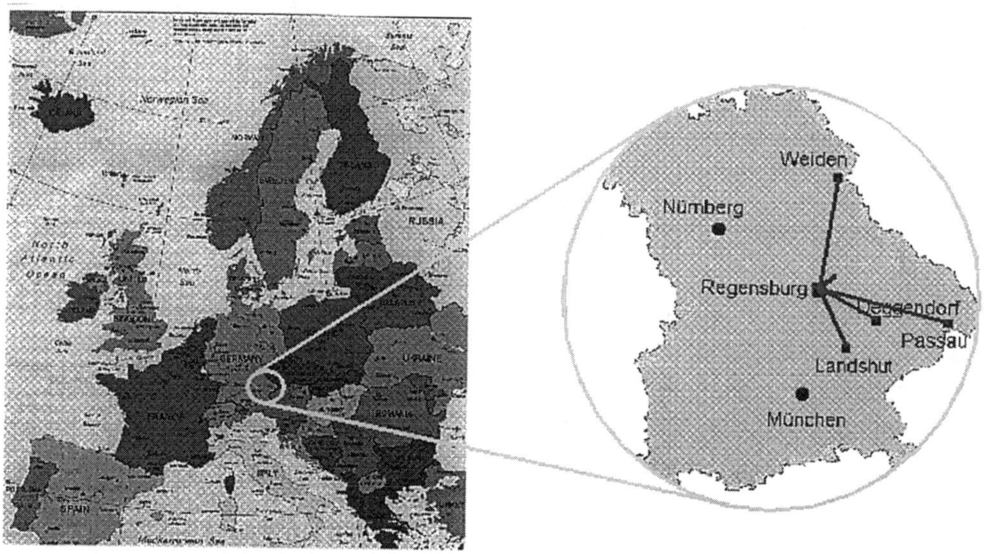

At present, a pilot project using the RETCAM 120 system in 5 major NICUs of Eastern Bavaria is in progress (figure 4). The problem is that although the overall savings will be superior to the costs of the system, the money comes from different sources and cannot be easily redistributed. So although the advantages are very evident, the realisation of the project may cause major problems. In the project, several questions shall be addressed. (1) Sensitivity, specificity, positive and negative predictive value of the method in the hands of (a) ophthalmologists and (b) trained nursery staff (2) Cost effectiveness (3) Ease of data transfer in a network system (4) Improved treatment protocols through analysis of the natural course from stored data (5) Comparative studies among different NICUs.

5. Future applications

In the pilot project, future applications will be tested. (1) documentation of the variability of the optic nerve head in health and in congenital optic nerve anomalies during the first years of life (2) Evaluation of the system in acute pediatric diseases with ocular involvement (e.g. shaken baby syndrome, papilledema associated with head trauma or other causes of elevated intracranial pressure) (3) Longitudinal studies of neuropediatric diseases with ocular involvement (e.g. neurometabolic diseases, early onset periventricular leukomalacia).

Multicenter studies without examiner bias of larger numbers of patients with even rare diseases will give new insights in the pathogenesis of complex entities. Development of even higher resolution cameras and optics, and of new software will allow improved evaluation of even more subtle changes.

Acknowledgements

We acknowledge helpful discussions with PD Dr. Segerer, Head of the Department of Pediatrics, St. Hedwig Hospital, Regensburg.

References

[1] Cryotherapy for Retinopathy of Prematurity Cooperative Group. Multicenter trial of cryotherapy for retinopathy of prematurity: one year outcome; structure and function. Arch Ophthalmol 108 (1990) 1408-1416.

[2] T. Tsitsis *et al.*, Diode laser photocoagulation for retinopathy of prematurity. Trans Am Ophthalmol Soc, 95 (1997) 231-6.

[3] V. Seiberth *et al.*, Transscleral vs transpupillary diode laser photocoagulation for the treatment of threshold retinopathy of prematurity. Arch Ophthalmol, 115 (10), (1997) 1270-5.

[4] V. Seiberth *et al.*, Diode laser photocoagulation for stage 3+ retinopathy of prematurity. Graefes Arch Clin Exp Ophthalmol, 233 (8), (1995) 489-93.

[5] J.A. McNamara *et al.*, Laser photocoagulation for stage 3+ retinopathy of prematurity. Ophthalmology 98 (5), (1991) 576-80

[6] H.M. Müller *et al.*, Structural and functional outcome after diode laser coagulation (DLC) of threshold retinopathy of prematurity (ROP3+). Invest Ophthalmol Vis Sci, 39(4) (1998) 399.

[7] F. Pohlandt, Augenärztliche Untersuchungen zur Erkennung einer Frühgeborenenretinopathie. Pädiatr Prax Klin (1993) 15:261.

[8] Joint Statement of the American Academy of Pediatrics, the American Association for Pediatric Ophthalmology and Strabismus, and the American Academy of Ophthalmology. Screening examinations of premature infants for retinopathy of prematurity. Ophthalmology 104 (1997) 888-889.

[9] The report of a joint working party of the Royal College of Ophthalmologists and the British Association of Perinatal Medicine. Retinopathy of prematurity: guidelines for screening and treatment. Early Hum Dev 46 (1996) 239-258.

Address for correspondence

Birgit Lorenz
Department of Pediatric Ophthalmology, Strabismology and Ophthalmogenetics
University of Regensburg
Franz-Josef-Strauß-Allee 11
93053 Regensburg, Germany
birgit.lorenz@klinik.uni-regensburg.de

The Impact of Telemedicine on Health Care Management
M. Nerlich and R. Kretschmer (Eds.)
IOS Press, 1999

ByOPHTEL: A Bavarian Project for Rapid Telemedical Exchange of Knowledge, Files and Skills between Practitioners and Hospitals in Eye Care

Manfred MERTZ
Department of Ophthalmology and Eye Hospital "Rechts der Isar", Munich University of Technology, Munich, Germany

Abstract. ByOPHTEL, part of the Bavarian initiative Bayern Online, derived its name from the European project OPHTEL, to which it is closely linked and which, in Bavaria, is more or less worked out and performed by identical persons and institutions. It provides a group of 7 practitioners in and around the city of Munich with the possibility of exchanging general ophthalmologic knowledge as well as patient-related information with anyone in the group, or with the related ophthalmologic, internal, resp. scientific centers at the TU Munich and the GSF Neuherberg. Connections are routinely performed in the asynchronous or in the synchronous mode, and all partners participate in the scientific projects Knowledge Based Information System, Glaucoma Monitor, and Diabetic Retinopathy Monitor-- as well as in the enhancement of a trustful patient-physician relationship ("second opinion") and a closer cooperation in out-patient and in-patient ophthalmical surgery and medical treatment.

1. Introduction: Basic and Historical Aspects of Tele-Ophthalmology

In ophthalmology, vision is the main field of interest. Vision is of the utmost importance not only for the patient, in the sense of preventing its reduction or even loss due to any disease, but also for the specialized ophthalmic physician. In nearly all diagnostic procedures, he needs optic equipment (such as biomicroscopes, "slit lamps", ophthalmoscopes) or secondary imaging sources (laser ophthalmoscopes, ultrasonography, radiology, nuclear magnetic resonance, electrophysiology, and perimetry). Further, in the therapeutic wing of ophthalmology (laser and microsurgery, microendoscopy), the handling of various imaging apparatuses is absolutely necessary, and this also holds true for all teaching purposes of students and physicians-in-training. Moreover, exchanging images-- instead of long, and even misunderstood linguistic descriptions-- must enhance efficacy in the necessary communication between practitioners and hospitals concerning diagnostic images and therapeutic outcomes of their common patients. Thus, ophthalmology presents itself as a medical speciality which must also gain maximum profit from **tele**-vision.

This explains why ophthalmologists were among the telemedical pioneers in Germany when the first large medical network was implemented in the eighties: the project MEDKOM [1-6].

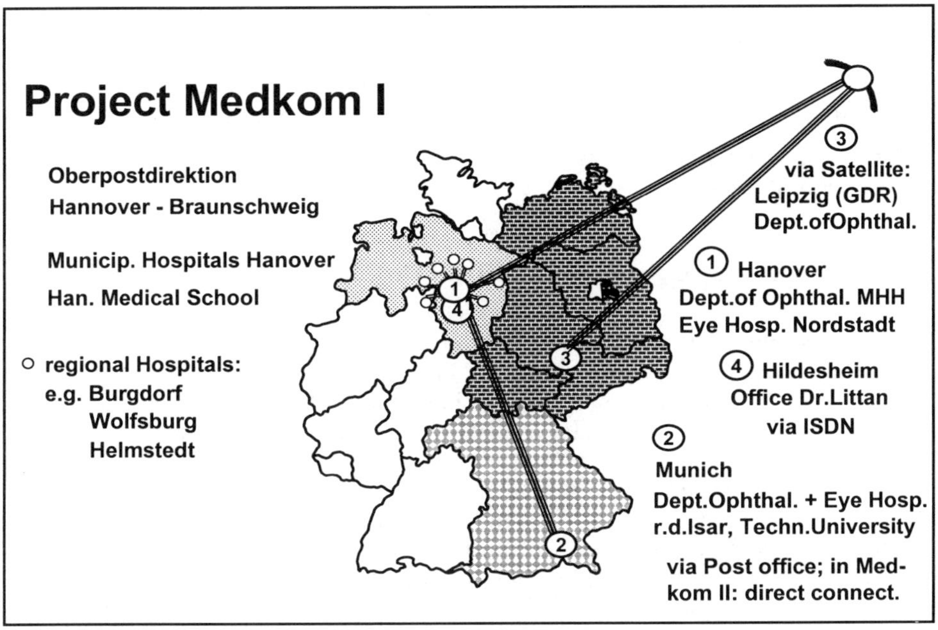

Fig1: The project MEDKOM was based technically on a broad bandwidth glass fiber net (VBN). Most of the participating hospitals were located in and around the city of Hanover, Lower Saxony. For single events and experiments, satellite connections were also used, e.g. in a conference and a tumor patient's examination „across the Wall" of the still existing GDR.

2. The Glorious Start of MEDKOM and the Famous Project´s Silent Death

The huge technical installations in the Department of Ophthalmology, Hanover Medical School, were completed in 1988. Immediately, there began a time of intensive communications over near and far distances. "Teleophthalmological rounds" were routinely performed with the Hanover Municipal Hospital, while single exchanges and experiments were run with a practitioner's office in Hildesheim (*ca.* 60 km.), and the Department of Ophthalmology, Munich University of Technology (*ca.* 600 km.). The usefulness of teleophthalmology was demonstrated most impressively when Prof. Lommatzsch, Karl-Marx-University in Leipzig, GDR, performed a satellite-based follow-up examination "over the wall" on a Hanoveran melanoma patient, whom he had treated with his brachytherapy one year before.

MEDKOM's suitability for ophthalmologic purposes originated from the rather high quality of the transmitted picture sequences concerning both spatial and temporal resolution. This was provided by the use of glass fiber technology; its analogous data transfer capacity was said to reach up to 144 Mbit/sec. At its best times, the project MEDKOM connected more than 30 hospitals and departments in Lower Saxony and elsewhere, including ENT and neurosurgery (from which it originated), hematology, pathology, dermatology, urology, and internal medicine [Fig. 1].

Nevertheless, MEDKOM collapsed immediately after the termination of the second project phase. What were the reasons why? The answer to this question proved to be essential for all following projects in teleophthalmology.

1. When financial support by the state had come to an end, nobody could efford the ongoing high costs.
2. Because of the lack of an easy and quick documentation technique, MEDKOM could not sufficiently meet the needs of both patients' file management and legal standards.
3. The high glass fiber/laser technology remained available only in municipal areas, while, at that time, it could not be spread to rural environments.

3. Teleophthalmology in the Digital Era: OPHTEL, ByOPHTEL and BAVARIA-SLOVENIA

The rapid development of digital data transfer in the nineties offered a chance to overcome the problems previously exhibited by MEDKOM [7]. The new common networks, such as the World Wide Web, would provide every point of the world with necessary information; and in medicine, advanced knowledge and skills would not continue to be the privilege of medical centers such as universities.

Therefore, on the European and as well on the national level, new projects were started. OPHTEL was founded to connect institutions and hospitals for eye care and internal medicine in Denmark, Great Britain, France, Italy, and Germany, under the administrative and scientific leadership of the Medis Institute (GSF) and based on the teleophthalmologic experience of the Department of Ophthalmology, Munich University of Technology [8,9].

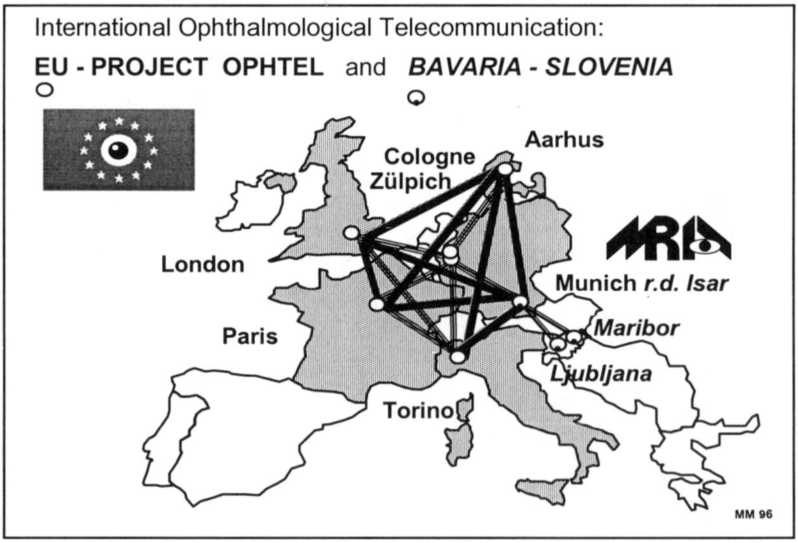

Fig. 2: The European project OPHTEL connects a number of university hospitals for eye care and internal medicine with scientific and commercial institutions. In Munich, University of Technology, it is also linked to the project BAVARIA-SLOVENIA (and to ByOPHTEL, see Fig. 3). The EU-project deals mainly with asynchronous communications while the Slovenian project is layed out for synchronous teleconsultations.

In order to optimize the outcome and to reduce the costs of the necessary developments, the project ByOPHTEL-- part of the larger project Bayern Online, supported by the state of Bavaria [10]-- was planned and executed in close connection [11].

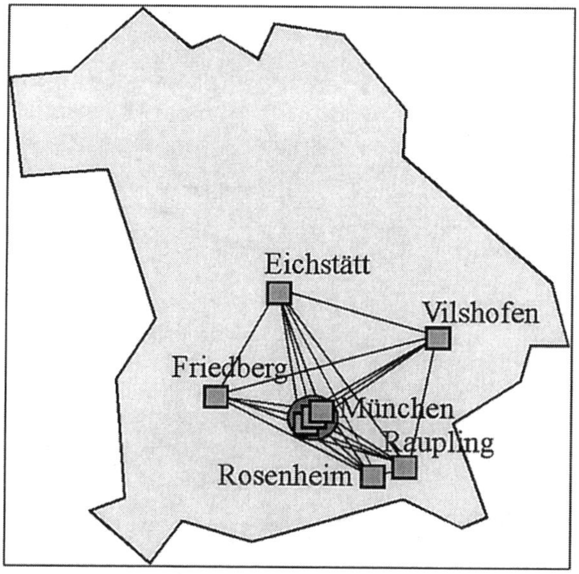

Fig. 3: The ByOPHTEL projects connects practitioners in their offices in the city of Munich and in approx. 60-90 kilometers distance range thereof, in more rural sites.

In parallel, the Munich hospital continued celebrating MEDKOM-like clinical communications of a modern kind with the Department of Ophthalmology, University of Ljubljana, Slovenia, and also with its teaching hospital in Maribor. These connections were also supported by the state of Bavaria, and they were technically based on at first 2 (now 6) basic ISDN channels (128kbit/s) [12], [Fig.2].

Because the experienced Munich department was very well integrated in all three of these projects, the fast-growing progress found an immediate exchange between all partners.

4. Synchronous and Asynchronous Telecommunication: Technical Remarks and Limitations

For technical reasons only, it proved to be necessary to strongly divide synchronous and asynchronous applications [Fig. 4]. As seen from the image quality side, the necessary change from analogous to digital communication technology began as a severe set-back. Spatial and temporal resolution through online connections dropped dramatically (approx. by a range of 1000). This forced the partners to decide whether their communication tasks would need high temporal *or* high spatial resolution. Slit lamp examinations and demonstrations with the aid of an operation microscope need at least television-like moving pictures [5], whereas the examination and classification of fundus images, e.g., in diabetic retinopathy, need the highest possible spatial (and colour) resolution power [4,13]. Moreover, the transfer data mass increases when an International Knowledge Based System is aimed to be created, and the more so if this system is also to be used for monitoring purposes [14]. Thus, each partner in the ByOPHTHEL user group had to decide which of the two possible technical solutions available-- synchronous or asynchronous teleconsultation-- would meet his actual individual needs in the best way.

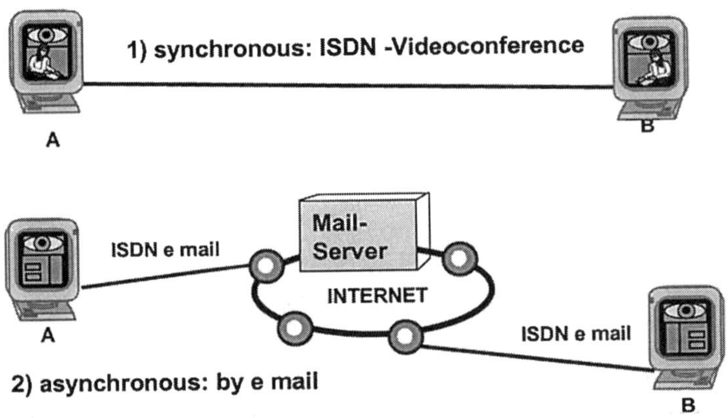

Fig. 4: In the ByOPHTEL project, synchronous as well as asynchronous communications are possible and in routine use.

5. Results

5.1 Clinical Structure and Telecommunication

In the long run, medical telecommunication cannot succesfully be performed only in a spontaneous manner. Planned, structured, periodically scheduled appointments for patient presentations and knowledge exchange proved to be better than spontaneous "emergency calls". For this purpose, a fax or an email letter announcing the kind of proposed questions should be sent one day in advance. In the Bavaria/Slovenia project, e.g., a *jour fixe* is arranged to take place every Tuesday noon for connections between Munich and Ljubljana, resp. Maribor. Naturally, there should be made an arrangement for real emergency cases, too.

5.2 ByOPHTEL: Exchange of Knowledge

As reported above, all members of the ByOPHTEL user group were intended to benefit from the Knowledge Based System to be implemented in OPHTEL. Therefore, they were integrated personally into the related data acquisition program from the very beginning. Also, they participated in data collection procedures for the glaucoma monitor [14]. Thus, the project ByOPHTEL overcame the traditional border between more practically- and more scientifically-oriented medical areas. One of the many subprojects of ByOPHTEL provided a striking example of the usefulness of this approach. A. Wegner, *et al.*, investigated the interobserver variability in the assessment of visual field defects in glaucoma. Perimetry, though a subjective psycho-physical examination method, had been estimated so far to deliver rather hard data for the diagnosis and therapeutic controle of glaucoma. Nevertheless, the comparison of the assessments of different members of the user group, to whom some hundred visual field printouts had been sent by email, resulted in a surprisingly low coincidence. Naturally, this result had to be taken into account when the glaucoma monitor was established [15]. Once again, it was proven that the teleophthalmologic connections between practitioners and medical centers should not be regarded as one-way streets.

5.3 ByOPHTEL: Exchange of Files

In different decisions, it is helpful for everyone to gain a collegue´s good advice, and this often holds true especially for the isolated situation of physicians in rural areas. Thus, it is one of the traditionally proclaimed aims of telecommunication to fill this gap by offering the chance of easily getting answers to acute, burning medical questions. Nevertheless, the history of telecommunication showed clearly that this technique is not reserved only to rare cases. More and more, patients also estimate the possibility to hear a "second opinion" in more common situations.

In both cases, consultation can be performed in the synchronous or in the asynchronous mode. Two of the user group members often search the telemedical contact with our university hospital in order to present patients online.

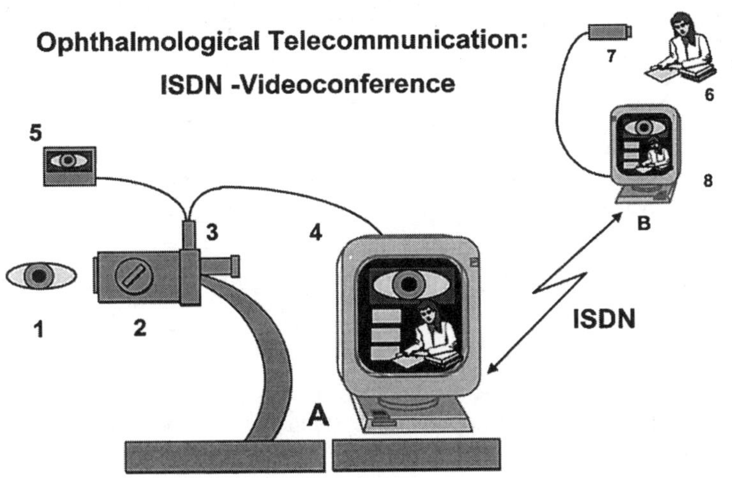

Fig. 5: An ophthalmological ISDN video conferencing system consists of a TV-camera (3) with control monitor (5) mounted at the slit lamp microscope (2). By this means, a patients eye (1) can be examined both directly (A) and from far distance (B). The computers A and B are connected via ISDN, and their screens (4,8) are showing both the near (ophthalmological) and the far image (the consulting partners face, 6, taken by a room camera, 7). This renders not only a good social contact possible but also an easy and quick documentation.

We then examine the patients' eyes biomicroscopically (from the distance), verify the diagnosis and-- if necessary-- the indication for ophthalmic surgery, and we talk with the patients concerning risks, appointments, etc.. In the postoperative phase, when the patient is back home, synchronous consultations are again useful for assessing individual follow-up therapy. This management is also a step to cooperatively enhance quality control.

On the other hand, the majority of the ByOPHTEL user group prefers the asynchronous exchange of files because doubtlessly this saves time, and it can be scheduled more easily. These advantages appeared very soon by the fact that members began to use the net not only centripetally, as an easy link to the hospital, but preferred the connections among themselves. This made sense, especially in the interactions between surgeons and their cooperating non-surgeons in the region, all of them now able to overview the complete files of their common patients at any time.

Nevertheless, if Internet data transfer is used, severe legal problems of data protection are still not solved sufficiently.

5.4 ByOPHTEL: Exchange of Skills

This is a specific domain for synchronous teleconsultations, especially among medical centers such as universities. The single practitioner normally does not have enough time available nor even interest in, e.g., observing the whole run of a difficult microsurgical operation in ophthalmology. Thus, most of the connections performed for the purpose of exchanging skills took place between the university departments of ophthalmology at both Munich rechts der Isar and Ljubljana. However, with the rapid development of out-patient surgery, this kind of teleconsultation will also be of growing importance. Guests will always be "present" in the operation theater (as will students and physicians-in-training), and I am sure that they will also participate in the traditional microsurgical courses of our hospital [16].

6. Outlook and Conclusion

When we remember the fate of the early telecommunication project MEDKOM, three reasons for the possible failure of all these efforts have always to be kept in mind:

1. Financial follow-up **must** be guaranteed-- by government or insurance groups, or both.
2. Documentation has to be easy and quick in order not to distract the physician's attention away from his patient, and it has to meet all legal standards.
3. For the protection of the patient's data while being transferred over a network, as well as when stored in a computer, security standards of a very high level have to be developed.

If all three of these problems find sufficient world-wide solutions very soon, ophthalmological telecommunication will be celebrated routinely for the rapid exchange of knowledge, files, and skills *like we are still used to perform it in the project ByOPHTEL.*

Acknowledgements

Twelve years of experience with ophthalmological telecommunication was gained in a strong and friendly cooperation with numerous scientists, physicians, and also administrators in the different projects, the leading persons of which I whould like to mention here gratefully.

OPHTEL: Toke Bek (Århus), Eva M. Kohner and G. Steve Aldington (London), Hans Biermann (Zülpich), Bernhard Waedlich (Cologne), Massimo Porta (Torino), Bernd Liesenfeld (Munich-Bogenhausen), Wilhelm van Eimeren, Gerd Mann, Gudrun Zahlmann, Wolfgang Piehlmeier (GSF Neuherberg), Marko Obermaier, Ian Ugi, Aharon Wegner, Alfred Schamburger (TU Munich).

ByOPHTEL, the user group: Klaus Dilger (Ingolstadt), Dieter Klaas (Friedberg), Lorenz Neubauer (Munich), Hansgeorg Kaatz (Munich), H. D. Walther (Raubling), Ekkehard Fabian (Rosenheim), Klaus-Dieter Schnarr (Vilshofen).

BAVARIA-SLOVENIA: Peter Dovsak (Ljubljana), Bojan Gracner (Maribor)

MEDKOM: Karl Hoffmann (Hannover), K.E. Littan (Hildesheim), Peter Lommatzsch (Leipzig), Hanns-Jürgen Merté (Munich), Hubert Poliwoda, Hans-Georg Layda (Hannover).

References

[1] M. Mertz, Ferndiagnostik und Fernkommunikation in der Augenheilkunde, *Klin Monatsbl Augenheilkd* **197** (1990) 79.

[2] G. Sterflinger, Überbrückt große Entfernungen: MEDKOM. Technische Universität München: *TUM-Mitteilungen* **1** (1991/92) 33-34.

[3] M. Mertz, MEDKOM, Telekommunikation als neues Mittel augenärztlicher Zusammenarbeit, *Klin Monatsbl Augenheilkde* **201** (1992) 393.

[4] M. Mertz and N. von der Ohe, Zur Fernübertragung dreidimensionaler ophthalmoskopischer Befunde, *Lasermedizin* **10** (1994) 8-14.

[5] M. Mertz and N. Schulte-Kellinghaus, Dreidimensionale Fernübertragung einer Spaltlampenuntersuchung über mehr als 1000 Kilometer. Jahrestagung der Vereinigung Bayerischer Augenärzte, Erlangen 1994 Jul 09-10. *Klin Monatsbl Augenheilkde* **206** (1995) 197.

[6] K.E. Littan, Telekommunikation zwischen augenärztlicher Praxis und Augenklinik, *Augenarzt* **26** (1992) 199-202.

[7] Deutsche Bundespost Telekom (eds.), Das ISDN-Anwenderbuch. 62 innovative Lösungen aus Wirtschaft und Verwaltung. ISBN 3-8203-0308-1. Darmstadt: Hoppenstedt 1994; S. 50-51.

[8] G. Zahlmann, S. Kluthe, M. Obermaier, M. Mertz, and G. Mann, Establishment and Use of a Teleconsultation Network in Ophthalmology. Proceedings IEEE Amsterdam Sept. 1997. CD-ROM 0-7803 (1997) 924-927.

[9] M. Mertz, G. Mann, G. Zahlmann, and M. Obermaier, Wissenschaftliche Rolle der deutschen Ophthalmologie im europäischen Telekommunikationsprojekt OPHTE,. *Ophthalmologe* **94** (1997) 523-528.

[10] Bayerische Staatskanzlei (eds.), Bayern Online. Datenhochgeschwindigkeitsnetz und neue Kommunikationstechnologien für Bayern. Das Konzept. Offensive Zukunft Bayern. Druckschrift RB-Nr. 02/95/07 (1995).

[11] G. Zahlmann, H.D. Walther, B. Liesenfeld, H. Kaatz, S. Kluthe, E. Fabian, D. Klaas, K.D. Schnarr, L. Neubauer, M. Obermaier, A. Wegner, M. Mertz, and G. Mann, Telekonsultationsnetzwerk für die Ophthalmologie - Erfahrungen und Ergebnisse, *Klin Monatsbl Augenheilkde* **212** (1998) 111-115.

[12] Siemens AG, Telemedizin ohne Grenzen. Hicom videokit in der Augenklinik rechts der Isar. Siemens AG (Hrsg.), Bereich Private Kommunikationssysteme, *Hicom Report*, Ausgabe März 1996. D-81359 München, Hofmannstr. 51.

[13] G. Mann, G.S. Aldington, T. Bek, C. Birkmann, H. Bornemann, K.D. Hepp, S. Kluthe, E.M. Kohner, B. Liesenfeld, M. Lungershausen, H. Mayer, M. Mertz, M. Obermaier, W. Piehlmeier, and M. Porta, Telescreening of Diabetic Retinopathy. *DNM (Diabetes, Nutrition and Metabolism)* **11/1** (1998) 89-95.

[14] G. Zahlmann, M. Obermaier, and C. Ritzke, Knowledge-based Monitoring of Glaucoma Patients-- A Conceptionists Approach. Medical Informatics in Europe (EFMI), 12th Internat Congress; Copenhagen 1996; Aug 19-22.

[15] M. Obermaier, A.Wegner, M. Mertz, M. Maier, and G. Zahlmann, Comparison of an One Step and a Two Step Approach of Artificial Neural Networks in Visual Field Evaluation. *Invest Ophthalmol Vis Sci* **38/4** (1997) 572.

[16] M.H. Emarah and M. Mertz, Telemedicine as Educational and Consultation Aid in Patient Management. Proc. of CATE 96, 1st Int. Conf. on Computers and Advanced Technologies in Education, Cairo, March 18-20 (1996) 97-100.

Address for Correspondence

Manfred Mertz
Department of Ophthalmology and Eye Hospital "Rechts der Isar"
Munich University of Technology
Ismaningerstr. 22
D-81675 Munich, Germany
E-mail: M.Mertz@lrz.tu-muenchen.de

The Impact of Telemedicine on Health Care Management
M. Nerlich and R. Kretschmer (Eds.)
IOS Press, 1999

Collaborative Telemedicine between Optometry and Ophthalmology: An Initiative from the University of Houston

Danielle BEAUREGARD, Jade S. SCHIFFMAN, Rosa TANG
University of Houston, College of Optometry, Houston, Tx, USA

Abstract: The University of Houston College of Optometry (UHCO) has developed a strong Telemedicine Optometry/Ophthalmology program. Patient care, clinical teaching and research benefit from utilizing Telemedicine technology. This initiative between Optometry and Ophthalmology is at the forefront of eyecare! Presented here: clinical teaching opportunities via tele-education including retinal, uveitic, neuro-ophthalmic disorders and glaucoma. Seminars introduce students to this technology and enhance their clinical experience through exposure to eye pathologies often related to systemic diseases. UHCO's affiliated clinics include multidisciplinary centers staffed by optometrists: the Frost Eye Clinic (HIV multidisciplinary care), Good Neighbor Health Clinic and Rusk School Health Promotion Project (indigent multidisciplinary care). These centers can converse on line with eyecare professionals. Large sites interested in low vision/visual rehabilitation include: The Institute for Rehabilitation and Research (TIRR), the Social Security Hospital (Lima, Peru), the Matagorda General Hospital and the Quentin Mease Hospital. These sites, do offer quality care but require visual rehabilitation programs provided by UHCO. These sites also provide exposure to pathology for the students. A residency program trains optometrists in Telemedicine. The research program focuses on optics and imaging necessary to diagnose glaucoma, diabetic retinopathy, and neuro-ophthalmic disorders through Telemedicine. UHCO supports the advancement of standards in tele-eyecare.

1. Introduction

The University of Houston is currently further developing and strenghtening its Telemedicine program. The Telemedicine interests of the University Eye Institute are manyfold and include patient care, teaching, and research. (1, 2)

Concerning the patient care domain, telemedicine has been incorporated in many aspects of our services and includes management of multiple offices issues, co-management between optometry and opthalmology issues and also consultations with ophthalmological sub-specialties.

Telemedicine has been brought into the graduate program with the Doctor of Optometry degree during the fourth and third year clinical education program using electronic data and videoconferencing. It is also a major emphasis at the postgraduate level where a Residency in Telemedicine and Neuro-Ophthalmology is currently offered. Additionaly, a resident/graduate student who is working towards a degree in Physiological Optics is specializing in Telemedicine.

The research interests of UHCO are centered on the development of a model for Tele-Ophthalmology research. Glaucoma is thus utilized as a model for the determination of imaging resolution and examination standards including clinical and technical protocols. (1,2)

2. Instrumentation

The University Eye Institute utilizes the Aethra software and hardware. This hybrid system combines both store-and-forward imaging as well as video-conferencing. Whiteboarding is also available. This feature has great interest especially in the review of fundus images, including optic nerve images, because clinician findings can be compared and the images annotated on the whiteboard. This allows tele-education to occur. The annotations may be saved on the image or discarded. Similarly, the system allows real time playing of video-clips of patient cases either at the main site or at the remote site.

Our system set-up uses a one chip CCD (charged-coupled device) Sony camera, mounted to a standard c-mount and to a slit-lamp. We also use a Sony Cam-corder for the capture of video-clips of either pupillary or motilities examination. (4)

Currently, we also use a non-mydriatic Topcon fundus camera. American Medical Development also provides, if desired, a direct ophthalmoscope or even a binocular indirect ophthalmoscope.

3. Patient Care

The University Eye Institute has been very involved in telemedicine for several years. (3) Since 1995, telemedicine has facilitated access to ophthalmology sub-specialty on a routine basis. Although, ophthalmology sub-specialists frequently direct clinics at the University Eye Institute, telemedicine is available to satellite clinics to triage and/or diagnose and manage those cases that require further expertise. Also the University Eye Institute may turn to other facilities for opinions suc as TIRR : The Institute for Rehabilitation and Research.

The typical interaction situations that may be encountered include management between multiple offices. Case one will review this situation. Similarly, case two brings up the issue of co-management and/or second opinion issues. Peer networking, continuing education, specialty consults and patient education are other situations which may encourage the utilization of telemedicine in optometry and ophthalmology.

In order to provide a direct link between the main campus and its satellites, the Good Neighbor Eye Clinic (GNC) has served as a pilot site. The following two cases originated from this site and constitute good examples of the type of applications that favor Telemedical interaction in Optometry.GNC uses a telemedicine system both as a teaching and archiving tool but also as a link to specialists if necessary.

Case 1 is that of a 15 year old Hispanic boy who presented to the University Eye Institute with an epithelial and stromal corneal infiltrate and a possible dendrite. The infection was diagnosed as a herpetic corneal ulcer by the optometrist in charge. This was later confirmed by the corneal specialist the following day who put the patient on Viroptic (Vidarabine 0.3%) and subsequently on prednisolone 1% topically to decrease the inflammation. The next day, the patient returned for a follow-up visit and it was agreed upon that follow-up over the week-end period would be necessary. Thus the patient needed to be assessed by the resident on call. This review of the case between the resident and the attending optometrist was done through telemedicine. The resident who was to be on call that week-end was at GNC and, through videoconferencing consulted on the case. Additionally, she was able to appreciate the level of epithelial and stromal involvement of the lesion through fluorescein pooling and staining. This was done by store-and-forward stills and videoconferencing images. Thus, the resident was able to manage the case.

This first case can be considered as a management situation between multiple offices via telemedicine. This case required interaction between two optometrists to be properly managed.

Case 2 is that of a 70 year old Hispanic female from Mexico who presented with a poorly controlled case of primary open angle glaucoma (POAG). The patient was being monitored in Mexico by an ophthalmologist who was treating her medically. She was on maximum topical therapy: Pilocarpine 2% BID, Trusopt 0.3% TID (methazolamide) and Timoptic 0.5% (timolol maleate) BID. The patient presented to GNC where store-and-forward still images and video-clips were obtained and sent for review by the ophthalmologist. The ophthalmologist requested to further assess the patient on video-conferencing and to perform a dilated fundus examination. The patient was weaned off the pilocarpine over a few days period. She was also given phenylephrine 2.5% to instill in both eyes starting 24 hours before the session. At the videoconferencing visit, the patient's iridocorneal angles were deemed to be significantly narrowed as compared to the gonioscopic examination in the miotic state. The ophthalmologist requested serial intraocular pressure measurements and to assess the patient face-to-face. It was determined that a prophylactic peripheral iridotomy should be performed because of the narrowed angles and the amount of optic nerve cupping : c/d = 0.9/0.9 in both eyes confirming the telemedical diagnosis. The patient was referred to the glaucoma specialist at the University Eye Institute for surgery. The patient underwent bilateral peripheral iridectomies. She is now taking Brominidine 0.5% (Alphagan) BID instead of Pilocarpine and is doing very well following surgery.

This case is a good example of co-management between optometry and ophthalmology and also demonstrates the importance of collaboration between the professionals.

4. Teaching Interests

The telemedicine teaching program focuses both on graduate and post-graduate education. The graduate program is that of the Doctor of Optometry. This four year program follows that of a bachelor of science degree. Two post-graduate programs concentrate on telemedicine. The first one is a clinical residency for optometrists concerned with telemedicine and neuro-ophthalmology and the second one is a post-graduate degree in physiological optics focusing on telemedicine.

At the graduate education level, the following three clinics are geared for third and fourth year optometry students and focus on three aspects of ocular pathology: retinal and uveitic diseases, diplopia and binocular visual disorders and neuro-ophthalmological disorders as well as low vision rehabilitation of brain injury patients.

The Telemedicine Retina Clinic had been active for three semesters and introduces third year optometry students to retinal diseases through interactive teaching. These students, are beginning in their specialty clinical training, and thus, are being acquainted with retinal and uveitic pathology. Examples of cases encountered include ARMD (age-related macular degeneration), diabetes, Fundus Albipunctatus, choroidal neovascular membranes, etc.

Uveitic entities are also encountered such as neuroretinitis from cat scratch fever, sarcoid retinitis, Behcet's disease and other uncommon ocular entities. The students have the opportunity to examine and question live patients as well as review photographic cases. A live interaction with the retina sub-specialist is available either by face-to-face encounter or through whiteboarding and videoconferencing. This clinic has been particularly successful at addressing the pathophysiology as well as other mechanisms involved in each disease entity. Similarly, the students are asked to familiaze themselves with the required adjunct testing such as fluorescein angiography, gallium scans, MRIs, cat scans, chest x-rays, lumbar punctures and other systemic laboratory work including blood work. This extensive introduction to the ocular pathologies in regards to systemic involvement provides the optometry student with a systemic outlook on the eye.

The second and third clinics of interest are : the Diplopia and Binocular Vision Disorders Clinic and the Neuro-Ophthalmology Clinic. These clinics are attended by fourth year optometry students. These students encounter strabismus and other oculo-motor anomalies as well as neuro-ophthalmic disorders. The Diplopia clinic is more concerned with diagnosis, rehabilitation and therapy whereas the Neuro-Ophthalmology clinic is more concerned with neuro-ophtalmology diagnosis and management.

Computer storage of electronic files on patients are used mostly as an adjunct to teaching as the specialists are available on site. Yet, interactive videoconferencing has been used to interact with other programs interested in education.

Store-and-forward technology allows the creation of video-clips of patients which can be utilized for teaching of extraocular muscles and other motor disorders. Weekly, patients with such disease entities are recorded and an electronic record is created. These cases serve as teaching cases for the telemedicine clinics. The visual browser also allows preparation of the teaching session in a ready-made available format. Each visual browser constitutes a teaching session on a particular topic where still images and video-clips can be obtained from the patient or scanned if desired.

The fourth clinic of interest is the Low vision/Brain Injury Rehabilitation Clinic. This clinic is orchestrated in conjunction with TIRR. This major institution has a low vision clinic staffed by the University Eye Institute. Telemedicine is new to this clinic and is currently being introduced. This clinic serves to train fourth year optometry student and optometry residents in the management of brain injury patients. Many of these patients have systemic or traumatic disease which result in ocular, psychological, and physical deficits. The ocular deficits are common and depend on the type of brain injury. In traumatic brain injury, the damage present is dependent on if it is open or closed-head injury and on the acceleration-deceleration induced in the trauma. In closed head injury, diffuse neuronal injury, contusion and mass effect from intracranial hemorrhage are encountered. Ischemia, brain swelling and excitotoxicity constitute other relevant causes. (5) These injuries, depending on the site, will have potentially sight devastating results. As such, a low vision evaluation is required and rehabilitation either through prisms, glasses or low vision aids such as telescopes and microscopes may be required. The level of cognition and the presence of neglect in the patient may influence the therapy. (5) Thus the need to familiarize the students with the whole disease entity including the physical therapy so that catering of the low vision services may be achieved more efficiently.

The intended format of telemedicine involvement is currently an educational session where discussion and/or consultation with specialists can be available. Images of a particular patient are captured on site and sent to the University Eye Institute for review from the involved faculty members. Subsequently a visual browser including the anatomy involved, the case history of the patient, the physical testing as well as the therapy and management of the case are put together. This seminar is really geared towards rehabilitation and concerns the patient as a whole. This also serves as an introduction to a patient and how he or she might present to an optometrist's office (example: pre-stroke symptoms) so the optometrist will be familiar with vision warning signals of potentially severe systemic conditions. Additionnally the rehabilitative management is emphasized.

The residency program is concerned with the clinical aspects of Telemedicine and includes introduction to the technology through participation in the affiliated clinical sessions such as the Telemedicine Retina Clinic, the Diplopia and Neuro-Ophthalmology clinics and the Low Vision/Brain Injury Rehabilitation. Patient care and introduction to telemedicine research are also favored. The resident has, as a requirement for completion of the Residency program, to create and pursue a research question.

5. Research Interests

The Graduate degree focuses on the physiological optics involved in telemedicine. Currently, research is geared towards resolution issues and utilizes glaucoma as a model. A preliminary project has recently been completed in cooperation with GNC. This project was aimed at determining the relevant parameters in the remote diagnosis of glaucoma. This project was an introduction to the thesis project currently underway.

UEI's involvement in telemedicine research dates to 1994 with the publication of a Telemedicine Master's Thesis using telemedicine to assess the feasability of diagnosing and treating ocular diseases through a satellite connection. (6) The results of this thesis indicate the feasability of Telemedicine in regards to optometric/ophthalmologic co-management. Subsequently, the research has centered on establishing a model for Tele-ophthalmological research. Glaucoma is being utilized to determine both imaging and examination standards and protocols.

The GNC project was born out of this model. (1,2) This pilot project is aimed at examining and comparing all modalities of telemedicine, including store-and-forward still images and video-clips with a conventionnal face-to-face examination in regards to glaucoma.

The GNC results have had a tremendous impact since they have allowed to determine some of the strenghts and weaknesses of the Telemedicine system including resolution issues. Currently, the cornea is very difficult to assess on a standard 640 x 480 pixels image. Thus the need for increased resolution. As research in dermatology has demonstrated (7), the use of a three chip CCD (charged coupled device) camera is better as both spatial and color resolution are enhanced. The GNC project used a one chip CCD camera. The spatial resolution is enhanced both in a monochromatic CCD camera and in a three chip CCD camera. In a one chip RGB CCD camera, the color measurements are not only unreliable but they also decrease the amount of spatial resolution available whereas in a three chip RGB CCD camera, prisms redirect the colored light signal into three different sensors thus maintaining the available spatial resolution to the level of a monochromatic camera. (8) It is suggested that increasing the resolution of the camera may increase the resolution of the cornea and that of the other ocular structures.

Similarly, high bandwidth connections seem to be more appropriate than low bandwidth connections for videoconferencing in eyecare. In the aforementionned study, only one ISDN (Integrated Digital Service Network) connection was available for videoconferencing which degraded the images, especially that of the cornea. However, the ability to take digital still pictures exists to enhance the exam.The follow-up study will provide a three ISDN line connection ameliorating this problem. This connection is already in place and is currently being used.

The project to be undertaken focuses on resolution issues for the analysis of the optic nerve in glaucoma.

Another project at hand concentrates on comparing the resolution and quality of digital fundus images of the optic nerve taken with the Topcon non-mydriatic fundus camera to that of 35mm images. This retrospective study is aimed at determining the extent of involvement of pixel size and resolution as well as color gamut have on the diagnosis of optic nerve images. This will serve as a baseline for the following studies. (9, 10)

6. Conclusion

Telemedicine potentially has a great number of applications. Standards for image resolution and electronic records and the protocols for obtaining these images are necessary. Additionnal clinical studies are also necessitated for particular conditions to provide quality and standardized care.

References

[1] SCHIFFMAN, Jade S. et al.: Telemedicine Enters Eye Care: Practical Experience. Journal of Ophthalmic Nursing and Technology. May/June 1998. 17(3) Pp. 102-106

[2] WHEELER, Terry. Tele-Ophthalmology: A Tale of Seven programs. Telemedicine Today. June 1998. Pp.6,8-9

[3] COUSOUNIS, Helen.: Telemedicine In The Trenches. Review of Optometry. January 15 1998.Pp.41-45

[4] FLOWERS, Charles E et al.: Teleophthalmology: Rationale, Current Issues, Future Directions. Telemedicine Journal. 1997. 3(1). Pp. 43-52

[5] BONTKE, CF et al.: Principles of Brain Injury Rehabilitation. In R. Braddom (Ed.), Textbook of Physical Medicine and Rehabilitation. Philadelphia: WB Saunders. Pp. 1027-1051

[6] CAPUTO, Michael P.: The Application of Digital Satellite Communications in Conducting Telemedicine. Master's in Physiological Optics. University of Houston. 1994

[7] LOANE, M.A. et al.: Effect of Camera Performance on Diagnostic Accuracy: Preliminary Results From The Northern Ireland Arms of the UK Multicenter Teledermatology Trial. Journal of Telemedicine and Telecare 1997. 3. Pp.83-88

[8] Edmunds Scientific 1998 Optics and Optical Instruments Catalog

[9] BRIGGS, Raymond et al.: A Methodologic Issue for Ophthalmic Telemedicine: Image Quality and Its Effect on Diagnostic Accuracy and Confidence. Journal of the American optometric Association. September 1998. 69(1). Pp.601-605

[10] THOMAS, James D.: Digital Archiving of Echocardiographic Images. Coronary Artery Disease. January 1995. 6(1). Pp.4-9

Address for correspondence

Danielle Beauregard
College of Optometry
University of Houston
4901 Calhoun
Houston, Texas 77204, USA

The Impact of Telemedicine on Health Care Management
M. Nerlich and R. Kretschmer (Eds.)
IOS Press, 1999

Web-based Teledermatology Consult system: Preliminary results from the first 100 cases

Hon S. PAK, Mark WELCH, Ronald POROPATICH
Walter Reed Army Medical Center, Washington DC, USA

Abstract: The TRICARE Region 1 Teledermatology Consortium has developed a secure web-based "store and forward" consult system designed to allow medical treatment facilities throughout the region to submit dermatology consults.

Realizing that there is very little objective data on teledermatology, we have begun to evaluate our system through the integration of questionnaires for patients, referring physicians, and consultants in addition to telephonic patient follow up. We report the preliminary data from the first 100 cases received in the first two months since partly deploying the web based teledermatology consult system in the Tricare Region I (Northeast United States). We primarily address system effectiveness(percentage of cases that required follow up to dermatology and/or primary care physicians, adequacy of evaluating pigmented lesions) diagnostic agreement, acceptance, effect on access to care, and educational value to the primary care physicians.

1. Introduction

The military medical department has a unique mission of providing all levels of medical care for the battlefields and peace-keeping missions anywhere in the world in addition to ensuring the health of all soldiers, family members, and retirees during peacetime. Hospital closures coupled with a decreased number of military physicians have left many health care beneficiaries without readily available access to specialty care. Beneficiaries are being asked to travel great distances, put their names onto waiting lists, or incur high out of pocket cost to see the medical specialists. As the northeastern United States military health care region (Tricare Region 1) consolidates to meet patient care goals, the need to provide rapid access to specialty care from geographically distant sites is essential. In recognizing these problems, the region has taken steps to meet the following goals:

1. Improve access to care especially for those in remote locations(i.e. World-wide deployments)
2. Improve delivery of dermatologic care by educating the primary care physicians.
3. Prioritize limited dermatology resources.

In order to continue to provide quality healthcare in the face of decreasing resources, Walter Reed Army Medical Center(WRAMC) is actively involved in several telemedicine projects to meet the above-set goals. In particular, the TRICARE Region 1 Teledermatology consortium has developed a secure system designed to allow medical treatment facilities throughout the region to submit dermatology consults. The system includes a password protected and encrypted World Wide Web connection to a dedicated Web server housed at

Walter Reed Army Medical Center, as well as a computerized patient record. Currently when the consult is entered into the system, dermatologists from the Walter Reed Army Medical Center (WRAMC), the National Naval Medical Center (NNMC), Malcolm Grow Medical Center, and the Uniformed Services University of the Health Sciences (USUHS) access the Teledermatology Web server from within their organizations (or even their homes), and complete their evaluation.

To date, many telemedicine systems have used T1 connections or live video connections, which are costly to deploy and maintain, limiting its acceptance on a wide scale. For the most part, it is not practical nor efficient to have dermatologists stop what he/she is doing and answer live video consultations especially if one is in different time zones. The live video conferencing requires synchronizing the schedule of three people: the patient, primary care physician, and the consultant. In recognizing the limitations of live video consultations, the NCA Teledermatology Consortium has developed a system which allows the use of existing technology to improve the existing consult system. The current consult system relies on movement of patients, not information, a more costly and inconvenient solution to both the provider and the patient. This web-based "store and forward" teledermatology consult system requires very little in expenditure outside of a digital camera. This store and forward web-based system allows asynchronous transmission of medical data, which is ideal in that it does not require the patient, the primary care physician, and the specialist to be available for the consultation at the same time. It uses the existing internet as the medium and a simple yet complete, user-friendly template as the electronic consult form. This system allows digital images, captured using COTS(commercial of the shelf) digital cameras, to be attached to the electronic consult form from the primary care physician, ensuring that appropriate and critical information is sent through secure channels. It gives the optimal amount of patient information to the dermatologist and allows almost immediate feedback for the management, treatment and disposition of the patient. This accomplishes two things: first it allows fast readily available access to dermatologists regardless of location(improving quality of care) and secondly offers education to the primary care physicians on the variety of dermatologic diseases they are encountering.

In the recent years, there has been an increasing number of studies being published in the dermatology journals that attempt to show the potential of teledermatology. Although most have been small pilot studies with very little hard or comparable data that points to the cost effectiveness or improvement in outcomes, there are many small studies which are showing close to 80% diagnostic agreement between in-person evaluation and teledermatology consultations. Furthermore, prior studies from Ft-Myer/WRAMC have shown that up to 50% of all teledermatology consults can be successfully completed without ever requiring the patients to travel to a dermatologist. In realizing that there are limitations to the teledermatology consult system and that it will never completely replace in-person dermatologic evaluations, we have begun to evaluate the system through the integration of questionnaires for patients, referring physicians, and consultants in addition to telephonic patient follow up. We report the preliminary data from the first 100 cases received in the first two months since deploying the web based teledermatology consult system in the Tricare Region I.

In doing this ongoing evaluation along with gathering comparative prospective data of teledermatology vs. in-person dermatologic consultations, we are attempting to optimize and ensure quality of medical care via telemedicine. Through the joint efforts of the Army, Navy and Air Force dermatologists and telemedicine experts in Tricare Region I, we hope that it will serve the entire Department of Defense medical system in the not too distant future.

2. Data

Data collection began 1 May 1998 and this preliminary summary represents the first 100 cases from referral sites to include eight surrounding primary care clinics and hospitals without dermatologists in Tricare Region I (from NY to VA). The Dermatology consultants were predominantly from Walter Reed AMC.

a. Workload

45% of the cases required no visits to the dermatologists; however, this actually represents a 15-20% decrease in the workload. This reduction takes into account the work/time for the dermatologist to do the T-derm consults. Seventeen percent required follow up visits to a dermatologist. Unexpectedly a large percentage(14%) required resubmission of images due mostly to poor photographic technique; however, most of the resubmissions came from two clinics and in May 1998 when the consult system was first put in place.

b. Diagnostic Agreement

There was only a 33% diagnostic agreement between referring physicians and dermatologists which reflect the lack of significant dermatology training for primary care physicians in the United States and explains the high referral rates to the dermatologists.

c. Biopsy Rate

Pigmented lesions are of a particular concern to most dermatologists due to a fear of mis-diagnosing a melanoma. This concern was reflected in the high biopsy rate of 50% for pigmented lesions. This percentage likely represents an overcall by the dermatology consultants. Overall, a biopsy was recommended in 23% of the cases.

d. Data-Questionnaires

We collected questionnaires to determine how the patient and the primary care physicians felt about the consult system before and after recommendations were given. The results are as follows:

1. Patients Questionnaire

From the 77 questionnaires which were available for evaluation, most patients initially felt that the teledermatology consult system was better able to meet their healthcare needs. In fact, most patients were satisfied with the process of getting access to dermatologists via Teledermatology.

2. Referring Physicians Questionnaire, Part I

From the 81 questionnaires available, the Referring physicians stated that they would have done the following if the t-derm were not available:
12% - they would have telephoned a dermatologist
7.5% - they would have treated the patient without consulting a dermatologist
79% - they would have sent the patient to a nearby dermatologist- This is because there is no incentive in the military not to refer a patient and represents an area for potential improvement.

3. Referring Physicians Questionnaire, Part II (After Consultant's Response)

Of the 45 questionnaires available, we found that only 27% of the cases required a physical visit to the primary care physician for follow up. The remaining 73% required only telephonic follow up.

Generally, the referring physcians were very satisfied but more importantly, they felt that they had improved their dermatologic knowledge. Most felt that the T-derm consult was better than a standard consult more than 70% of the time. This is probably due to the fact that the current standard consults do not allow for much feedback from the consultants.

4. Consultant's Questionnaire

It took on average 1/3rd the time(7.7 minutes v. 20 minutes) to complete the consultations using this system when compared with an in-person appointment.

In 70% of the cases, the dermatologists felt that the consult was of sufficient quality and quantity(information) to make a diagnosis and recommend a treatment plan. Conversely, in about 30% of the cases, the dermatologists felt that seeing the patient in person would have made them more certain of the diagnosis and treatment.

5. Patient Follow Up

4-6 Weeks after the consults were answered, we called the patients to see how they were doing. Fifty five patients were available for questionnaires. The results were astounding:
-47%(26) of patients did not get a call back from their primary care physician
-36%(20) of patients had to see a dermatologist. This means that the 27% of the cases in which biopsies were recommended were going to a dermatologist not to primary care physicians. Of those that saw a dermatologist,
-40%(8/20) saw a civilian dermatologist
-60%(12/20) saw a military dermatologist

6. Patient Satisfaction

Patients' final satisfaction was lower than expected especially when compared to the patients' initial satisfaction. In fact, Only 64% were satisfied with the consult system. Twenty one percent were undecided. Fifteen percent were not satisfied with the consult system. Of those that were not satisfied, there were two major groups.

The 1st group included those whose primary care physicians did not call them with the recommendations. The smaller, second group were those that accessed dermatologists via the Teledermatology system who were then told to go on a waiting list to see a dermatologist in person for their routine skin condition.

We also asked if the patient would have preferred to wait and see a dermatologist in person at a nearby medical center instead of getting access via teledermatology:

38% said yes
42% said no
20% were undecided.

This points out that the current teledermatology system will probably not replace dermatologists in the near future.

We then asked patients if this consult system saved or wasted time:

56% said neither
5%said it wasted their time
39% said it saved time (both in access time to see the dermatologist and in distance traveled.)

As expected, those that saved significant amount of time(at least 90 minutes or more) were those that lived > 1.5 hours away and had limited or no access to dermatologists.

3. Positives and Negatives

a. *Positive Benefits*

From the above preliminary data, the following appears to be some positive benefits of this teledermatology system:

- Immediate access for patients to dermatologists
- Prioritize dermatology resources
- Educating primary care physicians
- 15-20% workload reduction
- Low cost to deploy widely
- Generally well accepted

b. *Potential Negatives*

There are some not too insignificant potential pitfalls:

- There is a potential increase in morbidity with a high biopsy rate depending on who performs the biopsies especially if the biopsies were unnecessary.
- There are some minor technical issues. Not all clinics had LAN lines for internet access and training people with no computer skills was time consuming.
- There is also a shift in the workload for the referring clinics which is difficult to measure.

4. Lessons Learned

With our current teledermatology consult system, it became obvious that we needed to improve training in photography and setting the correct expectations. More specifically, we needed to let the referring physicians realize that it is their responsibility to follow up with recommendations. In addition, the patients also need to realize that they may actually have to wait to see a dermatologist in person .

We perhaps need to improve patients' access to dermatologists for those 13% that were found to need a routine follow up with a dermatologist via our teledermatology consult system.

We also need to develop clinical guidelines regarding if and who we should allow to perform biopsies and how to train them.

As expected, those that lived in remote sites without access to a dermatologist seemed to have the most to gain.

5. Cost Effectiveness

Cost Effectiveness was not one of our initial goals, however, it became an issue when it was time to deploy a teledermatology system. The issue of cost effectiveness is complex. As discussed above, there is a 15-20% decrease in workload for the dermatologist and probably some fractional increase for primary care/referring physicians. We also need to take into account this increase in biopsies and possible increase in morbidity as a measure of cost.

To fully and adequately evaluate cost effectiveness, we need an outcomes study which is resource intensive & time consuming. We are currently planning for such study.

6. Conclusions

What can we assume from our preliminary data?

- There appears to be a 15-20% workload reduction to the dermatologist.
- The patients seem to benefit the most from this consult system.
- The system is easy to deploy on a wide-scale with the correct emphasis on training.
- It is difficult to prove cost effectiveness of this system unless an outcomes study is done.
- Training the outlying clinics is essential.
- We need to set the right expectations and responsibilities for both the patients and referring physicians.

7. The Future

We will continue to collect on-going data from this operational web-based teledermatology consult system to confirm our preliminary findings.

We also started a study to evaluate minimal resolution requirements for teledermatology which started in August 1998.

We also began a study to evaluate diagnostic agreement between teledermatology consult system and in-person evaluation by the same dermatologist. This will also evaluate the various skin conditions to determine any limitations of our system- especially pigmented lesions. We will also evaluate biopsy rate differences and need for photographic standards.

Address for corespondence

Ronald Poropatich
Walter Reed Army Medical Center
Washington DC 20307, USA

The Impact of Telemedicine on Health Care Management
M. Nerlich and R. Kretschmer (Eds.)
IOS Press, 1999

Are Dermatologists in Private Practice Interested in Teledermatological Services?

Alexander GLAESSL, Roman SCHIFFNER, Thomas WALTHER,
Michael LANDTHALER, Wilhelm STOLZ
Department of Dermatology, University of Regensburg, Regensburg, Germany

Abstract: Diagnosing dermatologic skin conditions can be difficult, especially in pigmented skin lesions. Therefore, the consultation of an expert *via* teledermatology could prove vital. For this purpose, a rapid transfer of medical data including high resolution images is essential. This transfer can be performed with a variety of modern telecommunication technologies, including ISDN, highspeed-ISDN, Internet, and Intranet. As the levels of both communication software and camera-systems can be quite different, our survey investigated the equipment of 84 dermatologists in private practice. A questionaire was distributed on computer equipment, operating system software, and any image documentation systems used, as well as required telecommunications equipment and possible applications of teledermatology. This survey showed a response rate of 54% and proves that dermatologists in private practice are interested in telemedicine services. Most dermatolgists surveyed use Windows 95 operating software and 74% have access to modern ISDN modems or PC-cards. Dermatologists currently prefer applications with low-tech communication hardware and software requirements. Consultation of dermatological centers was the favored application with 59%. Our survey clearly demonstrates that a high percentage of dermatologists in private practice would use teledermatology. In our experience, for the excellence of this service an image documentation system is essential to provide the teledermatolocical expert with standardized images with constant illumination.

1. Introduction

Diagnosis and even therapy of skin conditions can be difficult, especially in pigmented skin lesions. Therefore, the consultation of an expert in a health care center via teledermatology could prove vital. In most situations, the rapid transfer of medical data including high resolution image data (still-video, live-camera) would be quite sufficient for this consultation. Transfer of medical data can be performed with a variety of modern telecommunication technologies such as ISDN, highspeed-ISDN, Internet, and Intranet. Communication is possible in the range between live video-conferencing and sending attached files *via* Email by standard software. For image acquisition, different camera-systems can be used, including live Web-cam, still-video, and "classic" slides which are scanned and sent by Email. Our survey investigated the equipment and the requirements of dermatologists in private practice prior to the launching of a teledermatological project.

2. Materials and Methods

84 dermatologists in private practice in Bavaria were contacted by mail. The questionaires were returned by mail or fax. The dermatologists answered questions about computer equipment currently available in their private practices, operating system software, telecommunications technical equipment and software, use of a (digital) image documentation system, and possible or desirable requirements for a teledermatological service.

3. Results

Our survey showed a response rate of 54%. In detail, 33% of dermatologists were younger than 40 years, 44% were between 40 and 50 years old, and 23% were older than 50. 60% of physicians who did not answer our questionaire were between 40 and 50 years of age, 21% were older than 50 years, and 19% were younger than 40 years.

4. Hardware

95% of the dermatologists use a computer system in their private practice and 60% have systems with modern Pentium-processors, whereas more than 25% still use 386- and 486-processors. Interestingly, 14% of the dermatologists do not know the technical details of their computer system. Details about the hardware equipment, i.e. the processors used, are given in figure 1.

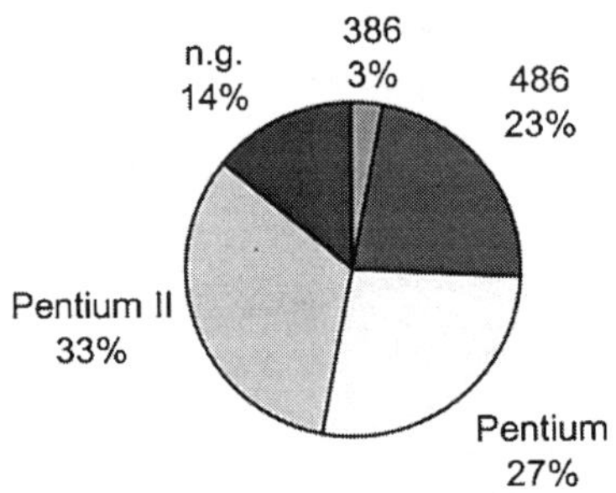

Fig. 1: Hardware equipment: processors used in private practice (n.g.= not given)

5. Operating system software

Most dermatolgists use Windows 95 operating software and some work with UNIX orApple. Older Win 3.x versions are only found rarely. Windows NT also seems to be a frequently used operating system software. Interestingly, 21% are still working with MS-DOS operating system software (fig. 2).

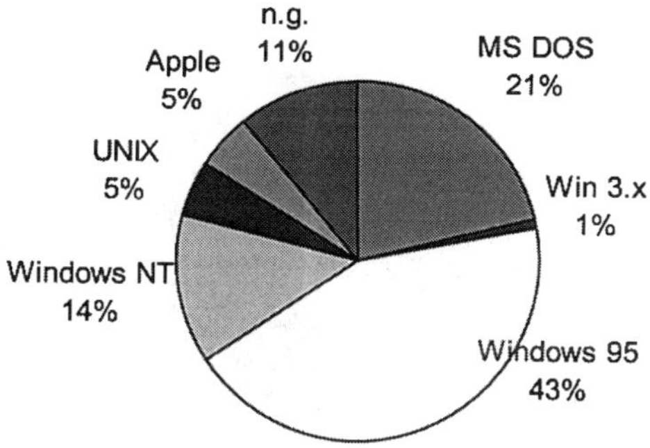

Fig. 2: Operating system software used in private practice (n.g.= not given)

6. Modems, Communication Software and Image Documentation System

74% of the dermatologists in private practice use modern ISDN modems or ISDN-PC-cards. Modems using analog standards are rarely found. Furthermore, detailed data on the general use of communication software and hardware were obtained (fig. 3). 56% of the physicians claimed to use Email on a regular basis. About 10% (in total 4 out of 45) of the dermatologists surveyed have installed their own Website in the Internet. The various medical software distributors used in private practice are shown in fig. 4. Data about employing digital image documentation systems and expert systems for pigmented skin lesions are shown in fig. 5.

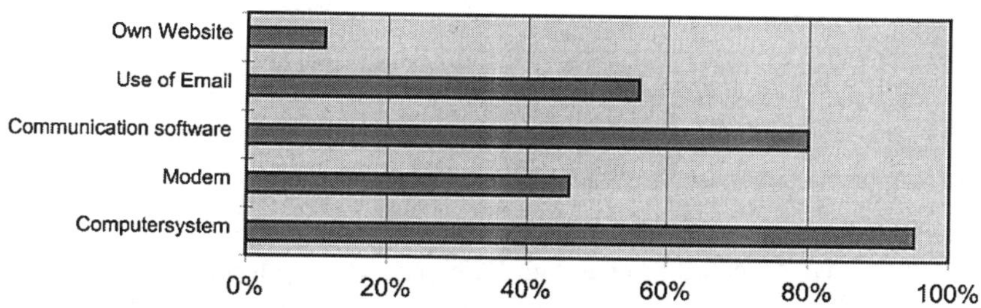

Fig. 3 General use of communication software and hardware

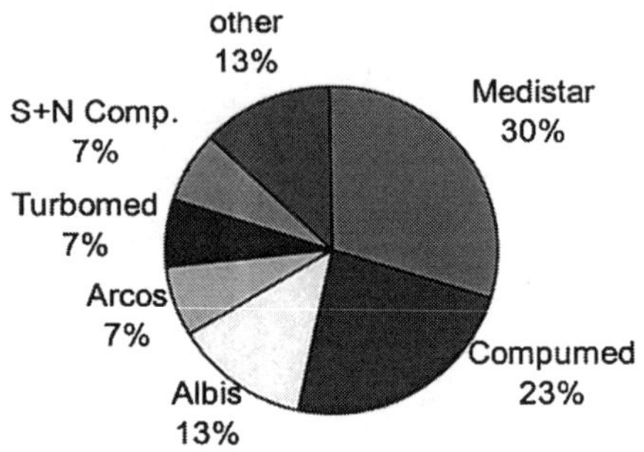

Fig. 4 Different medical software distributors used in private practice

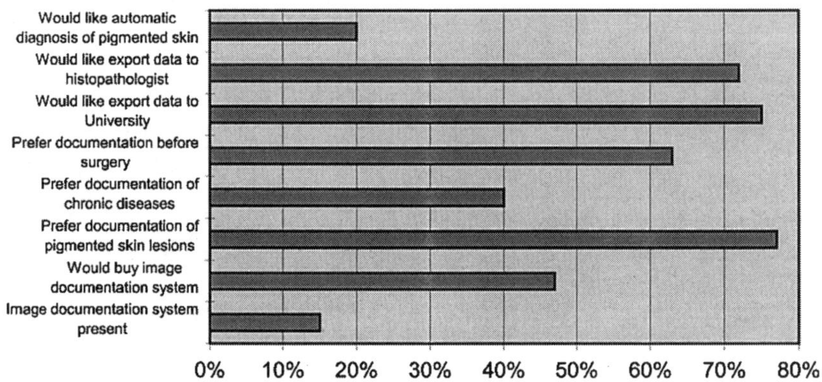

Fig. 5 The use of digital image documentation systems in private practice

7. Aspects of Teledermatological Applications

The questionaire proposed several aspects of potential teledermatologic applications and inquired about alternative possibilities of communication, e.g., teleconsultation, online/offline video-conferencing, attached emails (fig. 6). Figure 7 shows the dermatologists' intentions for teleconsultations, whereas figure 8 demonstrates further teledermatological prospects for the practicing dermatologist. With regard to the care of patients, 59% are responsive to teleconsultations with dermatological clinics, but only 36% with other practicing dermatologists (fig. 6). For scientific discussions and general dermatological topics, 82% intend to use telecommunication with dermatological clinics and 45% with other dermatologists (fig. 8).

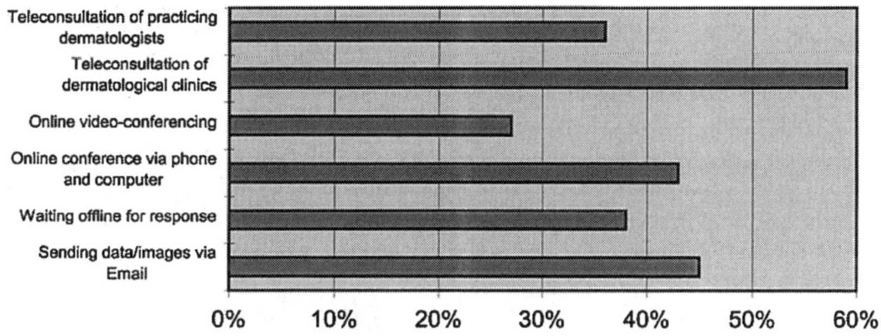

Fig. 6 Preferred ways of communication for direct care of patients

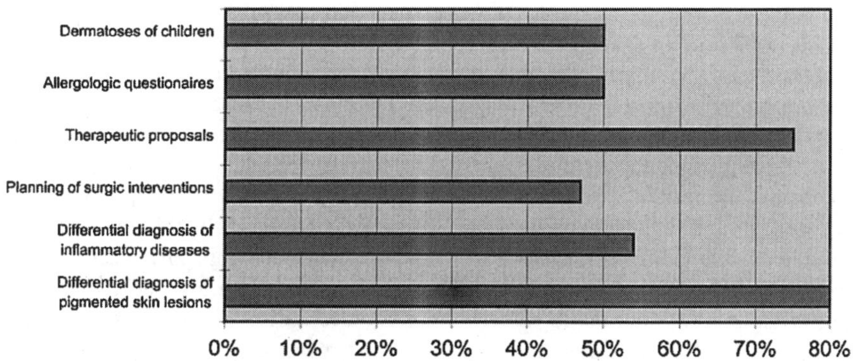

Fig. 7 Dermatologists' intentions for teleconsultation

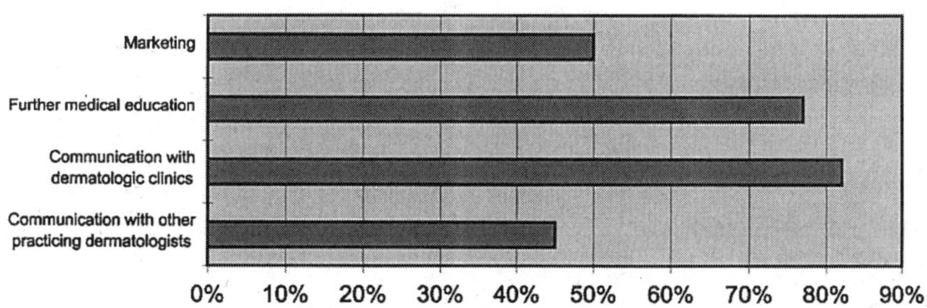

Fig. 8 Other intentions for electronic communication

8. Discussion

Diagnosing dermatologic skin conditions can be difficult, especially in pigmented skin lesions. Therefore, the possibility of consulting experts in health care centers seems very desirable. Our data demonstrate that dermatologists in private practice are interested in these telemedicine services. Although telemedicine is not suitable for solving every difficult question of geographically remote physicians, dermatology has a high potential for possible telemedical applications. As published in a study describing three independently designed telemedicine programs for underserved populations, dermatology emerged as the specialty most often performed by remote physicians [1]. An effective delivery of dermatological expertise through a video-conferencing link to a consultant dermatologist in a dermatological health care unit can be performed in geographically isolated practices [2].

According to our survey, dermatologists currently prefer applications with low-tech communication hardware and software requirements, such as standard ISDN hardware, sending images as attached files via Email, and offline-conferencing with standard communication software-- which confirms a recent study indicating that teledermatology is achievable by using a low-technology, low-cost approach [3].

However, our results do not agree with the conclusions of other authors, which indicate that a high proportion of dermatological conditions can only be successfully managed by realtime teledermatology [4]. According to our questionaire, teleconsultation of experts in dermatological centers is the favourable application. Towards this end, the quality of digital images-- especially of pigmented skin lesions-- is highly important when used in dermatologic health care centers for concordant diagnoses. Telephonic transmitted compressed images of pigmented skin lesions may be sufficient for expert consultation in less difficult cases [5]. In our experience, a high quality documentation system is needed to provide standardized images with constant illumination [6,7] because a reliable, reproducible and objective diagnosis with digital dermatoscopy (skin surface microscopy, epiluminiscence microscopy) in pigmented skin lesions is only possible if images were obtained with that constant illumination [6, 7]. For this purpose, it is necessary to use only camera systems which allow the acquisition of digital images without using automatic camera functions. Recently, Gilmour E et. al. [8] illustrated that telemedicine has the potential to diagnose and manage dermatolgic cases referred from primary care. Furthermore, it was shown that almost complete agreement between clinical and digital examination can be obtained for suspected skin cancers [9]. Telemedical services were also accepted by patients [10].

In conclusion, the results of our survey and our experience with pilot studies emphasize the need for telemedical services by specialized dermatologic centers for dermatologists in private practice, in order to both improve quality in practice and save time for patients in travelling to dermatological centers.

References

[1] S.A. Norton, A.E. Burdick, C.M. Phillips, and B. Bergman, Teledermatology and Underserved Populations, *Arch Dermatol* **133** (1997) 197-200.

[2] C.C. Lyon and P.V. Harrison, Digital Imaging and Teledermatolgy: Educational and Diagnostic Applications of a Portable Digital Imaging System for the Trainee Dermatologist, *Clin Exp Dermatol* **22** (1997) 163-216.

[3] P.V. Harrison, B. Kirby, Y. Dickinson, and R. Schofield, Teledermatology-- High Technology or Not? *J Telemed Telecare* **4**, supp. (1998) 31-32.

[4] M.A. Loane, R. Corbett, S.E. Bloomer, D.J. Eedy, H.E. Gore, C. Mathews, C. Steele, and R. Wootton, Diagnostic Accuracy and Clinical Management by Realtime Teledermatology: Results from the Northern Ireland Arms of the U.K. Multicentre Teledermatology Trial, *J Telemed Telecare* **4** (1998) 95-100.

[5] N. Provost, A.W. Kopf, H.S. Rabinovitz, W. Stolz, M. DeDavid, Q. Wasti, and R.S. Bart, Comparison of Conventional Photographs and Telephonically Transmitted Compressed Digitized Images of Melanomas and Dysplastic Nevi, *Dermatology* **196** (1998) 299-304.

[6] W. Stolz, R. Pompl, T. Burgdorff, A. Horsch, W. Bunk, R. Schiffner, A. Glaessl, G. Morfill, and W. Abmayr, Computerisierte Verlaufskontrolle und Bildanalytische Auswertung Pigmentierter Hautveränderungen, *Zeitschr Derm* **184** (1998) 170-175.

[7] W. Stolz, R. Schiffner, L. Pillet, T. Vogt, H. Harms, T. Schindewolf, M. Landthaler, W. Abmayr, Improvement of Monitoring of Melanocytic Skin Lesions with the Use of a Computerized Acquisition and Surveillance Unit with a Skin Surface Microscopic Television Camera, *J Am Acad Dermatol* **35** (1996) 202-207.

[8] E. Gilmour, S.M. Campbell, M.A. Loane, A. Esmail, C.E. Griffiths, M.O. Roland, E.J. Parry, R.O. Corbett, D. Eedy, H.E. Gore, C. Mathews, K. Steel, and R. Wootton, Comparison of Teleconsultations and Face-to-Face Consultations: Preliminary Results of a United Kingdom Multicentre Teledermatology Study, *Br J Dermatol* **139** (1998) 81-87.

[9] J.D. Whited, B.J. Mills, R.P. Hall, R.J. Drugge, J.M. Grichnik, and D.L. Simel DL, A Pilot Trial of Digital Imaging in Skin Cancer, *J Telemed Telecare* **4** (1998) 108-112.

[10] D.S. Reid, L.E. Weaver, J.M. Sargeant, M.J.M. Allen, W.F. Mason, P.J. Klotz, and D.B. Langille, Telemedicine in Nova Scotia: Report of a Pilot Study, *J Telemed Telecare* **4** (1998) 249-258.

Address for correspondence

Alexander Glaessl
Department of Dermatology
University of Regensburg
Franz-Josef-Strauss-Allee 11
93053 Regensburg, Germany
E-mail: alexander.glaessl@klinik.uni-regensburg.de

The Impact of Telemedicine on Health Care Management
M. Nerlich and R. Kretschmer (Eds.)
IOS Press, 1999

European Field Tests with HISTKOM Telepathology Equipment

Peter SCHWARZMANN, Bernd BINDER, Michael KÄSER, Rüdiger KLOSE
University of Stuttgart, Institut für Physikalische Elektronik, Stuttgart, Germany

Abstract. HISTKOM telemicroscopy equipment for telepathology is designed for the most challenging application in telepathology: intraoperational frozen section diagnosis. Adapted to this application, it is also excellently suited for all other telepathology modes requesting less sophisticated equipment. The technical concept and user interface are oriented to routine daily pathology. HISTKOM underwent heavy field-tests at several locations. The field-tests designs and the results of five of these are reported in this paper.

Telepathology will exploit its advantages in networks hosting participants requesting and offering services. The solution of the interoperability problem caused by different equipment from different suppliers within such a network will be a major task, the solution for which is in progress.

The new generation of HISTKOM equipment and software is designed in a modularized concept, allowing the integration of various hardware components from different manufacturers; thus special configurations can be realized easily. HISTKOM is offered as complete turnkey system, but can also be installed in yet existing configurations of the customer if they meet specifications.

1. Introduction

More and more services in *telemedicine*-- services in medicine offered at a distance-- have become realizable these days. This is due to the development of the tools of *telematics*-- an acronym for a merger of telecommunication and informatics. One of the most promising, but also challenging fields in this context is *telepathology*-- the provision of services in pathology at a distance.

One of the first publications of this new field appeared in 1987 [1] and until today a variety of modifications have developed, including those with a simple offline transmission of images for second opinion or educational purposes, applications with interactive discussion facilities on transmitted images, and finally online telemicroscopy to render full diagnoses in pathology from a distance. The most challenging application of the last modification-- online telemicroscopy-- is telepathology for frozen section diagnosis within surgical interventions with no pathologist locally present or without sending the removed tissue physically to the pathologist's lab.

This paper will be restricted in principle to the frozen section scenario with online telemicroscopy to render intraoperational diagnoses from a distance. It is obvious that the successful introduction and operation of this service in telepathology will also cover the needs of all other modes of telepathology, e.g., the request of a second opinion diagnosis, the exchange of image material for primary or continuing education, and database applications.

Part 2 of this paper presents the HISTKOM equipment applied in the evaluation studies and its performance within an ISDN telephone network. Part 3 compiles the results of several types of field tests, and Part 4 discusses the formation of future telepathology service networks. For illustration, Fig. 1 outlines the strategy for such a network to host institutions requesting and offering services in pathology, as well as tools to create and handle electronic investigation protocols appropriately.

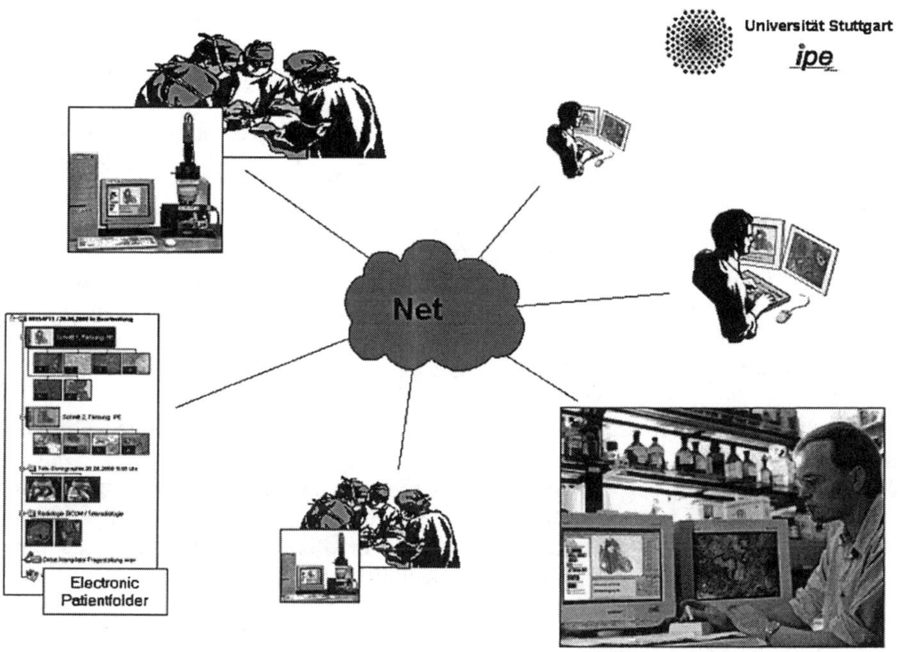

Fig. 1: Diagram of a service network for telepathology within the public telephone net, including remotely operable microscope stations at surgery locations, display stations in pathology labs to operate the microscopes remotely, and the electronic investigation protocol.

To remind nonspecialists in this field, a frozen section diagnosis scenario applying telemicroscopy will contain the following basic activities of the partners:

- During a surgical intervention, tissue is removed for immediate diagnosis to continue the intervention appropriately.
- The surgery team calls a pathologist equipped with a telepathology display station by telephone and asks for immediate diagnostic assistance.
- In an interactive procedure between pathologist and surgery team, the position and orientation of the section is determined in a macro image of the removed tissue. Then a frozen section slide is prepared by the surgery team and inserted in the telemicroscopy station in the surgery department.
- *Via* the net, a remote pathologist takes complete control of the microscope and inspects the slide as if it was under his own microscope.
- The pathologist transmits his diagnosis and information relevant for the adequate continuation of the intervention.
- An arbitrary number of frozen sections can spontaneously be prepared and diagnosed during the operation, if more tumor lesion is removed. Nowadays, this is not possible if the material is transported to the pathologist by courier.

- If no further frozen section diagnosis is necessary, the link between surgery and pathology is released, the intervention continued, and the pathologist may serve another surgery team.

In contrast to the scenario outlined above, the present procedure offers four alternatives:

- In large central hospitals, an in-house pathology department provides the frozen section service-- this is the gold standard.
- Small and medium-sized hospitals transport the removed tissue by courier to a nearby pathologist, accepting a delay of diagnosis due to the transportation time of up to 30 - 45 minutes.
- Small and medium-sized hospitals ask a pathologist to come in the for the time of surgery and pay for the traveling and wait time.
- No frozen section diagnosis is made at all with an increased risk of a second intervention after the final diagnosis of the embedded material. This situation is often found in medically underserved areas, especially in developing countries and remote areas.

In the last three of the four situations described above, telepathology can help to improve the quality of the service.

The new technique of telepathology with telemicroscopy allows the development and the installation of networks hosting participants who request and offer services in telepathology. From a technical point of view, such a network is in principle operable worldwide, provided that globally available nets are used, e.g., the telephone net and the Internet.

2. The HISTKOM Equipment

The development concept of HISTKOM was aimed at the construction of a telemicroscopy station with online capabilities in its operation, and which is oriented to the needs of daily routine pathology. It should be operated in inexpensive, globally available networks. The ideal goal was to provide the pathologist with a telemicroscopy tool for controlling a remote microscope as if it were present in front of him, with the only difference being that the microscope's field of view is inspected on a monitor instead of through the eyepiece of a real microscope.

From a technical point of view, such an idealized scenario can be realized by installing a broadband TV-connection of high quality together with a control channel to operate the microscope. This technically simple solution has been realized and evaluated in several institutions [1][2][3]. Unfortunately, these solutions have two severe drawbacks:

- The solution is really expensive concerning connection and data transfer. It is affordable only if operated within a campus with a dedicated TV-connection between surgery and pathology or within public-sponsored dedicated nets.
- Such a solution is only available at a few selected locations, not allowing the formation of general telepathology networks.

Another already existing technology with affordable costs-- video conference technology-- is not adequate for telepathology, as this technique cannot transmit the tremendous amount of detail in low-magnified histological sections in the requested quality. Due to the limited channel capacities of the telephone net for data transmission, video conference systems reduce the resolution in image details to maintain the high frame rate for a good video impression. In telepathology, however, the contrary approach makes sense: the frame rate may be reduced to maintain an extremely high quality of the single frame with respect to resolution and presentation of image details. HISTKOM follows the second approach without compromises.

Having in mind the above arguments requesting the application of inexpensive, globally available telecommunication networks, two main problem areas had to be solved in HISTKOM for a successful telepathology equipment:

- Telemicroscopy for telepathology can be applied economically only if based on narrow band networks (telephone, ISDN-telephone), which are available everywhere at affordable costs. The application of Internet technology has to be discussed carefully because of its restrictions with respect to warranted online capacity (see below).

- Telepathology equipment had to be developed to fit optimally without problems into the diagnostic procedures of a pathology lab. Secondly, the user interface has to reflect the pathologist's needs and must hide all confusing aspects of sophisticated computer facilities not necessary for the application-- the developer has to fit his program to the pathologist's needs and not vice versa.

The HISTKOM equipment is designed for standard PC-platforms and consists in principle of four basic components:

2.1. The Microscope Station

The microscope station is positioned at the location of the tissue to be diagnosed-- normally a surgery department. Its main component is one of the new types of computer controllable microscopes which allows the remote control of all relevant microscope functions. A connected 3-chip TV-color-camera allows the image material to be transmitted to the remote pathologist. For applications in pathology, the following microscope functions must be remotely controlled:

- x and y coordinates of the scanning table
- z-axis for focusing
- magnification (selection of objective)
- illumination of microscope
- Koehler setting of diaphragms
- autofocus.

A host computer controls the station and provides the TCP/IP interface for access to the specific interfaces connecting HISTKOM to a multitude of network types. Fig. 2 presents a photo of the HISTKOM microscope station.

2.2. The Display Station

The display station is located on the desk of the pathologist. It consists of two monitors, one for the microscope field of view and the other for the PC-host computer to control the remote microscope *via* the user interface. The host is equipped with a TCP/IP interface to connect it to another net- specific access interface. A two-monitor solution was selected to provide the pathologist parallel to the actual microscope field of view permanently with a full-frame macro image of the slide for orientation in it. Additionally, this screen contains the user interface for operating the microscope. As already indicated, the second monitor displays the actual field of view in the microscope (the virtual eye piece of the microscope) or, in the reviewing mode of archived investigation protocols, the selected screen shots made during the investigation procedure. Fig. 3 displays in detail this workplace of the pathologist and Fig. 4 presents the layout of a monitor with the user interface, combined with the macro image of a slide. The main parts of the functionality of the display station are explained in detail in the caption of Fig. 4.

2.3. Electronic Investigation Document (Patient Folder)

HISTKOM provides for the documentation, archiving, and mailing of an electronic investigation protocol containing text, graphics, and color image material of different sources. The design of this protocol meets the legal requirements. It includes, together with other information, the slide overview image with the areas investigated marked in color, and labels where separate images have been selected and archived as screen shots with higher magnification. The selected key images are included in full resolution together with text information, patient data, and diagnoses.

This protocol is designed to fit into the local database of HISTKOM, to be transmitted *via* software interfaces to the hospital information system (if necessary), and to be exchangeable with other partners in a telepathology network. In a separate transcoding process, the total investigation file can also be translated into the format of an HTML document. This can be mailed through the Internet and displayed by a receiver using one of the standard Internet browsers. No special HISTKOM hardware or software is necessary for this inspection procedure of the HTML investigation protocol. It is, however, the responsibility of the transmitting partner to care for data confidentiality. This facility is especially useful for second opinion, database, and education applications.

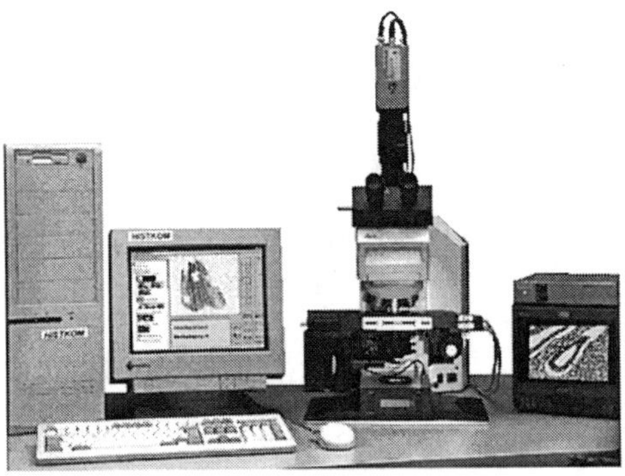

Fig. 2: HISTKOM microscope station in the surgery area, consisting of computer controllable microscope, 3-chip CCD-color-TV-camera, host-computer (PC), and control monitor.

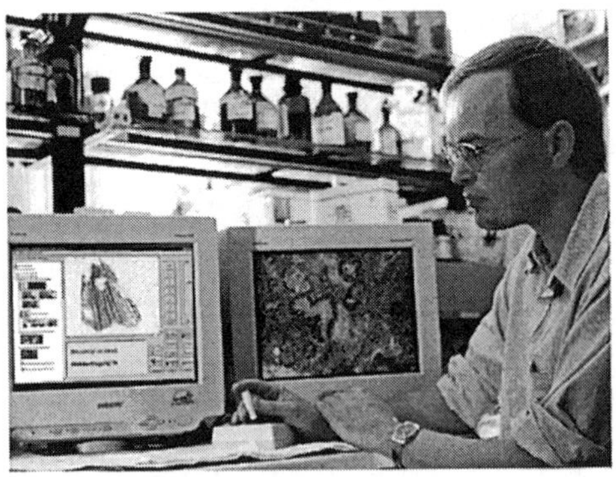

Fig. 3: Workplace of the pathologist (display station) with monitors displaying the macro image with user interface and monitor for the microscope field of view. Mouse and joystick control the remote microscope.

2.4. The Network Interface

HISTKOM uses TCP/IP as a universal internal protocol to connect to a variety of networks. This interface can easily be connected *via* available hardware and software interfaces to other networks, some of which will be regarded below.

In connection with the technical network problems, the problems of data confidentiality also have to be solved. HISTKOM provides three levels of data security:

- The inherent confidentiality of the switched ISDN telephone net (if ISDN is used), together with a scrambling technique if more than one ISDN channel is used in a system.
- An access control with chip cards authorizing and identifying the partners of a telepathology session.
- Coding the transmitted data by applying one of the technologies offered through registered trust centers.

The TCP/IP interface can connect *via* standard interfaces to the following types of networks:

- *The ISDN telephone network as the standard and preferred telecommunication link.* For this net HISTKOM offers the facility to bundle up to 8 ISDN B-channels (equivalent to 4 S_0-channels) to offer sufficient transmission capacity for a comfortable working environment, with an online impression for remote microscopy. ISDN is the standard network in the FRG and is also the agreed standard to be introduced in Europe. The cost of 8 bundled channels corresponds to that of 8 telephone connections if all channels are selected.

- *Local and wide-area ATM broadband nets.* ATM nets with high QS (Quality of Service) modes provide nearly ideal facilities for multimedia applications, as they provide a combination of switched connections (virtual link), variable bandwidth, and selectable modes of QS. Many governments in Europe have installed ATM networks for scientific institutions without charging them. Unfortunately, these nets are not yet available everywhere and are by far too expensive for telepathology if ordered separately by private persons.

- *VSAT net (satellite links).* This net is more expensive than the telephone net, but offers challenging opportunities to install worldwide links even to very remote and underdeveloped areas. These stations need no infrastructure, as a single satellite dish provides the connection to the telepathology network.

- *Internet.* Concerning costs and worldwide availability, the Internet offers ideal opportunities for telepathology. HISTKOM can also be connected to it. But for online telepathology, two severe considerations have to be made: first, the Internet gives no warranty for online application, as no data rate can be guaranteed. The online performance depends heavily on the momentary occupation of the net. In busy times, longer and unforeseeable interruptions may happen. If Internet connections can be applied with no other partners active in the net (local connections), online capabilities are possible. The other restriction of the Internet is the often insufficient data confidentiality inherent to this net, as only some software walls must be overcome (which is illegal, but cannot be avoided).

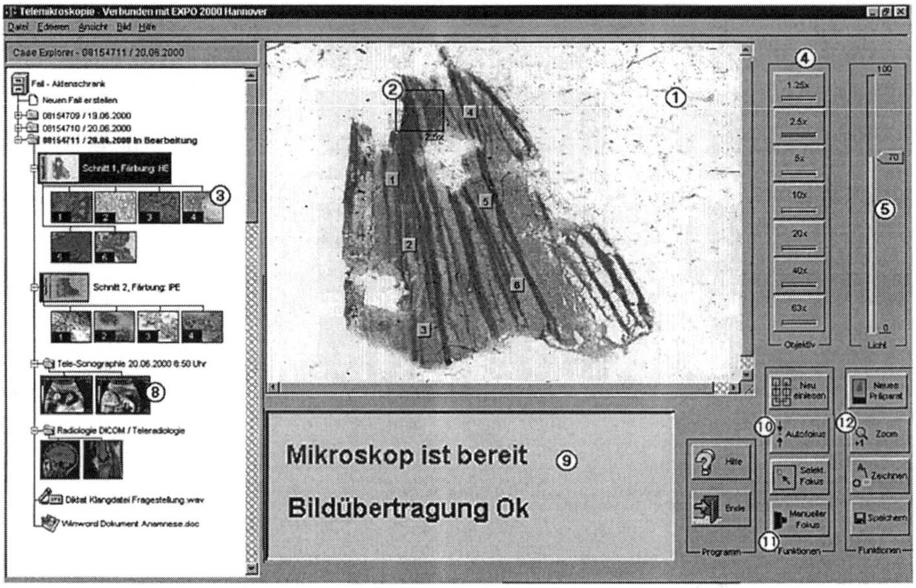

Fig. 4: Monitor layout for slide overview and user interface to operate the remote microscope. Out of the complete functionality set, a subset is listed below using the labels in the image.

1: Large overview of the total slide in high quality and resolution.
2: Window indicating the position and the scale of the actual microscope field of view displayed on the other screen.
3: Gallery and positions of all screen shots of key scenes made and archived in the investigation protocol during the diagnostic session.
4: Buttons to select objectives resp. the magnification of the microscope.
5: Control to set the microscope illumination.
8: Buttons to call other image material (e.g., US-imagery) of the patient folder or of another camera (e.g., video conference camera) on the screen.
9: Field displays information for presently active functions on the remote microscope and their status (e.g., busy (wait) or ready to accept new instructions). This field also accepts and displays text as patient information, diagnoses, and recommendations.
10: Button to request an autofocus procedure on the microscope.
11: Interactive control of the focus position (e.g., for focusing through a nucleus).
12: Button to request a zoom activity at the microscope (centering of an image detail and change of objective by one step).

3. Field Tests Carried Out with HISTKOM Equipment

The acceptance of telepathology equipment by pathologists depends on results of evaluation programs carried out under controlled conditions with routine test material. For this purpose, HISTKOM underwent a two-year test period with extended field-tests of different intentions. This partition reports the design, results, and conclusions of these tests.

Several of the technical tests, as well as the field-tests, were carried out as tasks of the EUROPATH project [4], a European program to promote telepathology. In this project, one task was dedicated to telepathology with telemicroscopy and investigated user needs, specifications for telepathology, implementation, evaluation, and demonstration of test equipment.

3.1. Tests to Evaluate Technical Performance

These tests included the system's stability and safety of operation, but before all its interoperability if operated in public networks connecting the microscope and the display station to public telephone nets. In this context, national and international ISDN network connections have mostly been tested between Stuttgart and a variety of locations, the most important of which have been in the FRG: Tübingen, Berlin, Münster, Munich, Bernburg; also in Europe: Oslo, Toulouse, Brussels, Budapest, and finally Kobe in Japan.

All technical tests demonstrated successfully the worldwide suitability of the ISDN technology. This was the case with a single-channel connection, but before all also with the dynamic bundling of up to 8 ISDN B-channels.

3.2. Field Tests Evaluating Diagnostic Capabilities

In total, 12 field tests have been carried out with about 1000 slides to evaluate the HISTKOM equipment with different intentions and operation modes. This partition presents the types and results of five representative tests in more detail. In all tests, the participating pathologists were responsible for the test design, the selection of the material, the evaluation, and the carrying out of the study. The intentions and essentials of these studies where:

- 3.2.1. Retrospective study with frozen section material and the restriction of the net connection to only one ISDN B-channel.
- 3.2.2. Retrospective study with frozen section material but with a connection to all eight ISDN B-channels.
- 3.2.3. Intraoperational frozen section service.
- 3.2.4. Telepathology applied to PAP-smear cytology.
- 3.2.5. Telepathology in an expert panel scenario in hematology.

A sixth study evaluated HISTKOM with retrospective embedded breast tissue material for differential diagnoses and grading. A seventh study within the British national continuing education program for pathologists tested HISTKOM for its suitability within quality assurance programs in pathology. Both studies have been carried out in the pathology department of the John Radcliffe Hospital in Oxford, U.K. and are included in this conference volume as a separate contribution [5].

3.2.1. Retrospective study with frozen section material and only a single ISDN B-channel active

This field test was the very first and was carried out with retrospective frozen section material of 109 consecutive cases of lung surgery. The study was performed by three pathologists from the Robert Bosch Hospital in Stuttgart, FRG. It was designed in a double blind manner: neither the participant selecting the cases and feeding the remote microscope nor the pathologists at the remote display station knew the diagnoses; they only received clinical information about the cases, as it was also available during the original frozen section diagnosis session. The study was not unblinded before its completion. Requested where the differential diagnoses. After unblinding, a panel of pathologists not involved in the diagnostic process compared the results of the telepathology mediated diagnosis with that of the conventional procedure made at the time of surgery, and finally with that of the reference diagnosis gained with the embedded material of the same case. Together with the diagnoses, data concerning the technical performance of the system and documenting the course of the session were also collected and evaluated. The main results of this study are compiled in Tables 1 and 2, below.

	Convent.	Telepath.
Correct	93.5%	82.3%
False neg.	1.9%	7.6%
False pos.	0.9%	0.9%
Postponed	3.7%	9.2%

Table 1: Comparison of diagnostic results of conventional and telepathology mediated frozen section compared to the reference diagnosis with embedded material.

Pathologist	Time consumed
1	40 min.
2	38 min.
3	63 min.
Conv. Diagn.	3 min.

Table 2: Time consumption for rendering a diagnosis for a frozen section preparation applying only 1 ISDN B-channel.

The diagnostic results of Table 1 demonstrate an increased number of postponed and false negative cases. As the image quality was rated excellent, the reasons for this deviation from the conventional procedure may be allocated to three reasons: the unfamiliarity of the pathologists with diagnoses on a TV-monitor, the reduced field of view of the TV-frame imagery, and finally the slower operation mode of the remote microscope due to the bottleneck of data transmission *via* a single telephone line.

It is obvious regarding Table 2 that the time consumption is too high for a routine application, due to the restrictions of the data transmission link. The consequence of this table is: to comfortably operate the telepathology system for rendering diagnoses, more than one ISDN B-channel has to be used. In the case of HISTKOM, the application of 4 S_0 ISDN channels (equivalent to 8 B-channels) reduces the time consumption by a factor of 8, resulting in a time interval of 4-6 minutes, which is quite acceptable. Operation with one channel can be accepted for rare cases and for second opinion applications, where only preselected slide areas are inspected.

3.2.2. Frozen section dignity diagnosis with retrospective material and 8 ISDN channels active

Two pathologists of the Institute for Pathology of the University of Tübingen carried out this study with retrospective frozen section material of 139 slides of breast surgery. Requested was only the diagnosis relevant for the continuation of surgery (dignity) and available were the clinical data before surgery. The observers were familiar with diagnosing on a monitor. Tables 3 and 4 summarize the main outcomes of this study.

	Observer 1	Observer 2
Correct	97.1%	95.7%
False pos.	0%	0%
False neg.	0%	1.4%
Postponed	2.9%	2.9%

Table 3: Comparison of the telepathology mediated dignity diagnosis with the reference diagnosis for 139 slides of breast surgery for two observers and 8 active channels.

	Observer1	Observer 2
Time Cons.	223 sec	144 sec
Stand. Dev.	92 sec	42 sec
Obj. Chang.	2.5	1.7
Stand. Dev.	1.6	0.9
Time Cons. Conventional	24 sec	24 sec

Table 4: Time consumption and number of changes of objectives per slide for the two participants of the study.

Fig. 5 (left diagram) outlines the development of the time consumption of the two participants during the study in graphical form. It is clearly seen that the two observers possess different levels of experience, which becomes obvious at several slides, where one pathologist consumed much more time than the other, who seemed to have come to his decision with the inspection of only a few key scenes of the slides. The right diagram in Fig. 5 (from another study) demonstrates the training effect in a much higher scale.

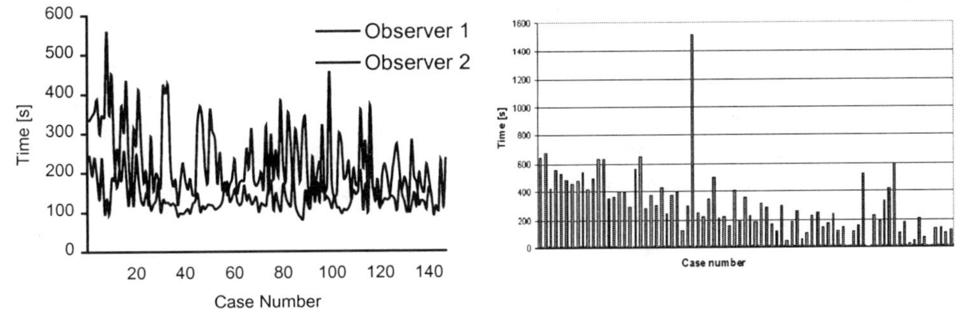

Fig. 5: Development of time consumption of the two observers of the study (left diagram). It is obvious that the two pathologists had different levels of experience enabling one of them to detect much quicker the key fields of view in the slide. Compared to study 3.2.1, the time consumption is quite acceptable. The right diagram from another study [5] demonstrates the training effect even more obviously.

The consequences of the results of this study are: 8 ISDN B-channels are sufficient in a frozen section scenario to render intraoperative diagnoses with acceptable time consumption. The image quality was rated as very good by both pathologists. Finally, the study demonstrated that familiarity with diagnosing on a screen, expertise, and experience influence evaluation time and quality. This has the consequence that the performance of frozen section diagnosis will exhibit a time-dependent characteristic during which the results improve by growing experience.

3.2.3. Study with intraoperational frozen section diagnosis

This study was carried out by the department of pathology at the hospital in Bernburg and the surgery department in Köthen, both in FRG. To meet the legal necessities at the introduction of a new procedure in medicine, for safety reasons a second pathologist was present in the surgery department rendering in parallel a diagnosis which was compared to that of the remote pathologist performing telepathology. Surgery was continued after consensus of both pathologists. HISTKOM was operated with the recommended 8 ISDN B-channels. The study included 47 cases of consecutive surgery of different organs. Table 5 summarizes the results; the reference diagnosis to which the telepathology diagnoses are compared is the final diagnosis with embedded material rendered after surgery.

Table 5: Results of the study for intraoperational frozen section diagnosis, compared to the reference diagnosis with embedded material. 47 cases of consecutive surgery at the hospital.

Correct diagnosis	78.7%
False positive	0%
False negative	2.1%
Postponed	19.2%

The high rate of postponed cases (which have been handled in this case by the second pathologist) reflects not only missing experience with the new technology, but also safety aspects with respect to liability to the patient, meaning that in cases with only minor doubts, the case was diagnosed as to be postponed. If the alternative would have been to continue surgery without frozen section diagnosis at all, the pathologist would evaluate the risk according to the consequences for the patient. About half of the postponed cases in telepathology would have been diagnosed by the pathologist in the conventional procedure.

As before, the image quality was rated as very good. The pathologist, however, would appreciate a further speed-up of image transmission.

The main results of the study can be summarized: at least during an introduction phase of telepathology equipment for frozen section service, postponed diagnoses will increase. This is due to the missing experience at the beginning and to the safety requirements in medicine, where doubts must be excluded as far as possible. The rate of postponed diagnoses will decrease as experience with the new tool increases. In cases with no pathology service available at all (remote areas, developing countries), telepathology will be the only opportunity, and will in any case be better than the present situation.

3.2.4. Study in telecytology with PAP-smear slides

The Laboratory for Clinical Cytology of the department of pathology at the Technical University of Munich carried out a study to evaluate the HISTKOM equipment for the remote screening of PAP-smears. At first glance it is not obvious why telecytology should perform in a different way than telepathology with histological sections. Some brief facts may illuminate the essential differences, which become most obvious in the PAP-screening situation. In short, the difference is the amount of data per slide to be transmitted. A short estimation may make this transparent.

If an area on a slide of 60mm x 25mm is assumed to be covered with deposited cell material, and the necessary resolution of the images is assumed to be 0.25 μm per image pixel (this is about the resolution of a 40x objective in the field of view), then about 40,000 TV-frames with 768 x 576 pixels are necessary to screen the slide completely. This corresponds to an information content for the slide of about 24 GByte. Assuming further an acceptable compression ratio of 20:1 and a channel capacity of 512 KBytes/s (corresponding to 4 ISDN S_0-channels), the transmission time for one slide would sum up to about 40 minutes! This is quite unacceptable. In contrast to PAP-smear cytology, where the slide has to be screened totally in detail with high magnification, histology needs only a few images of key locations, using low magnification together with a few fields of view with high magnification. The conclusion of this consideration is: telemicroscopy with narrow band transmission technique is not appropriate, at least not for conventional PAP-screening.
Ways out of this dilemma may be:

- Telemicroscopy stations for PAP-screening are connected to broadband links, which will become expensive if public lines are used.
- Higher image compression ratios can be applied.
- Telecytology is not applied in a prescreening scenario, where the whole slide is inspected, but in a scenario in which an expert diagnoses only alarms found and labeled in a prescreening procedure. These two levels of diagnosis correspond to the conventional procedure.
- Telecytology is applied in the upcoming new prescreening scenario, in which machines take over the bothersome task of prescreening and provide the pathologist only with a collection of alarms (presumably cancerous cells) found in the slide.

- Telecytology is restricted to slides not overcrowded with deposited cell material, as is mostly the case for fine needle aspiration preparations for example.

Having in mind the restrictions listed above, a study with prescreened PAP-smear reference slides, as they are used for continuing education and accreditation programs, has been designed. The slides contain two types of labeled areas: large areas with typical cell material and small areas containing only a few fields of view with diagnostic key cells. Fig. 6 illustrates the scales of the labeled field types with respect to the whole slide.

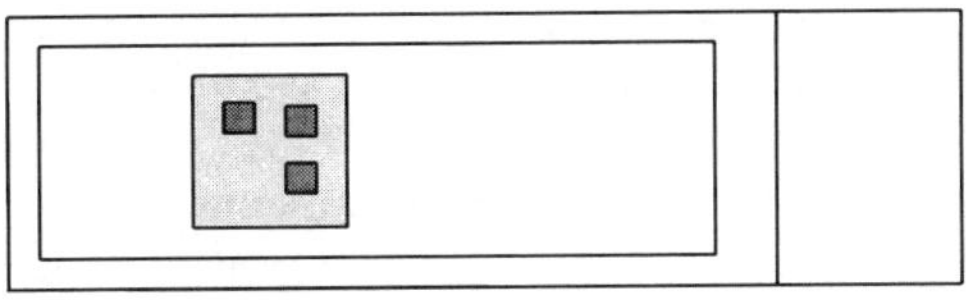

Fig. 6: The scale of the two types of labels on a slide used to guide the investigator to important diagnostic areas. The large labels (about 100 mm^2) request a search procedure to find the important events and the diagnosis step, whereas the small labels (about 1 mm^2) request only the diagnosis step.

Table 6 collects the results in the form of a confusion matrix, comparing the telemicroscopy diagnoses with the reference diagnoses of a panel. The figures in parentheses are for the results with respect to the small labels only, whereas the others also include the search process of the diagnostic session.

		Diagnosis by Telecytology				
	Class	Negative PAP I,II	Displasia PAP IIID	CIS PAP IVa	Carcinoma PAP V	Total
Re	I,II	45 (33)	2 (1)	1	-	48 (34)
fe	IIID	5 (4)	12 (8)	2 (1)	1	20 (13)
re	IVa	2 (2)	1	9 (3)	3 (3)	15 (8)
nce	V	2	-	3 (3)	13 (7)	18 (10)
	Total	54 (39)	15 (9)	15 (7)	17 (10)	101 (65)

Table 6: Comparison of results in PAP-smear diagnosis with telepathology applied and with the conventional procedure. Figures in parenthesis represent diagnoses based only on the investigation of the small marked areas, the other figures those made by screening the large marked areas.

The consequences of this very first study in telecytology for PAP-screening have been that with limited channel transmission capacity, the prescreening step is too time consuming. Expert diagnosis based on preselected alarms, selected by a cytotech or a prescreening machine, can be performed. The time consumption is still high, but growing experience with telemicroscopy will reduce it, as in the case of histology.

3.2.5. HISTKOM in a reference panel situation in hematology

The design of this study reflected the situation in which a hematologist or a practitioner consults an expert panel for a difficult case and a consensus diagnosis. The study, simulating a session in which six cases were presented, was double blind. The session was part of the "Seminar on Hematological Cytology of Acute Myeloid Leukemia" held in Haldensee, Austria by the expert group of the EORTC (European Organization for Research and Treatment of Cancer). The panelist, who brought with him six really difficult slides of blood smears for consultation and reference diagnosis, did not take part in the diagnostic process; neither did the panelist, who selected 10-25 fields of view to be transmitted and presented to the panel. The study was designed as passive telepathology (the consulting participant selects the fields of view and transmits the images). The panel discussed the cases and came to a consensus diagnoses. Afterwards, all other information-- including the later outcomes for the patient-- was unblinded to the panel.

After the study, the panelists were asked for their opinion concerning telecytology. Unanimously, all participants rated the image quality as excellent and suitable for hematology. They also stated that their diagnoses would have been the same as if they had used the microscope directly.

In contrast to the situation in PAP-smear screening, in hematology only a few fields of view, which may be selected by a physician, are sufficient. The selection of the interesting objects (leucocytes) is not difficult, but for their diagnosis the expertise of a specialist is requested. The final statement of the demonstration session was: telecytology is well suited for remote diagnoses.

3.3. Conclusions of the Field-Tests

Due to the limited space of this paper, the conclusions of the field test studies will be presented in the form of a few statements:

- The quality of transmitted images was rated by all participants as excellent and sufficient for diagnostic purposes.
- The high quality of the macro image and the tools for orientation in it were unanimously appreciated.
- For a comfortable working environment to render intraoperational frozen section diagnoses (not second opinion), an online impression of the image transmission and microscope operation should be provided.
- The compromise in online impression of 8 bundled ISDN lines was accepted.
- A high potential to reduce time consumption exists in a training period for pathologists to become familiar with the system and to exploit all of its opportunities adequately.
- In frozen section applications with no pathologist present at the microscope site, both partners have to agree in the new liabilities, as now the surgery team will make the frozen section preparation.
- The major challenge for the pathologist was not the application of the telemicroscopy technology, but the diagnosis from a monitor screen rather than from a microscope eyepiece.
- The field of view presented on today's monitors is reduced with respect to that of modern microscopes, if the same resolution is maintained.

4. Considerations for the Introduction of Telepathology Networks (suited also for immediate intraoperational diagnosis)

A broad and successful introduction and exploitation of telepathology, especially in the most challenging form-- the intraoperational frozen section service-- depends upon the solution of some yet remaining problems, some of which will be addressed in this partition. Their solution also offers new promising facilities realizable only with telepathology.

4.1. Technical Aspects of Installing Networks for Telepathology Services

As already mentioned, the technical tools for the realization of telepathology networks are ready (microscopes, cameras, data transmission facilities, display capabilities, software concepts). The challenge is to form out of this toolbox a system suitable for routine telepathology services. In this context, several points must be considered: the interoperability of systems in networks, the costs of operation, the availability of services, and legal requirements of the new technology.

First, the interoperability of systems in a telepathology network is addressed. It is unrealistic to design today standards for the development of conform telepathology equipment, because several systems are already on the market, or are near market. They are all incompatible with each other and allow no interoperability of participants in a net which is equipped with devices of different manufacturers.

A way out of this situation is to resign from a general standardization procedure and instead design interoperability tools to connect these systems, at least to an acceptable level. The EUROPATH project [4] of the European Union included a task to investigate these interoperability aspects in future telepathology nets. This working group will also be active beyond the end of the project. Within this interoperability group, whose members manufacture microscopes, telemicroscopy software, and complete telemicroscopy systems, further interoperability tools will be defined.

In a first approach, an interchangeable electronic investigation protocol in HTML format was defined, allowing its readability on any PC computer with a standard HTML browser. The second interoperability effort was the definition of a "Virtual Microscope Interface" (VMI), a collection of program calls to operate computer-driven microscopes. This interface allows manufacturers of telepathology equipment to connect to their systems microscopes from different manufacturers, and vice versa, allow microscope manufacturers to offer microscopes to different manufacturers of telepathology equipment. As the first network to operate telemicroscopy systems, the ISDN telephone net with the Euro-ISDN protocol was selected.

4.2. Medical Aspects of Interoperability and Liability

4.2.1. Standardization of medical diagnostic procedures

Future telepathology networks will cross national borders and therefore raise questions as to how the differences in diagnostic systems and different legal regulations can be handled. Within national efforts, unambiguous diagnostic systems for findings in pathology have been established-- as for instance, SNOMED and ADICAP-- and within the already mentioned EUROPATH project, transcoding systems to interconnect the notations of different coding systems have been developed. Not in all cases can such a transcoding be performed as a one-to-one relation.

4.2.2. Changes in liability in telepathology mediated frozen section diagnoses

In the case of the frozen section situation, with no pathologist present in the surgery team, another problem has to be solved by the corresponding chambers: in contrast to today's regulations, where the pathologist prepares the histological frozen section (palpation and detection of the location of the section), in the telepathology scenario, the surgeons team will take over this task, perhaps with interactive assistance of the remote pathologist. This difference in procedure will also influence the network of liabilities against the patient. It is the task of the corresponding chambers and legal bodies to find regulations for the new field of telepathology and its procedures.

4.2.3. New opportunities for services in pathology in telepathology networks

It is inherent in the development of telepathology networks that new services will be offered within them which would never get a chance for realization without such a network. This is because in routine pathology they would be requested only very seldom. Due to the potentially large community of participants in such a network, seldom-requested services may become economical and will improve diagnostic quality. Candidates for such services may be, from today's point of view:

- Expert panels for consultation in difficult cases.
- Data banks with reference case images for continuing education.
- Image evaluation facilities to quantify image contents.
- Quality control institutions to homogenize and to certify diagnostic procedures.
- Services offering diagnostic assistance to remote areas in the world. For instance, European pathologists may serve hospitals in medically underserved areas of Africa.

5. The Present Status of the HISTKOM System

HISTKOM is a joint development of the University of Stuttgart and the Deutsche Telekom AG, Bonn, who will market it. The first generation of HISTKOM equipment came into operation in 1995, and the second generation with improved functionality and versatility was presented at the MEDICA'98 in Düsseldorf.

HISTKOM relies in all hardware components on equipment available off the shelf and from different suppliers of all components. This is with respect to the microscope, computer equipment, and the telecommunication devices and interfaces.

The software is highly modularized in a toolbox, allowing also a fast adaptation to special conditions. This allows HISTKOM to be offered with a variety of modifications:

- As a complete system with hardware and software installed at the customer's location.
- As computer equipment with software installed to which an already existing microscope with the requested specifications is adapted.
- As software only, with installation into customer's environment if this meets the specifications of the HISTKOM components.
- As special configurations, adapted to already existing broadband communication links at the surgery and pathology sites.

It is in the HISTKOM concept that other applications in telepathology, such as, e.g., still image transmission for second opinion applications, archiving, or education, can be realized with the components of telemicroscopy development.

Besides installation of stand-alone systems, the Deutsche Telekom AG has launched a telemedicine network "Global Healthcare" (GHC) within which HISTKOM will take over the services for telepathology.

References

[1] R.S. Weinstein, K.J. Bloom, and L.S. Rozek, Telepathology: System Design and Specifications. *Visual Communications and Image Processing Conference II* (Proceedings). New York, NY, 1987.

[2] P. Schwarzmann, J. Schmid, C. Schnörr, G. Sträßle, and S. Witte, Telemicroscopy Stations for Telepathology Based on Broadband and ISDN Connections, *Arch. d'Anatomie et de Cytology Pathologiques* **43** (1995) 209-215.

[3] T.J. Eide and I. Nordrum, Frozen Section Service via the Telenetwork in Northern Norway, *Zentralbl. Pathol.* **138** (1992) 409-412.

[4] EUROPATH, EUROpean Pathology Assisted by Telematics for Health. EU DG XIII-Project HC 1038, 1996-1999.

[5] J. O'D. McGee, Clinical Trials of Robotic Interactive Telepathology Accuracy in the UK NHS Breast Pathology External Quality Assurance Scheme. EU DG XIII-Project HC 1038, 1996-1999.

Address for correspondence

Peter Schwarzmann
Institut für Physikalische Elektronik
University of Stuttgart
Pfaffenwaldring 47
70569 Stuttgart, Germany
E-mail: schwarzmann@ipe.uni-stuttgart.de

The Impact of Telemedicine on Health Care Management
M. Nerlich and R. Kretschmer (Eds.)
IOS Press, 1999

Economic Analysis of Teleradiology Applications with KAMEDIN

M. WALZ, R. BOLTE, K.J. LEHMANN, J. LÜTGEMEIER, M. GEORGI
Department of Clinical Radiology, Faculty of Clinical Medicine Mannheim
University of Heidelberg, Klinikum Mannheim, Mannheim, Germany

Abstract: The teleradiology system KAMEDIN (German Telekom), installed on HP-Unix- and NT-Workstations, was evaluated in different scenarios and a cost-benefit-analysis was performed. CT examinations were transfered from a PACS workstation (GE) to KAMEDIN using DICOM-3 protocol. Teleconferences were realized with an intensive care unit by LAN, with a radiology department at 5 km. distance by ISDN, and with an on-duty radiologist 22 km. away by ISDN. On average, 36 CT slices per patient were transfered. Overall costs (costs for hardware, software, support, ISDN-fees, and staff) were compared to possible cost reduction, mainly concerning transportation and films.

These three scenarios could be realized during daily routine work. Differing in their amount of transportation cost reduction, two applications (intensive care unit, radiologist on duty) showed a break-even at 1817, respectively 528 teleconferences/year. Improvement of cost-effectiveness can be obtained on the conditions that existing hardware will be used and that the automatic data transfer will be improved. Combining all optimisation factors, the break-even decreased to a minimum of 167, respectively 77 teleconferences/year. The optimisation of patient management is an additional-- but in this study, not yet counted-- advantage of teleradiology.

1. Introduction

In recent years, different concepts and systems of teleradiology applications have been realized [1,2,3,5,9,10,11,12,13]. In general, these systems are connected to local networks and to telecommunication networks using ISDN. While the DICOM-3 protocol has become an accepted, uniform standard for radiological images and for radiological workstations, in teleradiology different protocols and image formats are still used. Conversion to proprietary file formats and protocols sometimes causes troubles and diminishes the chance of communication between different systems. Furthermore, the cost-benefit-relation of a teleradiology system depends on the number of possible communication partners and on the realization of different kinds of data transfer within the same system (e.g., PACS usage, external image transfer, teleconference with PC or workstation, etc.).

The evaluation of economic efficieancy of telemedical applications is effected by many factors [4,5,7,9,11,12,14]. Besides the "hard cost factors", which can easily be assessed by monetary aspects (e.g., costs for hardware, software, and transport), there also exist a lot of "soft factors". Their assessment is much more difficult. The patient`s convenience, improvement of communication between sites, and fastening of diagnosis or treatment are some examples of soft factors. Presently, calculation of "break-even" analysis is mainly based on the hard cost factors.

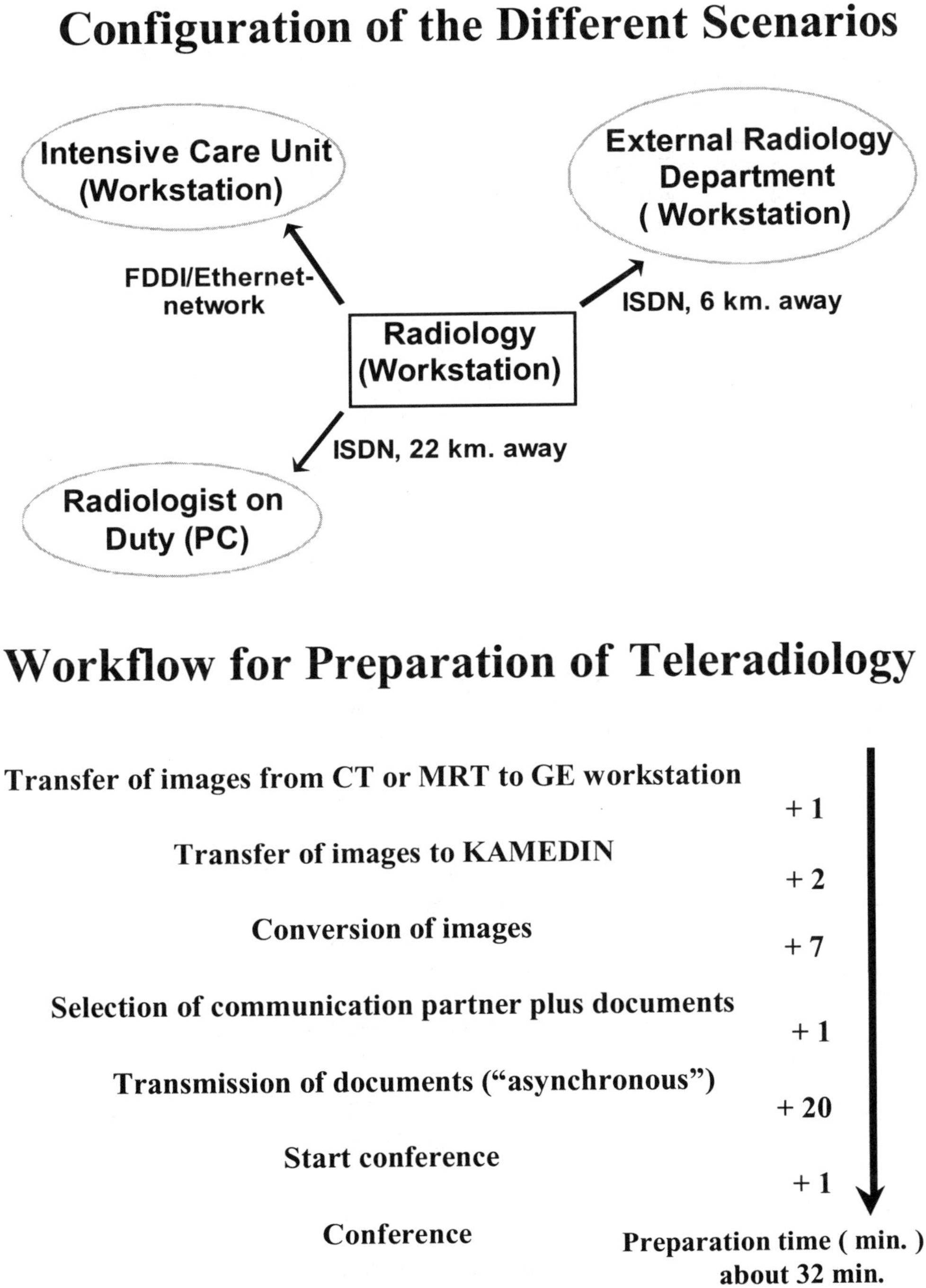

Fig. 1 a-b: Configuration of scenarios and Workflow for preparation of teleradiology conference.

In our study, a cost-benefit analysis of the new version of teleradiology system KAMEDIN (**K**ooperatives **A**rbeiten und rechnergestützte **Me**dizinische **D**iagnostik auf **In**novativen **N**etzen der Deutschen Telekom) was performed. For transmission of CT examinations, three different scenarios were realized (communication with an intensive care unit within the hospital, with an external radiology department, and with a radiologist on duty outside the hospital) corresponding to the main teleradiology application areas-- apart from emergency cases with predominantly therapy-related questions, as in neurosurgery (Fig. 1). Break-even analysis and optimisation calculation was done for each of the different scenarios.

2. Material and Methods

In a preliminary study, 50 teleconferences between KAMEDIN and the external radiology department had been evaluated (corresponding to Scenario II), showing that on average 36 CT scans had been transfered with a mean conference preparation time of 32 minutes (Fig. 1).

The CT examinations were performed on a HiSpeed Advantage Scanner (GE) and a Pace Plus Scanner (GE), and transfered to an Advantage Windows Workstation (GE). Data transfer from the Advantage Windows Workstation to a Kamedin Workstation was realized by DICOM-3 protocol. An integrated DICOM-server, developed by the Institute of Informatics V of the University of Mannheim, provided the data for the KAMEDIN format. Subsequently, this data was transmitted to the computers of the conference partners (Fig. 1). Configuration and function of the KAMEDIN workstation is almost identical to that described before [5]. Meanwhile, the DICOM 3 format (also used for server in its newest version) has been integrated in KAMEDIN; thus data transfer has been simplified. No legally accepted documentation is provided by the system. As a temporary, simple solution, fax transfer of report and paper documentation may be used.

In Scenario I, CT examinations were transfered to a KAMEDIN workstation on the intensive care unit within the hospital *via* FDDI/Ethernet-network immediately after the examination. The start of the teleconference was arranged by phone, according to the actual workload and urgency of therapy. In the conventional working scene, hardcopies were given to the ward and demonstrated in daily radiological conferences.

In Scenario II, CT scans were transfered *via* ISDN to an external KAMEDIN-Workstation in a radiology department 6 km. away, for immediate discussion of results between the CT radiologist and either the radiologist there or the physician. Before that, only a weekly demonstration at the external department took place.

In Scenario III, a teleconference was established *via* ISDN to a KAMEDIN-PC operated by a radiologist specialist on duty 22 km away. Subsequently, data transmission was performed by the radiologist in the hospital for discussion of results. Otherwise, the specialist had to come to the hospital for reporting, demonstration, and discussion.

These local scenarios represent some of the general, frequently-used teleradiology applications characterized:

In Scenario I, by

- Transport of patient to radiology department for examination in the same or in another hospital,
- Exclusive electronic (fast) transmission and discussion of images between radiologist and clinician, and
- Non-provision of hardcopies;

In Scenario II, by

- Transport of patient to radiology department for examination in a distant part of the hospital or in another hospital,
- Electronic demonstration and discussion between local radiologist and external clinician or radiologist,
- Continued provision of hardcopies and conventional conferences, and
- Applied only for improved, undelayed patient management and therapy;

In Scenario III, by

- Transport of patient to radiology department for examination in the same hospital, and
- Consultation of radiologist/expert at different locations, either by less experienced doctor in hospital or for centralized emergency service.

The third scenario is presently one of the main teleradiology applications, both in Germany and worldwide.

Evaluation time of the survey has been one week per scenario. The cost-benefit analysis was done in cooperation with the business consultancy UBG (CH-8820 Wädenswil). As "hard cost factors", the costs for investment (hardware and software), for support and maintenance (service, hotline, update, etc.), for the ISDN connection and transmission fees, and for staff and preparation time were evaluated. Possible decrease of patient transports, as well as reduction of costs for hardcopies and hardcopy transport, were combined as "hard benefit factors". Comparing the hard cost factors with the hard benefit factors, a break-even analysis was performed. The number of examination per year which is necessary to reach the break-even was investigated.

3. Results

Each scenario has successfully been adapted to a special local situation. Time for transmission of image data before the beginning of the conference took approximately one minute in Scenario I (FDDI/Ethernet clinical network). In Scenarios II and III (using both ISDN channels), the average transmission time was, respectively, 17 and 18 minutes. The total time from image transmission (using ISDN) through the end of the conference was 38 minutes (Scenario III). On average, 36 CT-slices per patient were transfered.

	Scenario I	*Scenario II*	*Scenario III*
Fixed Costs (DM):			
Investment cost, Deduction/Year,	8750,-	8750,-	7668,-
Support costs/Year	17188,-	17188,-	17188,-
Variable Costs/Examination (DM):			
Staff, Transmission fees	8,25	12,75	17,68
Hard Benefit Factors/Examination (DM):			
Reduced time	4,80	-	64,80
Hardcopy savings	14,73	-	-
Hardcopy transportation savings	3,00	2,40	-
Examination/Year to achieve "break even"	1877	no break even	528

Table 1: Cost and utility factors of Scenarios I-III.

Total fixed costs per year are 25.938 DM for Scenarios I and II, and 24.856 DM for Scenario III (using PC instead of workstation). The "net benefit" per case ranges from -10,35 DM (net loss) in Scenario II to +47,12 DM (net profit) in Scenario III; (Table 1 shows cost and utility factors of Scenarios I-III).

The analysis of the scenarios under the condition that the whole investment sum is necessary in each scenario shows a break-even at 1817 examinations per year for Scenario I and at 528 examinations per year for Scenario III (Fig 2). The net benefit per examination in Scenario I (14,28 DM) and Scenario III (47,12 DM) depends first upon how much time physicians can save compared to the conventional workflow in which they have to wait, e.g., for the radiologist driving to the hospital, finishing the examination, and producing his report. In teleradiology, they can return to the ward shortly after the examination and get the images and report there some minutes later. No break-even was achieved in Scenario II because the costs for each examination exceed the savings of the hard benefit factors per examination. The main reason for this is the missing reduction of transport costs for the physician, the patient, and the hard copies.

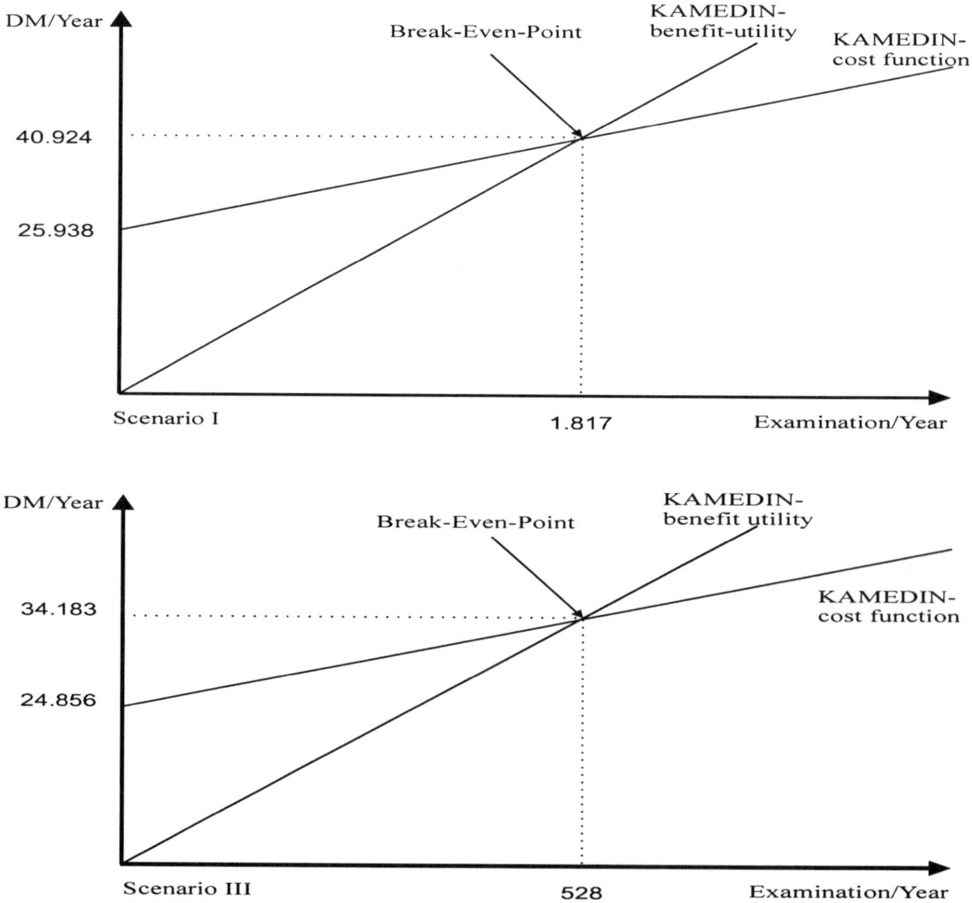

Fig. 2 a-b: Break-even-point for Scenarios I and III. Cost function: Sum of all costs per year and examinations. Benefit utility: Sum of all savings per examinations.

If existent hardware (e.g., PACS workstation or RIS PC) or one system for several applications can be used for teleradiology, a relevant decrease of costs is possible. The support costs may be reduced when system stability increases. Further cost reduction is possible if supervision of transmission is no longer necessary, and the whole process can be reduced to one manual interaction because the rest takes place automatically. Figure 3 shows the calculated cost reduction (hardware, support, and waiting time) for Scenarios I and III.

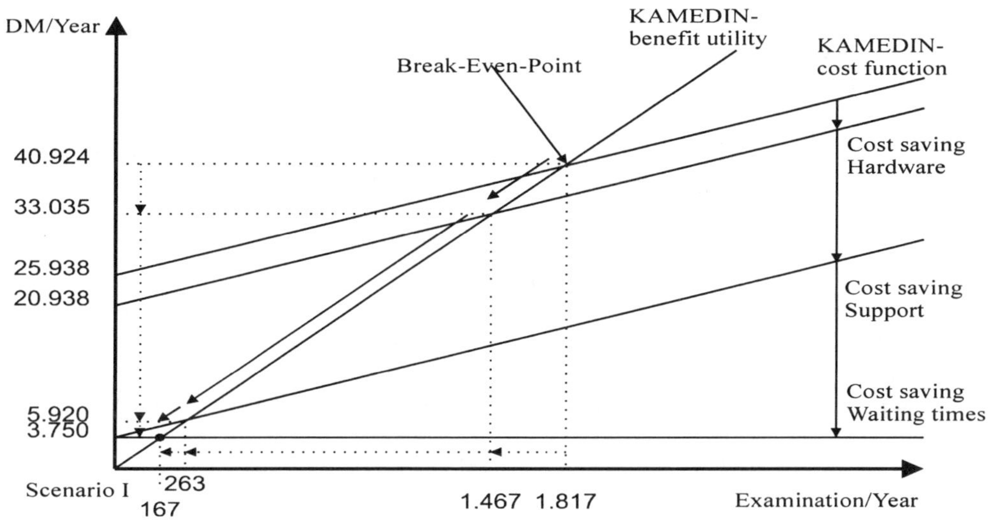

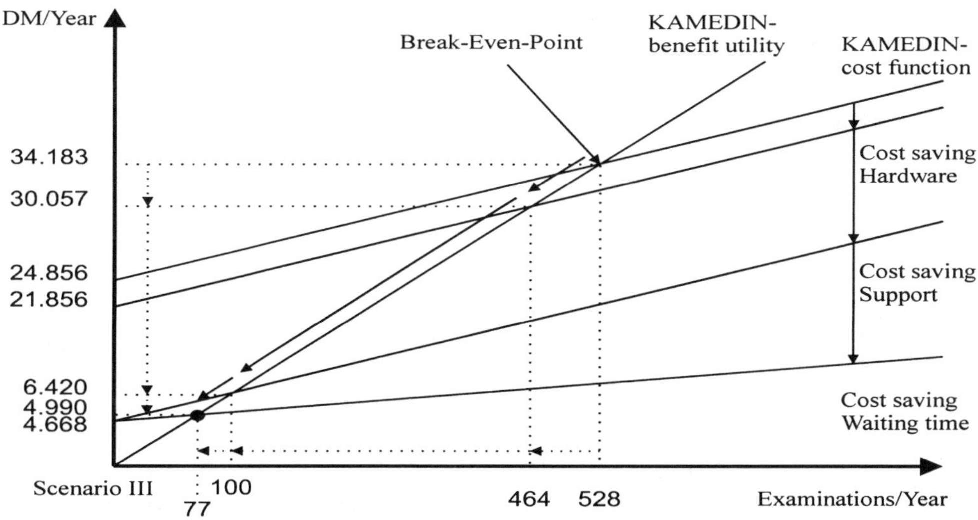

Fig. 3 a-b: Optimization chances in break even analysis of Scenarios I and III. Cost function (sum of all costs per year and examinations) versus calculated benefit utility (sum of all savings per examinations). Cost saving was calculated by possible reductions of costs for hardware, support and waiting time for physicians.

The break-even of Scenario I drops from 1817 examinations per year to 1467 examinations per year by minimizing hardware costs, and drops to 613 examinations per year due to reduced support costs. Automatic supervision of the transmission process alone is able to decrease the break-even to1152 examinations per year. Combining all optimization factors, the amortisation of the KAMEDIN system would be possible with only 167 examinations per year. A comparable calculation for Scenario III shows a decrease of the break-even from 528 examinations to 464 (hardware reduction), 100 (support reduction), 411 (waiting time), and 77 examinations (combination of all factors) per year.

4. Discussion

Although technical conditions for the broad use of teleradiology have improved in recent years, regular radiological teleconferences are still rare. An accepted medical image format for PACS has been defined (DICOM 3), whereas standardisation of transmission protocols in teleradiology is not yet achieved (but on the way). Furthermore, teleradiology systems with specialised or additional functions often require new hardware. However, additional hardware or software is not always necessary. Table 2 shows a summary of our opinion as to which kind of system is suitable for each kind of application (3). Here, the expression "offline" refers to asynchronous, and "online" to synchronous, communication.

Suitability of Teleradiology System Types in Different Application Areas

	Offline Communication	Online Communication	Video Conference
emergency consultation	+	++	+
expert consultation	++	++	+
demonstration/discussion	-	++	+
image and report distribut.	++	0	0
radiological reporting	+	+	+
education	+	++	+
research	++	+	0

++ = very suitable, + = suitable, 0 = not necessary, - = not suitable

Table 2: Suitability of teleradiology systems (offline = asynchronous versus online = synchronous versus teleconferencing systems) for different application areas.

A major improvement is possible if teleradiology software can be integrated in already existent workstations, e.g., of a PACS or PCs under continueing guarantee of data security and system stability. Systems like KAMEDIN, which can be run on PCs (Windows NT) or workstations, allow flexible use and enable integration into existent hardware. Nowadays, an extended DICOM network may also be used for external image communication. Confidentiality and report documentation must be provided in these cases, too.

The economical analysis shows that the break-even will not be easily achieved with a stand-alone teleradiology configuration. It seems to be nearly impossible to reach the minimum numbers of, respectively, 1817 and 528 examinations per year for each scenario. The economical success of a teleradiology project highly depends on the amount of cost reduction for transport of patient, hardcopies, physician, and radiologist. These factors can become more important in other application areas than in the evaluated scenarios, (e.g., in neurosurgery by avoidance of expensive and possibly unnecessary patient transportation, or in rural areas with a low supply of medical expertise and high distances to medical centers). Scenario II, as an example of conferences between a radiological center and an external radiology department, may become profitable under other local conditions, e.g., if hardcopies can be saved or the clinical demonstration takes place only electronically. In the evaluated scenario (II) there is no break-even, due to the missing replacement of hardcopy or transport costs; this is because the necessary EDV infrastructure in clinical departments, and also the process of acceptance and adaptation to digital workflow, are not yet fnished.

Optimisation chances for the system`s economy in Scenario I (intrahospital radiological–clinical conference) and Scenario III (radiological conference with distant expert) depend on one side upon the reduction of hardware and support costs. On the other side, the drop-off in investments by using already existent hardware or software, and the realization of an automatic data transfer almost without staff involvement, improves the economical situation. Looking at the evaluated conditions even two years ago, the break-even by usage of specialised teleradiology systems can be achieved with a realistic number of examinations, and there exist many local conditions and scenarios which will probably show better cost-utility-curves [2,4,7,9,11,12,13,14]. Additionally, nowadays secure and less expensive simple DICOM-based image communication between distant sites can be established at many radiological departments and offices. The most important remaining obstacles for teleradiology in Germany are legal handicaps, including liability, missing-- to telemedicine adapted-- reimbursement regulations, and the uncertainty of medical professionals about the maintenance of good patient care by establishing telemedicine under cost pressure [6,8,10].

References

[1] A.D. Perednia and A. Allen, Telemedicine Technology and Clinical Applications, *JAMA* **273** (1995) 483-488.

[2] J. Reponen, S. Lahde, O. Tervonen, E. Ilkko, T. Rissanen, and I. Suramo, Low-cost Digital Teleradiology, *Eur. J. Radiol.* **19** (1995) 226-231.

[3] M. Walz, K.J. Lehmann, R. Loose, R. Bolte, M. Schinkmann, and M. Georgi, Evaluation of New Teleradiology Systems: Concepts, Application Areas and Requirements. In: H.U. Lemke, K. Inamura, M.W. Vannier, and A.g. Farman (eds.), Computer Assisted Radiology. Elsevier, Amsterdam, 1996, pp. 549-553.

[4] P.A. Halvorsen and I.S. Kristiansen, Radiology Services for Remote Communities: Cost Minimisation Study of Telemedicine, *Brit. Med. J.* **312** (1996) 1333-1336.

[5] R. Bolte, K.J. Lehmann, M. Walz, R. Loose, J. Lütgemeier, F. Seibert, C. Busch, M. Schinkmann, and M. Georgi, Radiologisch-medizinische Desktop-Konferenzen-- Klinische Evaluation des Teleradiologiesystems KAMEDIN im Routinebetrieb eines radiologischen Instituts, *Aktuelle Radiologie* **6** (1996) 199-202.

[6] M. Walz, B. Wein, K.J. Lehmann, R. Bolte, M. Kilbinger, R. Loose, R.W. Günther, and M. Georgi, Ziele, Anforderungen und Rahmenbedingungen der Teleradiologie: Eine Bestandsaufnahme, *Radiologe* **37** (1997) 260-268.

[7] D. Heckermann, V. Wetekam, W. Hundt, and M. Reiser, Advantages and Cost-benefit Analysis of Various Teleradiology Scenarios, *Radiologe* **37** (1997) 285-293.

[8] R. Bolte, M. Walz, K.J. Lehmann, T. Hothorn, C. Brill, L. Hothorn, and M. Georgi, Teleradiology: Results of a Questionnaire of German Radiologists, *J Telemed Telecare* **4 S. 1** (1998) 69-71.

[9] M.C. Davis, MR Teleradiology Network Serving Remote Imaging Centers, *J Digit Imaging* **11 S. 1** (1998) 88-92.

[10] G.W. Boland, Teleradiology: Another Revolution in Radiology?, *J Digit Imaging* **11 S. 1** (1998) 93-95.

[11] G.H. Bowers, E. Steiner, and M. Kalman, Implementing Teleradiology in a Private Radiology Practice: Lessons Learned, *J Digit Imaging* **11 S. 1** (1998) 96-98.

[12] T.K. Wu, J.L. Liu, H.J. Tschai, Y.H. Lee, and H.A.T. Leu, An ISDN-based Telemedicine System, *J Digit Imaging* **11 S. 1** (1998) 93-95.

[13] U. Engelmann, A. Schröter, U. Baur, O. Werner, M. Schwab, H. Müller, M. Bahner, H.P. Meinzer, E. Borälv, and B. Göransson, The German Teleradiology System MEDICUS: System Description and Experiences in a German Field Test, *Eur. J. Radiol.* **26** (1998) 219-225.

[14] C. Ruggiero, Teleradiology: A Review, *J Telemed Telecare* **4** (1998) 25-35.

Address for correspondence

M. Walz
Institut für Klinische Radiologie
Klinikum Mannheim gGmbH
Theodor-Kutzer-Ufer
D-68167 Mannheim, Germany
Phone: +49 621 383 2276
Fax: +49 621 383 3817
e-mail: *km22@rumms.uni-mannheim.de*.

The Impact of Telemedicine on Health Care Management
M. Nerlich and R. Kretschmer (Eds.)
IOS Press, 1999

WWW-Based Access to Radiological Patient Data: Two Years of Experience

Björn BERGH[1], Roland FELIX[2]
[1]*Dept. of Information and Data Processing, Medical Centre of the Johann Wolfgang Goethe-University, Frankfurt am Main, Germany*
[2]*Strahlenklinik and Poliklinik, Charité-Campus Virchow-Klinikum, Medical Faculty of the Humboldt-University Berlin, Germany*

Abstract. This paper describes the theoretical concept behind, the technical implementation of, and the experiences created with a self-developed system to access radiological patient data by WWW-technology. *Materials and Methods*: The WWW-system interfaces the RIS *via* HL7 and the PACS *via* DICOM. Core components are a secure Web-Server and an underlying database system (DB). The DB contains all relevant information from the RIS and thumbnails of corresponding images archived in the PACS. After authorisation, the user receives this information in the form of dynamically generated Web pages. By mouse-clicking a thumbnail, the original DICOM-image is sent. It is displayed with a helper application (DICOM-Viewer), allowing all kinds of image manipulation and post-processing. *Results*: Determined advantages of the system were: platform independence, security features, a fixed link of image and report, universal availability, and simple usage. The only critical issue was performance. Cost savings could be seen in: a reduction of DICOM workstations, employment of all available hardware, and reduced training and teaching efforts. *Conclusions*: The author believes that a WWW-based concept is the only feasible approach which is in the same way technically possible, clinically acceptable, and financially affordable in order to grant a variety of users access to radiological data-- although improvements in performance have to made by, e.g., closer implementation of those systems to the RIS and PACS architecture, and by employing high-grade image compression.

1. Introduction

With the rising budgetary restrictions in the public healthcare sector, the demand for cheap and effective solutions, especially in the expensive area of medical technology and informatics, is continuously increasing. Many hospitals have therefore investigated the capabilities for deploying Internet technology in a hospital environment. The advantages of this approach are currently leading to the development of many distributed information systems based on the WWW (World Wide Web) in different types of organisations all over the world, the so-called "intranets".

When the Charité University Hospital (Campus Virchow-Klinikum, Berlin, Germany) planned the establishment of a Digital Radiology and a PACS in 1994, some basic objectives were defined which should be respected by all means. The overall goal was to achieve the universal availability of all patient-related radiological data not only for all users on the campus, but also for users in associated hospitals and practitioners. Hence, one core element is a hospital-wide distribution of images and reports in conjunction; this should be fulfilled by a system with an open architecture on the basis of established standards like HL7 (Health Level 7) and DICOM (Digital Imaging and Communications in Medicine). Furthermore, the system was supposed to cover all legal and security aspects, as well as the respective diagnostic needs of different clinical users. In addition, cost effectiveness had to be one of the major concerns in the whole project. At that time, it was already clear that the integration of a large number of UNIX-based viewing stations would exceed the available budget, while not sufficiently satisfying the integration of images and reports as well as security aspects. Therefore, WWW-technology was chosen as the general platform for integration and access. Since at the beginning of the project there was no suitable product available on the market, it was decided to try to solve the issue by starting hospital-based development. The present paper describes the theoretical concept behind, the technical implementation of, and the experiences had with this system over the past two years.

2. Material and Methods

2.1 General Concept for the Retrieval of Radiological Patient Data

The establishment of viewing facilities for radiological images on a broad basis in a large hospital is a very costly procedure. Hence, to avoid misspending it is important to adjust necessary investments precisely to users' needs. To keep costs at the lowest possible level, we therefore developed a concept which includes three different levels of review quality in conjunction with costs and associated with specific user groups (comp. Fig. 1).

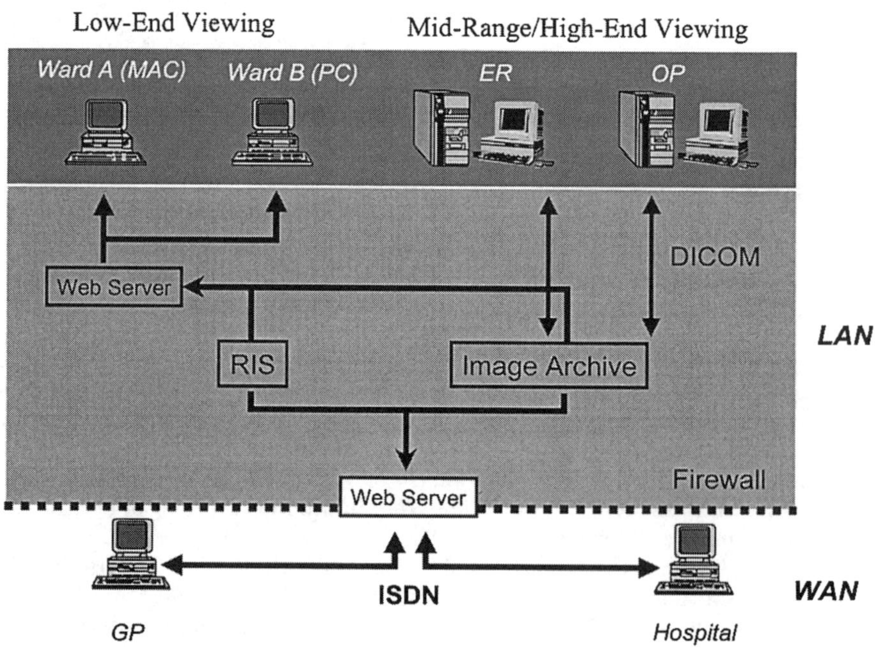

Figure 1.

High-End Viewing (HEV): High-End Viewing is intended to provide facilities for primary diagnosis in radiology. These workstations have to fulfil all medical needs and requirements to perform softcopy reading of radiological examinations. They will mainly be UNIX workstations with high-end graphic cards and high-brightness/contrast monitors. All kinds of image post-processing are available. These stations will only be used in the radiology department and work on the basis of DICOM.

Mid-Range Viewing (MRV): These workstations are also intended for primary diagnosis, but by clinical user groups. Identical to the HEV, they have to provide diagnostic image quality and hence employ the same monitors and graphic cards; however, post-processing is not available unless for specific clinical requirements. These WS will be located at strategically important points inside the hospital (e.g., ICU, ER, one on each ward, etc.) and also make use of direct DICOM connections.

Low-End Viewing (LEV): All users inside and outside the Charité with any kind of computer have access to the radiological images in conjunction with their respective reports *via* a WWW-based system. Image display is accomplished with a helper application in the browser. When the clinical user feels that the image quality is inappropriate for his purposes, he can walk to the closest MRV workstation to display the images in full quality. The principles of the LEV will be described in more detail in the following sections.

2.2. Concept and Technical Design of the WWW System

Core components of the solution are a secure WWW server that handles access control, dynamic generation of the WWW pages, and data transmission, as well as an underlying database which stores the data itself. The system is also connected to the RIS (Radiology Information System) as well ass the PACS, and interfaces with both to provide WWW access. We used Oracle RDBMS, especially for Windows NT and Sun Solaris 2.x, as the database system [10].

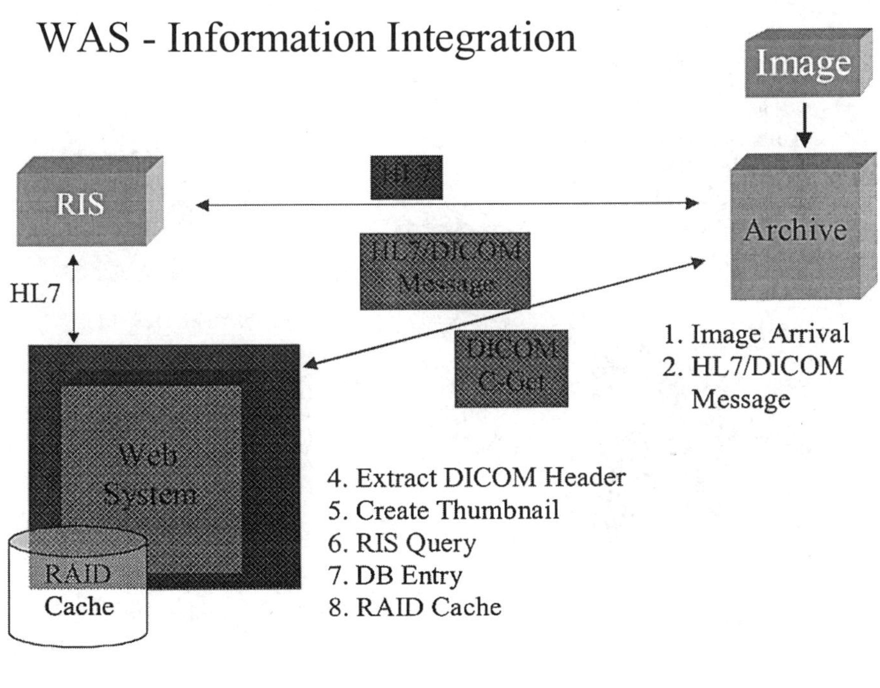

Figure 2.

For the WWW-DB gateway we switched from writing our own Perl CGI programs to employing the Oracle WebServer option, which provides a very easy and secure interaction between WWW client, Web server, and the database, as well as rapid application prototyping. Both components are in the following discussion called a "WWW-Access-System" (WAS).

2.2.1. Information Integration

As soon as an image arrives in the digital image archive, an HL7/DICOM message is generated which is sent to the WAS (comp. Fig. 2). The message contains, in addition to general demographic data, specific DICOM-related information to further facilitate the process. After the WAS has received this message, it uses the DICOM information to perform a DICOM C-Get and thus fetch the image. From this image, a thumbnail (128x128 pixels) is created and stored locally in the WAS-database, together with the demographic information. Then the WAS performs an HL7 query to the RIS based on the patient and examination ID to retrieve additional information on the examination performed (e.g., report, procedure, clinical information) and adds it to that information already in the database. The original image with full resolution is stored locally in a "first in-first out" RAID cache inside the WAS, to provide immediate access in the first days after image generation.

2.2.2. Information Retrieval

Analogous to the process of information integration, information retrieval consists of multiple steps (comp. Fig. 3). After authorisation, the user arrives at a selection template where he can enter his search criteria extended by wildcards (comp. Fig. 4).

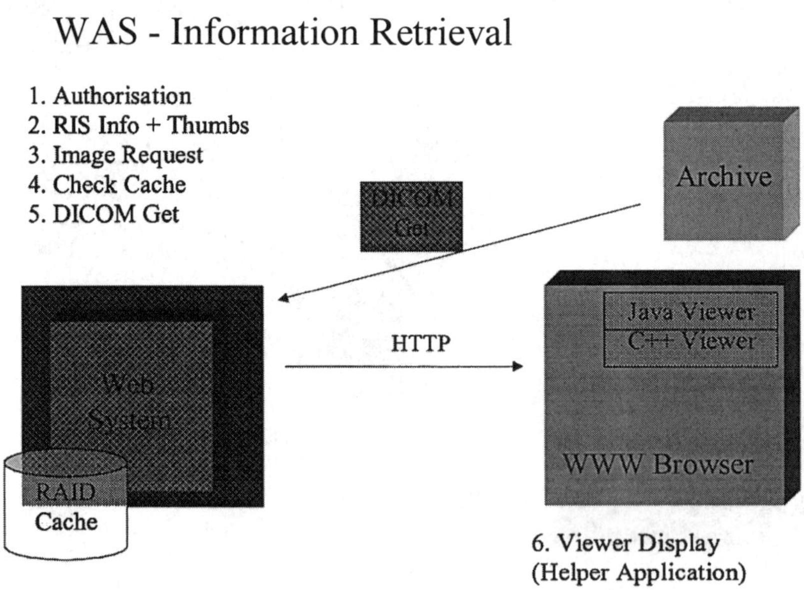

Figure 3.

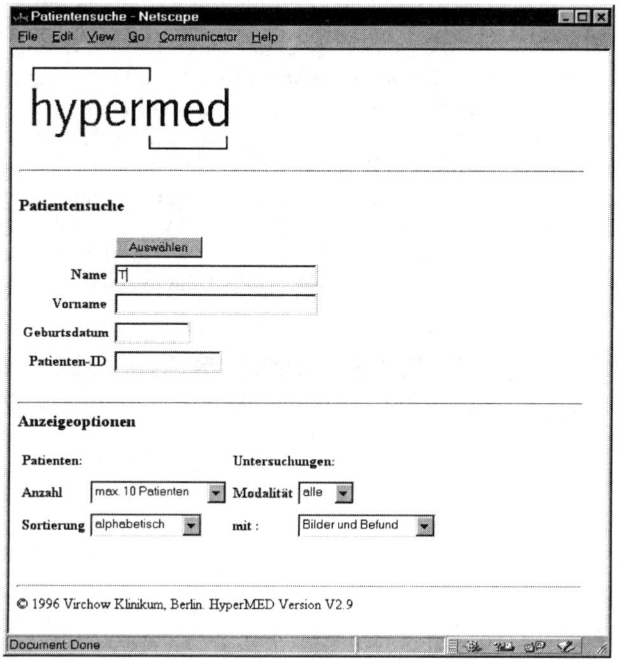

Figure 4.

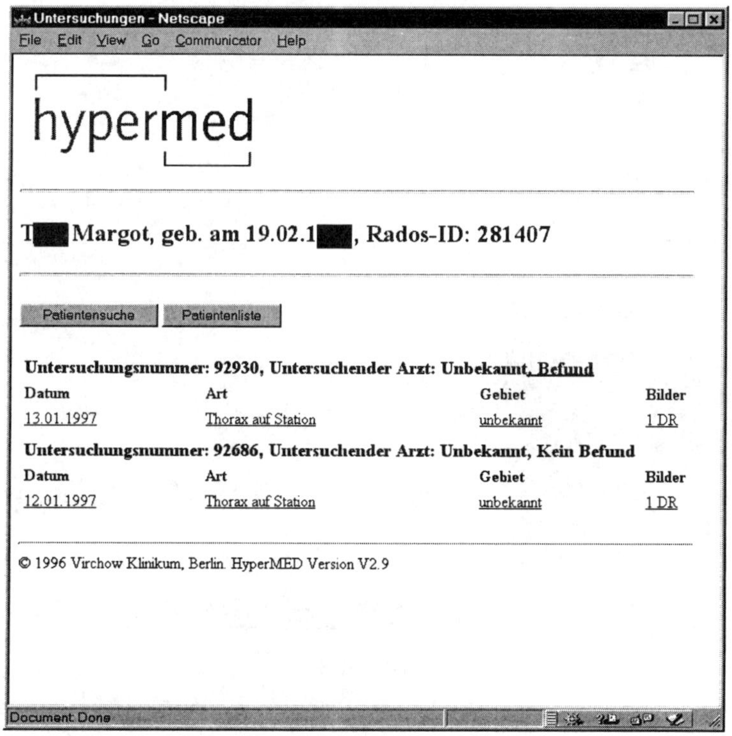

Figure 5.

Upon receiving the menu with different matching patients and thereafter the submenu for the desired patient, a user can select the specific examination of interest (comp. Fig. 5). By doing so, available information in the database is packed into a dynamically generated WWW page which includes general information from the RIS and existing thumbnails, as well as a link to the respective report (comp. Fig. 6). This page is transmitted *via* HTTP. By mouse-clicking the report hyperlink (in German: Befund), the report is sent as an HTTP document. When the image thumbnail is clicked, the WAS first checks if the image can be located in its local RAID-cache. If so, then no communication with the archive is established, but rather the image is retrieved and directly forwarded to the user. If not, then the WAS initiates a DICOM C-Get to the image archive and fetches the original DICOM-image, which is then copied to the requesting customer.

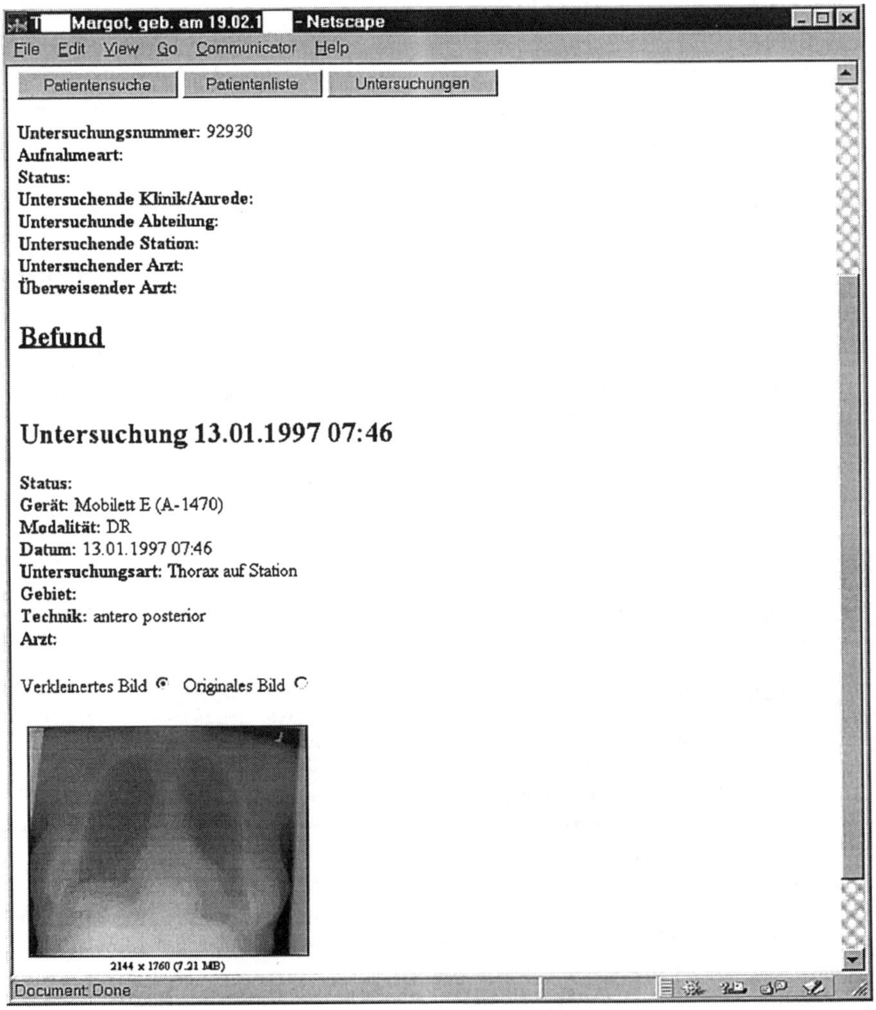

Figure 6.

In either case, the user has the choice between the image in its full original resolution or as a reduced alternative (half the size) to decrease loading time (comp. Fig. 6, in particular the buttons "Verkleinertes Bild" and "Originales Bild" above the image thumbnail). Upon arrival of the image on the user's computer, the DICOM file extension starts a Helper application which is installed on the local PC (comp. Fig. 7). By employing this DICOM viewer, the user can perform all kinds of image manipulation and post-processing in the same way he could if the image had been retrieved *via* a direct DICOM communication.

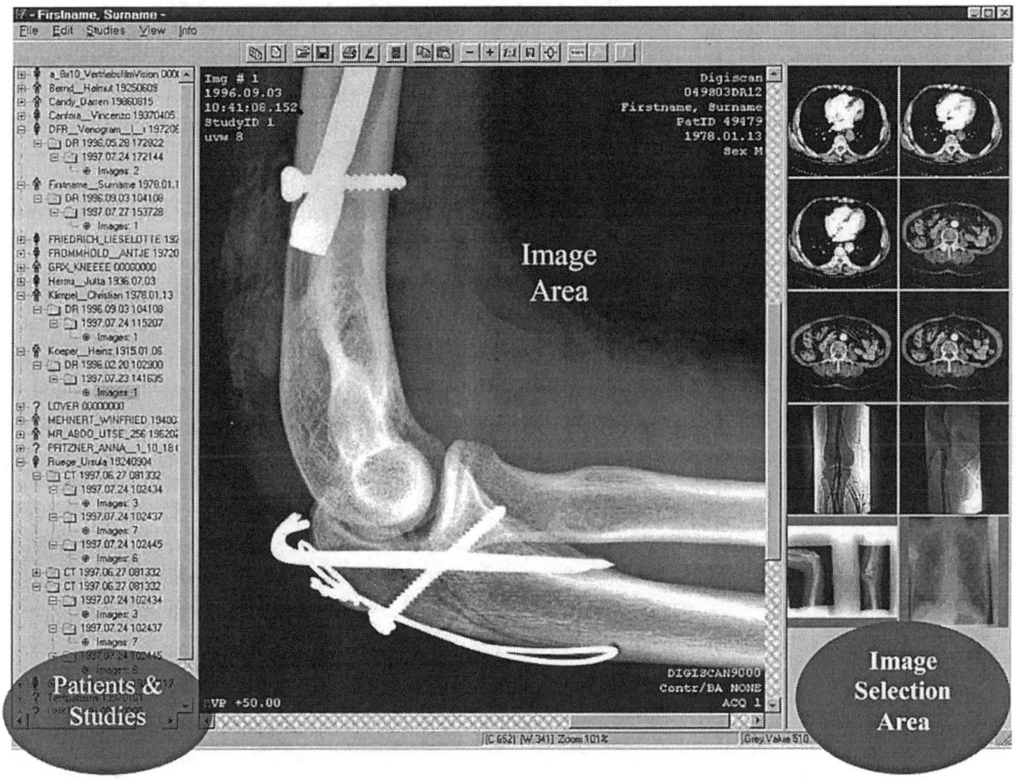

Figure 7.

2.2.3. Security Aspects

The access to documents is of course restricted. Each user has to be registered and perform a login with password control. Once admitted to the system, access is not restricted for users residing on the campus itself. Users from outside the Charité always have a specific role, which entitles them to access only their own patients' information. Internal access from the campus intranet is possible as well as from anywhere else. External communication is enabled *via* ISDN lines which are connected to the hospital LAN (local area network) *via* an ISDN router. A phone number check is performed.

2.3. Other Components

Some other components which are integral parts of the general surrounding IT infrastructure and which have a particular relevance to the present issue will be described briefly in the following:

- Concerning the employed network, the Virchow-Klinikum has a 155 Mb/s ATM-backbone (Asynchronous Transfer Mode) for high speed broadband communication, connecting all buildings up to the floor level and partly with direct connection to the information sources or display devices. This is moreover true for the connection between the radiological imaging modalities, reading workstations, and the image archive with the campus network. Most front-end PCs at the different wards, however, are still connected *via* 10 Mb/s Switched-Ethernet.
- An HL7 communication server (CAI-net) was installed to allow for the communication of data between all the different departmental subsystems, including the RIS, the PACS, and the WAS.
- The exiting RIS is a RADOS system based on MUMPS. Due to the fact that this system has originally been developed in cooperation with the Virchow-Klinikum, the source code was available and the RIS underwent a variety of changes over the past years, including the implementation of HL7 interfaces.
- A digital image archive development project (PACS) was started in 1995 in cooperation with an industrial partner. The majority of the imaging modalities have in the meantime been connected to the archive *via* DICOM, either through a proprietary or a standardised interface to the RIS. The archive itself currently consists of a main archive server (HP), 85 GB RAID, and 185 GB MOD Jukebox.
- A Windows-compliant helper application has been used for the display of images, i.e., a dedicated ACR/NEMA and DICOM viewer (comp. Fig. 7). This was also developed by the Virchow-Klinikum, since there was no Windows-based viewer available which met the radiologists' requirements at the beginning of the project. The viewer is a 32-bit-programme for the display of medical images running under Microsoft Windows platforms. The implementation was realised in C++. The main aim during the development and conception was to create a programme which can be intuitively handled, and which allows fast visualisation and effective processing of medical image formats.

To assess the results of the achieved implementation work, investigations using interviews, questionnaires, and technical measurements were undertaken.

3. Results

The solution as described above has now been operational for about two years within various wards with great success. The advantages of the presented WWW access system are numerous in different terms.

3.1. Technological Aspects

From the technology point of view, one of the principal advantages of WWW-based solutions is platform independence, which is particularly useful within non-homogeneous hospital environments like that in the Charité, where a mixture of different hardware platforms are installed. All available hardware components (PC, MAC, UNIX etc.) can be employed as long as they support the use of standard WWW browser technology. Development of a specific extra client is unnecessary, since any available WWW browser-- as long as it supports the HTML features utilised to structure the delivered pages-- can serve as a client. This obviously also avoids unnecessary support and maintenance efforts on the user's side.

The development process is very short, since the only work is converting document contents into HTML format.

Due to the general evolutionary process in the Web technology sector, one can always make use of the most advanced features. This includes in particular security features, which naturally have huge importance within a clinical environment. In addition, the WWW-based system helps to provide solutions for technical problems which otherwise could hardly be solved in a standardised manner. This is most of all true for access control and the integration of images and reports. Both issues are only vaguely addressed in standards like, e.g., DICOM. It is expected that with further development of WWW technology, especially JAVA, more advantages may become obvious.

The only major technological disadvantage that could be found was the overall performance of the system and its individual components. The performance measurements that were undertaken with uncompressed chest x-ray images (8 MB/image) indicated the following results. When only a single user accessed the WAS and the images still resided in the local Web cache, retrieval time was reasonable in comparison to a standard retrieval procedure using an ordinary DICOM workstation. However, if the images had to be fetched from the image archive using the DICOM procedure for the interconnection, waiting time increased by a factor of three. In the event that ten concurrent users were asking for images to be transferred, the transmission time was multiplied by a factor of five when loading the images directly from the cache, and increased by a factor of 20 when the images had to first be retrieved from the PACS.

Another issue which demonstrated unforeseen problems was the security policy. Whereas it was easy to give users located outside the LAN a dedicated role and to restrict their access only to patients which had been referred by them to the hospital, it was almost impossible to define clear rules for the access policy inside the hospital. We have tried different models, including representative groupings and distribution matrixes, but none of them showed fully satisfying results.

3.2. Usage

The clinical users pointed out two main advantages. The first one was the general availability of all images on almost any computer just minutes after the images had been acquired in the department of radiology, or through other devices located in their respective departments. Doctors whom were working as consultants for other departments especially appreciated the fact that they could log-in from almost any computer independent of their actual physical location, using the same password and working within the same user environment. Also, for clinical units in which an immediate action is necessary (ICU, ER) and where it sometimes took minutes or hours until images were available in the conventional way, the introduction of the WAS marked substantial progress.

The second main feature that the users appreciated was ease of use. In particular, the fact that the system was so similar to the desktop browsers with which they were familiar significantly increased their acceptance. This effect became even more obvious, since in the past users were very often confronted with abstract, uncomfortable user interfaces and had to relearn use procedure with every software upgrade or update. Another advantage was also seen in the fact that the user interface would only change in conjunction with general modifications in the development of WWW browsers.

Quite interesting results could be achieved concerning judgement of the quality of those images delivered by the WAS. These results were mainly influenced by the specific computer and graphical systems (primarily monitor) which were used to display the images, but also strongly influenced by the clinical specialities of the respective doctors. In general, it can be said that in around 85% of the cases, users found the WAS sufficient for their clinical needs, as long as the images were transmitted in full resolution. Furthermore, they claimed that even the quality of the reduced image was appropriate for their purposes in around 40% of the cases. This was mainly true for cases where CT and MRI images marked the major part of the images that had to be reviewed. The main advantages of the WAS illustrated above led to the situation that users, when asked whether they would desire more mid-range stations on their wards or whether they would like to use the WAS, uniformly preferred the WAS.

The only critical issue of importance which was remarked upon was performance. In particular, for digital radiography and computed radiography images (which may have up to 28 MB), users required a significant acceleration in transmission. Some users also noted that those big images were quite difficult to handle with their hardware and in particular RAM equipment, but it was assumed that this situation could be changed easily.

3.3. Economic Aspects

Although we did not perform a sophisticated cost-benefit analysis, there already exist some areas in which clear economic benefits can be determined. By employing WWW-based access systems, the amount of mid-range workstations, which are very costly, needed to establish a digital environment decreases significantly. This alone may save, depending on the size of the hospital, some million EUROs. Furthermore, all available hardware may be used and no additional software purchases are needed. The easy use of the system saves time and thus avoids money-consuming training programs and teaching periods. Due to its association with general computer development, all changes in the standard browser will in the same way apply to the clinical users' GUI.

An additional factor which reveals huge potential is the administration and support of the multiple clients in a hospital. The employment of WWW technology already assists this effort substantially, although the DICOM viewer still had to be installed and updated in the present system. With the migration towards a JAVA-based viewing tool, even this aspect could vanish, so that in a foreseeable time period the installation and support effort for clients, at least from the radiological viewpoint, could tend towards zero.

4. Discussion

Given the universally rising impact of Internet technology, and in particular WWW technology, on the development of the information technology sector, it could be anticipated that over time a deployment in the healthcare sector would take place, especially since increasingly tighter budgets request cheap and effective solutions. A variety of working groups and hospitals have over the past years invested in WWW technology to integrate different systems and components. The majority have undertaken efforts to facilitate the distribution of radiological images and reports by those means. There exists a variety of publications which demonstrate the principal differences in the approach, conceptual design, and technical implementation possibilities for a WWW-based access to radiological data, interfacing RIS as well as PACS components [1,3,4,5,7].

The inherent implications, as well as general advantages, of WWW-based systems have been described extensively, and most of the authors-- including ourselves-- agree fully concerning the fundamental benefits in use and cost-benefit, including the legally important integration of images and reports as well as security features. The majority of existing studies describe mainly technical implementation approaches and their general advantages. Only a few have investigated more thoroughly exact performance behaviour in a real-time environment and in hospital-wide usage. However, the results described above concerning the retrieval performance of the WAS indicate a principal weakness in this field. Since performance is a vital factor in a hospital, we believe that this problem has to be addressed more intensely. To better understand the relevance and importance of these effects, one has to refer to the differences in technical implementation of systems developed by hospitals as well as by industrial companies which are available on the market.

Among existing systems, one can determine major conceptual differences concerning the *access strategy* and the *image quality* which is delivered to the end-user.

In terms of access strategy, most systems are based on a concept that does not allow queries into the DICOM archive. The images are actively routed by the image archive to the Web-system and stored there locally, mostly on a RAID device. Routing is performed on the basis of a set of pre-defined criteria. Images are then available for a certain time span which only depends on the size of the attached RAID-system. With the influx of new images, old ones are deleted following a "first in, first out" principle. The main disadvantage of these systems is that there is no way for the user to retrieve images after they have been erased, if not using a dedicated DICOM workstation. In this sense, these systems can be called "non-interactive". In the majority of cases, these projects involve multiple Web servers to suit the needs of different clinical user groups and to decrease the workload for an individual server. On the other side, this implies an increased burden for the image archive server, which then has to perform multiple routing operations. This also creates the situation in which a variety of images have to be routed more than once, whenever they are needed by more than one user group.

The opposite is the "interactive" system [5], to which the Berlin system also belongs [10], wherein the user has full access to all images stored in the image archive. Only this can be considered a permanent extension of the dedicated PACS workstations. A crucial aspect in this case is the additional workload for the archive server. This also results from the auto-routing procedures which the image archive has to perform for each image entering the PACS and each image which has to be forwarded to the WAS, in accordance with the increasing number of users who directly access the image archive and order examinations. The precise amount of those operations is almost unpredictable, and therefore resulting changes in performance can hardly be anticipated. This situation occurs due to the fact that in a conventional PACS environment, the amount of users is more or less known through the number of existing workstations, whereas in the case of a Web system it can be extremely variable. The exact number of concurrent users-- which is the important digit-- can usually only be defined after the installation of a system under real-life conditions. In addition, an extension to multiple Web servers is also very often difficult due to conceptual reasons.

Concerning image quality, one can find two different main approaches. A first group of systems always only provides 8-bit images, whereas a second group uses instead the original DICOM image bit-depth, which ranges from 10 to 24 bits. In the first case the images are usually sent in a GIF (Graphics Interchange Format) or JPEG (Joint Photographic Expert Group) format, frequently employing the JPEG compression mechanism, which was originally designed for 24-bit colour images. Browning, *et al.* [3] report using JPEG images and describe a transmission time of up to five seconds for 8-bit images at a 75% quality level. Since our system used the full DICOM images, which are at least twice the size of a respective 8-bit image, the performance results seem to be comparable. The major disadvantage of using 8-bit images is that only a small part of the originally available image information is maintained and visible, and changes in the window and level settings cannot be made as they can for a full DICOM image. The degree of this drawback becomes clear in the case of CT and MRI images. The alternating display, e.g., of a CT examination of the chest in a soft tissue, a lung, or a bone window setting is only possible with full bit-depth, but never with an 8-bit image. The clinical value of 8-bit images is therefore extremely restricted and we decided not to use them at all. On the other hand, one may argue that the 8-bit image reflects the image as it was at the time of diagnosis. This is true only if the PACS archive stores images in the appropriate status, which is usually not the case. Mostly, the 8-bit image is created immediately before transmission to the Web system, if not there alone.

Bearing in mind the advantages and disadvantages of different approaches discussed above, the authors still consider their initial choice-- to develop an interactive system using the full bit- depth of images-- to be the right one. Instead of gaining performance by using 8-bit images and non-interactive systems, we believe that there are other possibilities that are more valid and promising for increasing the overall performance of Web systems. The first is the inclusion of the enormous potential of wavelet-based image compression. Other authors [6,8] have demonstrated such possibilities, and with the current work undertaken by the JPEG 2000 Consortium to standardise the usage of wavelet algorithms, a deployment in radiology seems soon to be possible-- especially since the DICOM committee is accompanying these efforts. By using wavelet compression, an acceleration of the whole image transmission chain between the image archive and the user's viewer could be achieved.

The comparison of the transmission times for images coming directly from the cache and for those that have to be fetched from the archive indicates that the underlying DICOM connection significantly prolongs the transmission. According to these results, an optimisation could be possible by circumventing this part of the connection. This can be achieved through a modified system architecture wherein communication is handled on a lower level by using, e.g., concepts like CORBA or Active-X [2]. A tighter integration of the Web components and the image archive is a mandatory precondition to implementing such a system. This requires a close cooperation to resolve what is less a technical than a logistic problem, since very often both products belong to different owners.

To summarise, the authors believe that a WWW-based system is the only suitable approach which is in the same way technically possible, clinically acceptable, and financially affordable enough to allow a large number of users access to radiological patient data. The conceptual design chosen for our implementation has proven to be the right one. In an appropriate combination with DICOM workstations, it satisfies all clinical needs. For users gaining access *via* WAN connections, it can be recommended today without any restriction. Inside a LAN, the current limits in performance should be addressed by implementing a system technically closer to the PACS architecture, and by using a sophisticated image compression mechanism.

References

[1] E. Bellon, J. Wauters , J. Fernandez-Bayo, M. Feron, K. Verstreken, J. Van Cleynenbreugel, B. Van den Bosch, M. Desmaret, G. Marchal, and P. Suetens, Using WWW and JAVA for Image Access and Interactive Viewing in an Integrated PACS, *Med Inform* (London) **22:4** (Oct.-Dec. 1997) 291-300.

[2] W.D. Bidgood Jr., Y. alSafadi, M. Tucker, F. Prior, G. Hagan, and J.E. Mattison, The Role of Digital Imaging and Communications in Medicine in an Evolving Healthcare Computing Environment: The Model is the Message, *J Digit Imaging* **11:1** (Feb. 1998) 1-9.

[3] G.C. Browning, Y. Liang, K.A. Buckwalter, R.A. Kruger, and A. Aisen, World Wide Web Interface to Digital Imaging and Communication in Medicine-Capable Image Servers, *J Digit Imaging* **9:4** (Nov. 1996) 178-184.

[4] A. Gropper, S. Doyle, and K. Dreyer, Enterprise-Scale Image Distribution with a Web PACS, *J Digit Imaging* **11:3 S1** (Aug. 1998) 12-17.

[5] C.J. Henri, R.K. Rubin, R.D. Cox, and P.M. Bret, Design and Implementation of World Wide Web-Based Tools for Image Management in Computed Tomography, Magnetic Resonance Imaging, and Ultrasonography, *J Digit Imaging* **10:3 S1** (Aug. 1997) 77-79.

[6] J.A. Maldjian, W.C. Liu, D. Hirschorn, R. Murthy, and W. Semanczuk, Wavelet Transform-Based Image Compression for Transmission of MR Data, *AJR Am J Roentgenol* **69:1** (Jul. 1997) 23-26.

[7] C. Mascarini, O. Ratib, G. Trayser, Y. Ligier, and R.D. Appel, In-House Access to PACS Images and Related Data through World Wide Web, *Eur J Radiol* **22:3** (Jun 1996) 218-220.

[8] D.F. Schomer, A.A. Elekes, J.D. Hazle, J.C. Huffman, S.K. Thompson, C.K. Chui, and W.A. Murphy Jr., Introduction to Wavelet-Based Compression of Medical Images, *Radiographics* **18:2** (Mar-Apr 1998) 469-481.

[9] U. Tachinardi, S.S. Furuie, N. Bertozzo, L. Moura, M.A. Gutierrez, and C.P. Melo, Hypermedia Patient Data Retrieval and Presentation through WWW, *Proc Annu Symp Comput Appl Med Care* (1995) 551-555.

[10] J. Thomsen, C. Zielinski, D. Emmel, B. Bergh, L. Kleinholz, and R. Felix, A World Wide Web Based Access to Clinical Patient Data. In: R.F. Kilcoyne, J.L. Lear, and A.H. Rowberg (eds.), Computer Applications To Assist Radiology, *Proc. SCAR 96* **8** (1996) 358-363.

Address for correspondence

Björn Bergh
Dept. of Information and Data Processing
Medical Centre of the Johann Wolfgang Goethe-University
Theodor-Stern-Kai 7
60590 Frankfurt am Main, Germany

Remarks

The first author of this paper changed his employer during the preparation of the manuscript. His current status is reflected as indicated on the title page. Nevertheless, all presented work has been undertaken and performed at the Charité-Campus Virchow-Klinikum Berlin.

The Impact of Telemedicine on Health Care Management
M. Nerlich and R. Kretschmer (Eds.)
IOS Press, 1999

Southern Health Board – Advanced Telematic / Telemedicine in Healthcare Services in the South West Of Ireland

U.M. O'SULLIVAN[1], Jack SOMERS[2]
[1]*IT/EU Projects Manager, Southern Health Board, Cork, Ireland*
[2]*Management Services Officer, Southern Health Board, Cork, Ireland*

Abstract: The Southern Health Board has been involved in Telematic Healthcare services for the past number of years. Our involvement in a number of EU funded projects has given us extensive experience and expertise in this area. The primary focus of our telematic applications is optimising health services delivery with a particular emphasis towards people who are isolated due to social and physical boundaries and limitations.
Our main projects are:

NIVEMES (Network of Integrated Vertical Medical Services) includes the exchange of medical information between urban centres and isolated communities including those at sea, rural, elderly and disabled persons.

RISE (Remote Information Services for the Elderly) focuses on the enhanced healthcare services of the elderly and disabled through the use of telemedical applications.

HEALTHLINE To strengthen the successful outcome of Telehealth implementation by specific projects in the EU by providing the expert Training and Information dissemination services to providers, beneficiaries and the general public, using the Telehealth systems and infrastructure applied by those projects

KATE (Killarney & Telecom Éireann) the SHB in conjunction with the Information Age Town Project in Killarney are working towards benefiting the local community through the innovative use of Information and Communication Technologies.

TASTE (Technology Assessment in Telemedicine) An EU funded trans-national initiative aimed at developing a methodology for assessing medical technology, particularly in the area of Neurosurgery.

FECV (Forward Emergency Control Vehicle) An European Space Agency project through which we are developing an advance communications vehicle for major emergence/event management through Satellite linkage to SHB systems.

The increasing cost of the delivery of healthcare is a major concern for all governments within the EU. The spiraling cost of the hospital sector is a common policy problem and one of the difficulties of effecting major change. Almost every country in Europe is struggling to reshape its hospital services, particularly in the large cities where medical science has far outreached hospital buildings that are inappropriate, inefficient or in the wrong location.

The hospital networks of the future will have fewer beds than those of today, as lengths of hospital stay reduce and ambulatory surgery increases. The big breakthroughs in diseases like cancer will only happen if governments can draw together the many threads that make up their health services and encourage them to work together.

Over the next decade, we believe that a small number of European centres will emerge as pre-eminent in these highly specialised fields and as a consequence attract patients from across the community as well as professionals for training. The quality of healthcare and equity of access remains a huge challenge in all countries. Quality varies enormously. Clinical audit systems are developing well and they will throw light on poor or inadequate performance.

How Information Technology and Telecommunications respond to these challenges will play a significant role in achieving the new models of healthcare required. In the hospital hence the increasing development of digital information and media for diagnostic and therapeutic care has led to increasing demands for systems that can store and manage this information. This is a considerable advance on the existing traditional Hospital Information Systems.

Through a number of Projects both EU funded and of our own initiative the Southern Health Board is addressing these challenges. We have been involved in Telematic Healthcare services for the past number of years. The primary focus of our telematic applications is optimising health services delivery with a particular emphasis towards people who are isolated due to social and physical boundaries and limitations.

1. Description of the Environment

The Southern Health Board area of healthcare responsibility is the South West Region of Ireland incorporating the counties of Cork and Kerry. It is perhaps the most varied of areas encompassing populous urban areas such as Cork City with approximately 250,000 citizens, average size towns of population 5,000 to 15,000, small rural villages and islands with residents of between 50 and 300 people.

The area is a major tourist attraction due to the scenic farmlands and river valleys which contrast with the wild sandstone hills of the south west, and above all there is the magnificent coastline scooped and fretted by the Atlantic into great bays and secret coves strewn with rocky headlands. These aesthetic delights are in themselves some of the contributory factors to the isolation of some of the population of the region. The Ring of Kerry for example is unequalled as a place of great beauty and the hair-raising cliff edge roads add to its mystic. However it is not appreciated when the journey is a medical emergency or a trip for neo-foetal monitoring in the middle of winter.

With an overall population of 546,400 in the region the age profile is as follows:-

Provision of Acute Hospital care in the region is based at two primary centres, Cork University Hospital a high-tech Class One Trauma Centre and Tralee General Hospital where we have Regional Specialist Services, supported by two smaller general Hospitals at Bantry and Mallow. There is also a network of 21 Community Hospitals which provide locally based health support services to the community.

Of the 546,400 citizens in the region, the majority of the population are entitled by virtue of Government Tax deductions from wages to subsidised healthcare and a smaller number have private medical insurance. In the region 183,000 people are entitled to free medical care due to age, health or economic circumstances. These people are assigned to a local GP for primary care and a capitation fee is paid to the GP under the National General Medical Payments System. This category of patient forms a General Medical System [GMS] panel at the GP Surgery.

Attendance at hospital clinics are by appointment and usually the patients have to travel from the remote rural areas to the central hospitals for specialised diagnositc services such as X-Ray, Ultrasound and dermatological assessment.

Accident and emergencies are dealt with by the A&E departments at the hospitals with patients being transferred by air or land ambulance services. In more remote locations initial assistance is given to the patient by locally based General Practitioners [GPs] or Public Health Nurses [PHNs]. Examples of this are outlined further in this chapter.

2. NIVEMES Network

NIVEMES (Network of Integrated Vertical Medical Services) includes the exchange of medical information between urban centres and isolated communities including those at sea, rural, elderly and disabled persons.

Developments through NIVEMES of GP linkages, HIS integration and the continuing development of medical device interfaces, have presented opportunities to complement and expand emerging technologies and to translate these technologies into achievable service initiatives. For example, the use of the electronic patient record and the integration of medical devices have led to the development of Virtual Patient Clinics focussed on the elderly in the succeeding and complementary project (RISE)

Amongst many tangibles in relation to services, the NIVEMES project has developed a number of added value aspects to the System. In particular the facility to Electronically 'Tag' messages ensures greater security of the confidential patient record. Clear identification of Sender, Recipient, etc., gives accountable audibility of the transaction.

Prior to this, when x-rays or ultrasound images were physically posted between sites, once the film left the remote site it was dependent on providence and goodwill in almost equal measure to arrive at its intended destination. Prior to the advent of NIVEMES the only reliable way to have the x-ray diagnostically evaluated at the central hospital was to send the patient to that central hospital for their x-ray in the first place.

POPULATION OF THE CORK / KERRY REGION 546,400

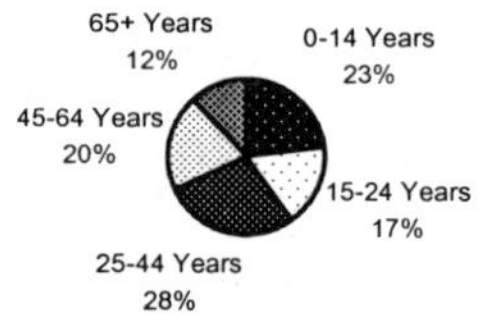

Through the use of NIVEMES System this unreliable method is no longer necessary and the efficiency leads not only to cost savings [far fewer repeat events due to misplaced film] but also to more timely diagnosis, immediate integration of the event into the patients record and far less inconvenience to the patient as a person.

The NIVEMES System is also an important improvement at a time when the International Shipping Industry is rapid adopting new standards and technologies for communication between ships and shore e.g. GMDSS. Extending the scope of NIVEMES services is in line with increased flexibility demands, and will most certainly provide for the long-term survival of marine and island communications systems like NIVEMES that are based on the use of digital equipment.

Two scenarios for testing/demonstrating the ship node were agreed. These relate to the physical aspect of network connectivity and the limitations of the existing networks.

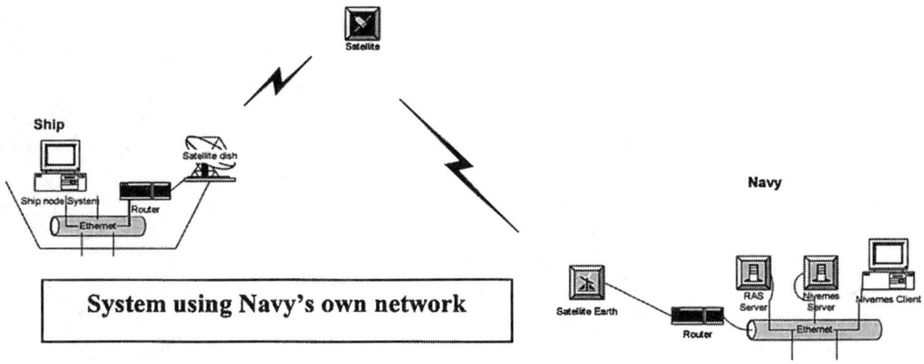

Scenario 1: This involved connecting the Medical facilities at the Naval Base to the ship node using the Navy's existing LAN Network. This was later extended to extend transmission back to the A&E department at Cork University Hospital

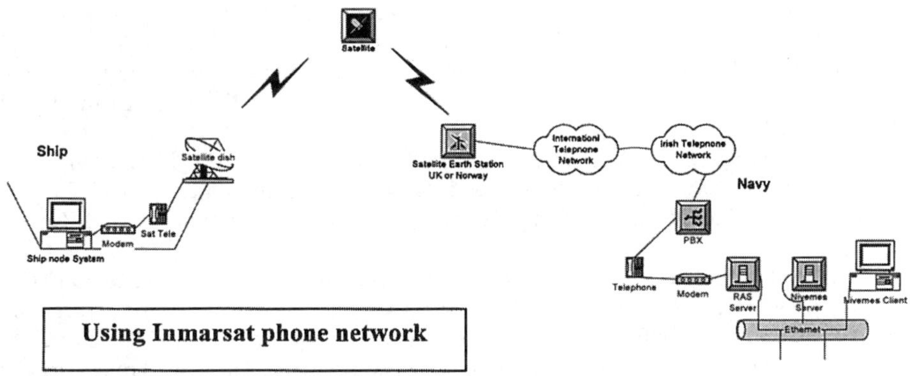

Scenario 2: This involved connectivity using the INMARSAT phone network. In this occasion the physical connectivity was different but the system verification process was the same.

For the purpose of demonstration in both scenarios a PC, an ECG unit and a digital camera were used.

3. Caherciveen Community Hospital

Located 2 hours from Cork and 1 hour from Tralee, Caherciveen Community Hospital is the first hospital built specifically as a community Telemedicine mode. Therefore NIVEMES in particular, and other Telemedicine and ICT initiatives had a particularly important role to play in its establishment and development and are integral to its sustainability. The main user group of this hospital are the elderly but the availability of Telematics e.g. Transmittable Ultra Sounds and X-Rays at local level will be of benefit to the local population as a whole [8731 (1530 aged 65+)].

Prior to the launch of Telemedical Services at the purpose built unit in Caherciveen Community Hospital, people had to travel to Tralee for routine X-rays, post-operative monitoring, ECGs, ultra sounds in addition to general specialist clinics.

For example Neo-foetal monitoring could only be done at Tralee General Hospital [40 miles away over mountainous terrain], a deterring journey for 'mothers to be', X-rays meant a trip over the same terrain and then a comparatively long wait for results.

In fact on the day of the Official Opening an ambulance arrived at the hospital to take two elderly patients to Tralee General Hospital for X-rays and was told that they were not needed as the patients, both in their 70s, had been X-rayed in Caherviveen.

The main funding for this project, IR£400,000 was raised locally through various fund-raising activities. There was also a contribution of IR£100,000 each from The Southern Health Board and the Irish Government. The hospital has a high nationwide profile as it is situated in the constituency of the Irish Minister for Justice, Equality and Law Reform John O'Donoghue T.D.

4. RISE

RISE (Remote Information Services for the Elderly) focuses on the enhanced healthcare services of the elderly and disabled through the use of telemedical applications. ***KATE*** (Killarney & Telecom Éireann) the SHB in conjunction with the Information Age Town Project in Killarney are working towards benefiting the local community through the innovative use of Information and Communication Technologies. The synergy created by the RISE and KATE Projects has resulted in the establishment at Killarney of the first Virtual Out Patient Clinic.

We are making Killarney a Virtual Co-ordination Centre (V.C.C.). This will enable the provision of seamless, co-ordinated, shared healthcare and community services for everybody living in the Killarney district using modern Information & Communication Technologies (ICTs).

Through these ICTs we plan to introduce at Southern Health Board sites and at strategic publicly accessible points e.g. Cyber Café, facilities for Tele-Access to the Board's services. We envisage that the bulk of this traffic will be local but provision will also be made for transfer of the caller to more definitive services available only at Tralee or Cork. As technology develops these initial tele-services may be upgraded to multi-media services.

Another innovative area using ICTs is the integration of General Practitioners (GPs) into the Southern Health Board system. This provides for easier booking of clinic appointments, tests etc., and the more efficient dissemination of patients' results back to their local GP.

The V.C.C. is being augmented by the implementation of Ireland's first 'Virtual Out-patient Centre for the Elderly', where elderly people in Killarney are able to 'virtually attend' specialist clinics in Tralee and Cork whilst still physically in Killarney. In essence this will bring specialist care to Killarney instead of people always having to travel to Cork and Tralee.

At present in Killarney the Southern Health Board have services at many locations. These locations have PSTN lines direct or on to Key Systems or small PABXs. This caused inconvenience to the general public when they rang the wrong location as they could not be transferred and they had to incur the cost of another call. It can also be applied to communication with other Southern Health Board locations at Tralee and Cork.

The solution to this has been the provision of a Direct Dial In (D.D.I.) Service to all the Killarney Southern Health Board sites with the functionality of call transfer and voice mail between the locations.

During the development use is being made of ICT Services and equipment such as multi-media, health telematics, smart cards, alarm systems and portable computers for the provision of an integrated suite of services including:-

- Telemedicine
- Homecare Support
- Teleservices such as Entertainment, Human Communication and Special Interest Groups support.
- Home System Aspects.

HEALTHLINE is being developed to strengthen the successful outcome of Telehealth implementation by specific projects in the EU by providing the expert Training and Information dissemination services to providers, beneficiaries and the general public, using the Telehealth systems and infrastructure applied by those projects.

HEALTHLINE has three levels of Training; Health Informatics, NIVEMES support and RISE Support.

HEALTHLINE also provides Organisational Services

Though it may seem very basic this type of information is essential to Health Professionals working in all areas but most particularly in remote areas. Subjects will include:

Induction

With a staff of over 8,500 there is a large turnover of staff and it is important that everyone can immediately identify whom they need to contact within the Southern Health Board in relation to a specific matter. This will explain organisation structure and procedures.

Board Minutes

Training Services

Information about the various Training Services available to staff, not only those directly available through HEALTHLINE but also those provided both in-house and out-sourced.

Internal Vacancies

Internal vacancies will also be advertised and applied for through HEALTHLINE ensuring that all staff have timely information about the post(s).

Nurse Education

A strong emphasis in SHB User Requirements was placed on Nursing Education, access to quality information, communication and peer support. A lot of work was done in the above filtering and expanding of user requirements but the steering group felt this was worthwhile as to choose the best subjects would greatly improve the chance of success for Healthline in the SHB. A strong emphasis was also placed on user involvement in the Healthline group with, where available, the use of existing expert groups/committee to shape and validate the project.

Nurse Study Days

These are held about once a month and cover current topics such as Nursing Policies and Procedures, Best Practice, New devices, New drugs, etc. hese days are organised by the the Cork and Kerry Nurse Education Committee User Group which has a membership made up of Nurse Managers and Tutors from General, Midwifery, Psychiatry, Community, Mental Handicap, and representation from the Southern Health Board. The Aims and Objectives of the Committee are twofold: Post-basic Nurse Education and Developments in Nursing. The group will implement and validate the HealthLine Nursing Education "Study Days" component of HealthLine.

Information Services for Nurses

The Nurse Library Users Group will be the main source of material for this section. This group is a cross-sectional user group of nurses and students entitled to use the library as staff or students of University College Cork, staff of Cork University Hospital, Erinville Hospital, and St. Finbarr's Hospital. The primary concern of the group is to identify and improve where necessary, information services for nurses. During the validation phase in HealthLine, the group will update library users on the HealthLine technology available and provide necessary training on the use of this technology. Finally, the group will receive feedback from users and feed it back to the central SHB HealthLine Project Team and Steering Group.

Diabetic Patient Care

In the Cork and Kerry region there are three full-time employed diabetic nurses. These nurses communicate and share information with each other. In the main they co-ordinate all services to diabetic patients in their care area. This group will contribute to HealthLine by contributing articles, postings and other materials relating to diabetes.

HIV/AIDS Services Information

The HIV/Aids User Group is a multidisciplinary team consisting of nurses, doctors, a pharmacist, a counsellor, a dietician and the voluntary groups who are involved in this area. This group cares for all patients (except children) with HIV and Aids in the Southern Health Board region. This group will give advice and validate the HIV/AIDS for Nurses courses delivered by HealthLine as well as contributing relevant material to the services content aspect.

Midwifery Care

Since 1991, the midwives in Cork have been meeting as an educational committee. They are a mixture of managerial, tutorial and working midwives. Because of their various roles, they have access to midwifery information of all types for use in HealthLine. This group will source and make available information on midwifery care for HealthLine.

Continence Management

Building on the material collated in conjunction with the RISE project and the efforts of the Board's Continence Advisor we will provide material for support of the remote based Health Professionals in relation to Continence and Incontinence. This will include:-

- Catheters – Types, Usage, FAQs.
- Cause and prevention
- Pelvic Exercises
- Caring for the carer
- Related services.

Health Education and Promotion

The Southern Health Board currently compiles and distributes a wealth of Health Education and Promotion material. Through HEALTHLINE greater availability of this material could be achieved. Subjects include:-

- Nutrition
- Smoking Cessation
- Weils Disease
- Meningitis
- Head Lice
- Living with Arthritis

Support for Telematic Systems – RISE and NIVEMES

The Southern Health Board has a number of remote sites which use the NIVEMES system and a number which are in the process of having the RISE system installed. With an ever-expanding network and increased demand for access to telematic services by their remote workers they need additional support for telematic applications and remote diagnostics– more than those available through their Help Functions. HEALTHLINE will be their means of providing this support not only through the Remote Training Aspects detailed elsewhere in this report but in provision of additional services starting with the following areas.

Telematic Systems Overview

An overview of the NIVEMES and RISE telematic systems with links to more detailed information. NIVEMES targets remote populations and RISE is aimed at caring for the elderly in the information society particularly those isolated by geographics or socio-economics, so use of the Internet, such as HealthLine proposes is a most appropriate means of support.

Medical Devices

HEALTHLINE will provide a vehicle for information about Medical Devices used in conjunction with NIVEMES, RISE and for remote diagnostics in general. There will be information on

- best practice in usage,
- updates on devices available and
- discussion fora.

Software Updates

Remote workers can be informed about updates in Telematic Applications Software. They can also be informed about new applications and systems and where they would be most effective and appropriate. This will be particularly useful for General Practitioners who are not employees of the Southern Health Board but who may wish to avail of the services provided through these applications.

FECV – Forward Emergency Control Vehicle

In April 1982, in a report advocating the use of satellite communications in emergencies, Jerry FREIBAUM of NASA Headquarters stated, "The unpredictability of locations and time of need mandates that the communications system must be able to operate anywhere at any time. Similarly, because human survival and property damage are directly affected by response time, high degrees of mobility, reliability and availability must be inherent to the system. This equates to a requirement to operate despite breakdowns of terrestrial systems due to weather, explosions and saturated 'phone systems".

The FECV is specifically designed to meet the needs of "high degrees of mobility, reliability and availability" in a way that is "affordable" in all economies. In particular, it addresses the demands for rapid deployment and intervention in the "Golden Hour"; the first

60 minutes of any major emergency/disaster in which medical treatment is most critical to the preservation of life and limb.

The design of the FECV results from the Southern Health Board's own extensive experience of major emergency and disaster management and its own initial familiarisation with both the supply and demand sides of the market for such vehicles. Similar vehicles currently available are mostly designed for military use and are, therefore, too expensive, too large and too sophisticated for most healthcare and other relevant organisations. In contrast, the FECV combines an optimum level of technological sophistication with low cost. The FECV is also significant in its integration of terrestrial and satellite communications. This combination enables the establishment of communications immediately upon arrival on-site and before SatComs can be established. Thus, maximum advantage is taken of the Golden Hour.

Training

To successfully implement all of the above, in addition to non-telematic changes in work patterns and processes, we had to undertake a major training initiative. The challenges that telematic applications presented in terms of Training had to be recognised and addressed. An essential aspect of finding the optimum training plan was taking account of the opinion of those who are trained and their managers. The comprehensive and detailed Software Manual is suitable for indepth application training over an extended period of time or for use as reference material in a non-emergency situation. Given that the majority of End-users are located at remote sites or on board ship the training for these persons had to be equally remotely accessible. It must also be remembered that these personnel, who in the majority are neither medically or IT qualified, will most likely be using the systems 'under pressure' in a stressful emergency situation.

To address this problem with alternative training delivery mechanisms, we needed to develop an approach to 'remote training'. This remote training can be used to supplement an existing channel (e.g. providing "real person" question and answer support to compliment a CBT application) or as a stand-alone alternative.

In some cases a complete introduction to ICTs was necessary such as basic PC use including:-

- Introduction to PC
- Introduction to 'windows'
- Basic Keyboard skills
- Mouse use skills
- Creating, saving, finding, modifying and deleting files
- Familiarisation with ICTs
- Printing

Training in the use of the telematic system at each site comprises:-

- The Multimedia Health Record Module
- The Administrative Module
- The Reports Module
- The Medical Aids Database Module
- The Ship Node Module

Training in the actual use of some some of the devices or their adaptations for use with telematic systems also had to be organised, planned and delivered. It was necessary to consider not only the initial contact training but also the on-going support which the user will require over the longer term. This will apply not only to difficulties which may arise and to software developments but also in the event of additional devices being integrated into the systems.

The telematic system however is more than Software. Its real strength and usefulness is in the range of services it facilitates, aimed at a number of target groups such as Hospitals, Insurance Organisations, Maritime Industry e.t.c. All these users need to be instructed on the best possible way of running the services, in order to acquire not only a cost efficient installation but also the best possible management of the system.

There are a number of Services Organisational and Procedural Issues which each of the sites identified as being of significance in respect of designing their Training Plans. These include:-

- Staffing Structure
- Staffing Level
- Training for the 'Remote' Trainers
- Tools for the Trainer
- Training Request Procedures
- Training Schedule Procedures
- Internal Systems Requirements
- Preparing the 'students' for training
- User/Manager Feedback
- Track the Results
- Impact on existing Training/Support Services
- Cost of Training/Support Services

In addition to the above it was/is essential to track the results of the training. These results will provide valuable feedback on the effectiveness of the training, required resources, etc. number of sessions per user to complete training. Long-term Training issues such as content, scheduling, duration, etc, can be better planned when these opinions are evaluated.

5. In Conclusion

The changing demographics of the population in Europe with an ever increasing elderly population will present new and difficult challenges to healthcare providers. The requirement to maintain and support the elderly in their own communities is critical to the provision of these services. The important questions of equity of access will also pose major questions for governments. The social policy of supporting rural development cannot be taken in isolation from the provision of healthcare services.

It is clear that one of the newest and most innovative mechanisms in support of new models of healthcare delivery is Telemedicine. Apart from the important aspect of medical care delivery which has been demonstrated in telematic projects, the development of systems based on digital acquisition of medical data will play a key role in the move towards the measurement of clinical outcomes and evidence based medicine.

The constantly evolving I.C.T. area is presenting the system designers with new affordable technologies. The liberalisation of the Telecommunications Industries have compressed distances and time. The opening of gateways to globally accepted and standardised E-mail systems will mean great savings and added flexibility for telehealth systems.

Now that, through telematic R&D projects, such those we've just skimmed through, telemedicine has matured in effectiveness and efficiency with concrete medical impact, it is important and timely to ask whether telemedicine may have a role in developing countries.

Developing countries face particular problems in the provision of medical services, which relate to the lack of capital, facilities and systems. Roads and transportation are inadequate and difficulties in transporting patients are often encountered. For countries with limited medical expertise or resources, telecommunications can provide a solution to some of these problems. The continued development of telematic systems as a compressed global network for text and multimedia communication has the potential to influence and shape new models of healthcare delivery globally and we for one [sic] can't wait to be part of it.

For further information on the above or any other areas of interest please contact us at:- Ursula O'Sullivan or Jack Somers, Southern Health Board, Wilton Road, Cork, Ireland. Tel +353-21-922990;Fax +353-21-923773; E-mail osullivanu@shb.ie or somersj@shb.ie Or visit our website www.shb.ie

Address for correspondence

U.M. O'Sullivan
IT/EU Projects Manager
Wilton Road
Southern Health Board
Cork, Ireland
Tel +353-21-922990
Fax +353-21-923773
E-mail: osullivanu@shb.ie
somersj@shb.ie

The Impact of Telemedicine on Health Care Management
M. Nerlich and R. Kretschmer (Eds.)
IOS Press, 1999

Remote Communities Services Telecentre Project

Carl W. ROBBINS
Faculty of Medicine, Memorial University of Newfoundland
St. John's, Newfoundland, Canada

Abstract: The delivery of teleservices to rural communities is challenged by the high cost of infrastructure and maintenance. This is compounded if land-based telecommunication links are absent or if bandwidth is limited, as is the case in many areas of the world.

The concept of the Remote Communities Services Telecentre (RCST) is a shared-use facility that can be implemented in rural and remote communities to provide telelearning, telehealth, communications, and information access services. This can be through conventional telephony or cable or, as more likely in remote regions, through the use of a shared wireless facility using satellite.

This model is being implemented as a wireless network in the Province of Newfoundland through collaboration between the Telemedicine and Educational Technology Resources Agency (TETRA) of Memorial University and a number of partners. Private sector partners in St John's include Collaborative Network Technologies Inc. (CNTI) and FutureWorks Inc. Partners in Ottawa include Telesat Canada, QTECH Hybrid Systems, and the Communications Research Centre. Funding support has been provided by the Canadian Network for the Advancement of Industry, Research and Education (CANARIE); Operation ONLINE of Newfoundland and Labrador; and the European Space Agency.

The Newfoundland partners were part of the Team Canada exhibitors group at the G7 Information Minister's Summits in 1995 (Brussels) and 1996 (Johannesburg). The TETRA Centre at Memorial University has previously been involved with international telehealth and telelearning projects in Africa and the Caribbean.

This presentation will discuss the RCST project as a model for widespread implementation in the belief that many rural communities world-wide which currently lack adequate wired telecommunications, will opt strategically for a wireless solution given technologic and economic realities.

The concept of the Remote Communities Services Telecentre (RCST) is to provide a telecommunications resource facility in small remote communities that have limited communications infrastructure. Such communities are found throughout the world, in lesser-developed and developed countries. In Canada, these communities tend to be in the north. The Telemedicine and Educational Technology Resources Agency (TETRA) of Memorial University has considerable experience in the delivery of services in education and health to such northern Canadian communities.

1. RCST Concept

The concept is to work within four scalable dimensions providing optimal flexibility. Services are provided as a set of core telelearning and telehealth applications with additional small business and government information applications. The technology is adaptable to the resources and the requirements of the target community.

Geographically, within the community, the concept is applicable to a single facility or to a network of connected facilities within a region. Connectivity at this secondary level would rely on local wireless systems or land-based telecommunications systems. A critical factor is the integration of human systems to support the technology in its assessment, planning and design, implementation and testing, staffing, training, evaluation, and maintenance and support of the system.

2. RCST Consortium and Funding Sources

The RCST consortium consists of a number of partners and is supported by a number of granting agencies.

Telesat is a Canadian satellite communications company and acts as prime contractor for the partnership. TETRA has been providing, for the past twenty years, telelearning and telehealth services within the Province of Newfoundland. It has experience with a number of international applications and maintains a full-scale telemedicine centre at the Health Sciences Centre, Memorial University. FutureWorks Inc. is a Newfoundland company applying technology for rural and remote communities around the world. Collaborative Network Technologies is a technology-management company with extensive experience in the design and implementation of telecentre facilities for rural communities. QTECH Hybrid Systems has developed an innovative system for the delivery of government information via kiosk to remote telecentres. The Communications Research Centre, within Industry Canada, is a premier research facility for wireless communications with over forty years' experience.

The RCST project has received major funding from the European Space Agency; the Canadian Network for the Advancement of Research, Industry and Education (CANARIE Inc.); and Operation ONLINE, a public sector corporation designed to enhance the development of information technology in Newfoundland and Labrador. The collaborating health regions in Newfoundland and Labrador, primarily the Health Labrador Board, the Western Health Care Corporation, the Central East Health Care Institutions Board, and the Government of Newfoundland and Labrador are also contributors to the project.

3. Responding to the Environment

Much of rural Canada is faced with the challenge of delivering health and education services to relatively small populations spread over great distances and Newfoundland and Labrador is no exception. Transportation and communications efforts can face harsh environmental conditions. With a landmass of 405,740 sq. km, incorporating 111,390 sq. km for the Island of Newfoundland and 294,330 sq. km in Labrador, and with a population of 570,000, the province has a small population density indeed. These geographic realities are compounded in the north by severe weather conditions, particularly in the winter. Transportation by sea faces the annual northern icepack, which is brought to the shores of the province by the cold Labrador Current. Transportation by land in Labrador is made difficult by limited highway infrastructure; therefore, the snowmobile is the primary source of transportation during the winter months. The use of helicopters carries high cost and is sensitive to varying weather conditions.

Communications infrastructure, although developing quickly, is limited particularly in Labrador so that there is varying access to acceptable bandwidth for any type of communications other than telephone.

4. The Health System

The health system in the province faces a number of changes, along with social change ongoing in the rural areas of the province. A strategy of regionalization over the last few years has meant a reforming of health system governance to a relatively small number governing boards. The recruitment and retention of health professionals has always been difficult in the more rural and remote parts of the province. To help address this problem the government has recently begun a pilot initiative entitled the Multidisciplinary Service and Teaching Unit (MDSTU) Project in three communities. The concept is to use health resources in these communities for a wide-range of educational services, thereby broadening the base of health services and attracting professionals with an additional interest in academic activities. The RCST initiative is designed, in part, to complement this initiative in the health system by enabling direct teaching and consultation in a real time mode between these communities. The intent is to use the experience of rural practitioners in the teaching of students in the medical and nursing school at Memorial University of Newfoundland.

There is a twenty-year history of using telecommunications for education and health services in the province. TETRA has developed a provincial network of some 200 audio-conferencing sites in 150 communities.

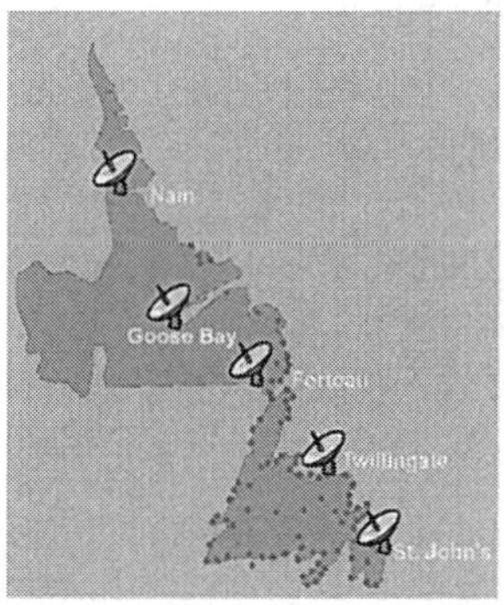

Figure 1: Newfoundland and Labrador

Many of these sites have used audiographics, and some 130 sites have been upgraded with computers to permit the storage of images and interaction between teacher and student with the manipulation of images, including animation. Clinical services over the years have included the use of links for teleEEG, teleimaging, and teleconsultation in primary care and psychiatry.

5. The Communities

The communities to be serviced by the RCST Project include Goose Bay, Nain and Forteau in Labrador and Twillingate, on the Island of Newfoundland (See Fig. I). Goose Bay is a community of some 8,000 people with a mixed population of Caucasian, Innu, and Inuit. It has a major role as a military base with substantial defense employment and regular NATO training activities. It has a large airport, a gravel road to Quebec, and a summer ferry service. The regional hospital, a centre for consultation services to coastal communities, has identified its needs as access to specialist services in St. John's and an ability to serve the remote coastal communities from a distance.

Nain has a population of approximately 1,200, mainly Inuit. There is high unemployment and transportation is by air, relying on a gravel airstrip and summer ferry. A new school is currently under construction and there is a modern health care centre. The identified needs are a full spectrum of network services in health, education, and community service.

Forteau, situated on the southern coast of Labrador, has a regional population of approximately 2,500, and an industry of mixed fishing and tourism. There is a health care centre. It has identified primary needs in advanced access to information services and business communication, but telelearning and telehealth will also be components.

Twillingate is a community in a region of approximately 5,000 people on the northeast coast of the Island of Newfoundland. It is serviced by a regional hospital. The economy has suffered major hardship with the collapse of the northern cod fishery. It has good road access to the rest of Newfoundland and is served by a regional hospital some 80 km away (Gander). Its primary needs have been identified as infrastructure for the teaching of health professionals, continuing, education and consultation.

The human systems component includes extensive needs' identification in the communities being served and the development of community participation by advisory committees. The system has been designed to enable application in a flexible way from a narrow (i.e. health) application to a broad-based application, inclusive of health and education and community development goals.

6. The Technology

The infrastructure to be employed in support of the telehealth application will include an Intel Team Station featuring an Intel Pentium II processor based PC with easy to use videoconferencing software, a wireless keyboard and mouse, a pan/tilt/zoom camera, an integrated audio system, and a large monitor. Medivision VisiTran image capture, store-and-forward application software will be used. The examinations will be performed using an AMD-2500 general examination camera with high resolution, power zoom, frame capture, and image polarization. The AMD-2015 ENT scope, which combines a high performance otoscope, short sinus scope, and an oral exam, will be used for ENT examinations. Applications in radiology, pathology, psychiatry, and cardiology are anticipated. From the more remote sites primary care teleconsultations will take place.

Other applications will include telelearning, enhancing the current resources of the TETRA site; access to government services for community members utilizing the QTECH kiosk; business and community information and Internet access.

7. System Evaluation

An evaluation system has been developed for the project that will parallel to the formal evaluation system identified for the MDSTU Project. Additionally, evaluation objectives have been established for the technologic infrastructure for system operations and for individual applications in each of the sites.

Address for correspondence

Carl W. Robbins
Faculty of Medicine
Memorial University of Newfoundland
St. John's
Newfoundland Canada

The Impact of Telemedicine on Health Care Management
M. Nerlich and R. Kretschmer (Eds.)
IOS Press, 1999

"HausTeleDienst" - A CATV-based Interactive Video Service for Elderly People

Karl A. STROETMANN, Thomas ERKERT
empirica *Gesellschaft für Kommunikations- und Technologieforschung mbH*
Bonn, Germany

Abstract: Since 1991, 17 elderly persons (aged 75 to over 90) in 15 households have been connected *via* TV-videophones to a service centre. A standard CATV network was modified to support a reverse channel. This has been world-wide the first fully interactive broadband video communications project implemented in a real setting and operating over an extended period of time. The overall *aim* has been to prove the ability of frail elderly and mobility-impaired persons to live independently, and to demonstrate strategies for reducing the load on social and health care service resources. Service components include remote care; information and assistance; emergency, counselling, training and exercise services. Practical experience, both from the side of the service provider and that of the users, is discussed. Simplicity of technical design and ease of handling contributed to a feeling of being empowered by the technology. In addition, the very personal and close relationship to the staff-- which was strongly supported, not inhibited by the video communications-- was a major factor in acceptance of the service. It proved a highly successful activity with a great potential for the future: In different contexts with newer technology, market trials are underway to commercialise this service.

1. Introduction

In the pilot service set up since 1991 in Frankfurt am Main/Germany, 17 elderly persons (aged 75 to over 90) in 15 households (a few have died in the meantime) have been connected *via* specially developed videophones to a service centre located in a residential care centre. The clients are connected to the service centre using a standard cable-TV network. This network was modified to support-- on a frequency band not used by CATV-- reverse channels to also carry analogue audio and video signals from the client to the service centre. The quality of the video pictures-- thanks to the broadband technology used-- was of high TV quality. The service centre uses a special one-way mirror onto which the picture of the elderly person calling is reflected and behind which the camera transmitting the picture of the service person has been placed. This results in a very high quality "face-to-face" or "direct-eye-contact" conversation, which has proven very important for a congenial communications atmosphere.

A number of services were developed and implemented during the pilot phase. All clients had the same high-quality communications facility with the same service centre personnel, but unfortunately, due to technical limitations, did not have direct communication with each other. However, a three-party conference call with an outside expert could be arranged.

The services, named "*HausTeleDienst*" (HomeTeleServices), are run by the *Frankfurter Verband für Alten- und Behindertenhilfe e.V. (FV)* in Frankfurt/Main Germany; it is a social care and services organisation providing the majority of sheltered housing, old person's homes, and daycare facilities in the city. In addition, it provides telephone alarm services to over a thousand clients in the area.

To our knowledge, this is indeed world-wide the first fully interactive broadband video communications project implemented in a real setting and operating over an extended period of time.

2. The Service Concept

The services in Frankfurt have the overall *aim*

- of proving the ability of elderly and mobility-impaired persons to live independently, and
- of demonstrating strategies to reduce the load on social service resources required to support this.

Investigation of current service provision and consultations with various providers of care services led to a number of service "components":

2.1 Active Information and Care

This service component was expected to be most useful for those elderly (the vast majority) living alone and who are, therefore, prone to depression and withdrawal. As this group is also often cut off from normal levels of contact with people outside their homes, the regular video and speech contact with service centre personnel provides a minimum support level by acting as a vital social link.

2.2 Remote Response to Emergency "Alarm Service"

Clients who know or fear that they may be in a situation difficult to handle can call the service centre and receive reassurance and help. This service component is an advancement on traditional phone-based emergency intercom systems, providing the opportunity of a visual assessment of clients' needs and their actual situations.

2.3 Remote Care on Demand

The users benefiting from this service are mainly family members who care for elderly and disabled relatives in their homes. In many cases, even short periods of absence are hardly possible or involve great difficulties, reliance on others, or stress and risk. Since care-givers are often unable to ask someone else to come to their homes, remote care can provide care-givers with some relief from their 24-hour jobs.

2.4 Information and Assistance

The aim of this service is to support continued competence of the elderly in mastering everyday problems. Clients are helped in filling out forms, in understanding complex bills, and with a whole range of organisational tasks-- including, for instance, arranging senior citizen vacations.

2.5 Remote Access to Expertise, "Counselling Service"

The counselling service is designed to give clients opportunities to put questions to experts on specific topics, helping them gain access to information relevant to their needs. Appropriate experts are those in fields of which regular service staff cannot be expected to gain detailed knowledge, such as law, specific rights to state benefits, or detailed dietary plans.

2.6 Training and Exercise Service

This service component covers a large range of training types, including communication training, memory training, and physical exercises. Those receiving some forms of psychotherapy can be given short refresher sessions of exercises in the intervals between full personal sessions. These services can also be offered in part using videotapes.

2.7 Support for Carers

The system enables service staff to provide support for non-professional care-givers who have to carry out tasks such as bathing, or changing clothes. Correct care techniques are often unknown by family care-givers with no training. Remote advice can enable them to fulfil even more difficult tasks.

Although the service concept consists of different service components, it is necessary to note that these components are based on regular and close contacts between the service providers and the pilot clients. Based on these relationships, needs could be identified which would otherwise not have been discovered by regular staff. Personalised help could be offered, creating a feeling of security and integration.

3. Evaluation Results

3.1 General Service Usage Patterns

Overall, the average usage pattern by all households taken together was almost eleven calls per day, i.e., the majority of people had video connections with the service centre daily.

A sizeable minority of calls (39%) lasted less than five minutes. 16% of the calls lasted between 5 and 10 minutes and 22% between 15 and 30 minutes. In 9% of all cases, contact between client and service centre was established for longer than half an hour, some of them reaching up to an hour and a quarter in length. A trend towards a slight increase of conversation time was observed.

Analysing the development of the number of calls in comparison with the overall length of contact reveals that the length of calls increased relatively fast in the beginning, as clients got used to the system. This high level was reached early, and since then the figures have changed only slightly. The clients' need for contact is high. The average duration of all calls was over 11 minutes; this number has since then varied only slightly.

Given that intensive human relationships are involved in the pilot service, one main concern in the research was to find out if there is any evidence of discrimination for or against individual clients. With the exception of 3 participants, all other pilot clients can be regarded as frequent users. They differ only in the regularity of their calls. Some call twice or three times a day. This consumes three-fifths of the total speaking time of the service providers. Others call very regularly, once a day. The average connection time of this group is 12.3 minutes, only half a minute shorter than the group described before. A third group of frequent users calls on average every second day. The group of infrequent users contains a total of 3 users. As expected, the calls of these infrequent users are less extensive than calls by frequent users. At 4.23 minutes, one person in this group exhibited the shortest average connection time. It is worth pointing out that a trend for increasing call length was observed not only for those clients who frequently call the service centre, but also for those who could be described as infrequent users.

Interview data revealed no evidence of any significant discrimination of specific users. Those who used the service infrequently did so of their own accord. The duration of calls can be regarded as an indicator for the intensity of the conversation, as well as for the quality of all contacts. In both respects, the results are very positive and promising for a future regular service.

3.2 Service Provider Experience

The picture component of the integrated alarm service enables the service provider to assess an assumed or real emergency situation much better. Such a videophone-based emergency system is far superior to a regular telephone-based emergency intercom system. In an emergency situation, it helps to create a feeling of security while emergency services are on the way.

Most of the calls made by clients could be associated with the active information and care service component. The ongoing and regular possibility to ask the service provider whenever there is a need seems to be especially important to the elderly. The service persons believe that this service element is the most important one for the pilot clients. Many senior citizens obviously just need someone to talk to when they feel isolated and/or lonely.

The remote-care-on-demand service also has a high potential. This service component offers a real and direct help to the relatives. It allows them to continue a "normal" way of living by offering a secure way of caring *via* videophone. This element also enables relatives to get advice, e.g., with specific care techniques.

Although the counselling service was very time-consuming in preparation, it is a useful source of help for elderly people, enabling them to get in touch with expertise which they would not get if experts had to visit them in person. It reduces the fear of asking experts, because the well-known service person can lower inhibitions by mediation between the experts and the elderly.

The training and exercise lessons were frequently joined by several of the pilot clients. Remarkable improvements could be observed in the case of a lady who frequently joined memory training exercises. The physical fitness training motivated people to do some additional exercises at a senior citizens' club; i.e., the service animated them to leave their home and to search for new contacts.

This very positive effect could also be observed in other situations, e.g., due to regular meetings in person (supported by transportation services of the service provider) of all participating clients, or to the arrangement of meetings outside the home through video communications. One lady who lost her husband was helped in reorganising her life, gaining a new sense of order and commitment (through a regular early morning call), and was supported in establishing new outside contacts.

The service provider staff and the service provider organisation summarised their experiences with the new service as follows: "The video-based *HausTeleDienst* fills a serious gap in social services". Fast and effective help is possible. One of the biggest advantages of the new system is to reduce unnecessary travel time, thereby allowing for more or better services with the same personnel resources. During regular service hours (research funds did not allow a 24-hour service), an opportunity for communication exists. This ongoing connection leads to a close relationship to the clients, enabling the service personnel to activate and motivate the elderly. A feeling of security can be conveyed. The close and regular contacts lead to a measurable improvement in personal health and well-being.

A wide range of services is thinkable, supporting the work of regular out-patient caregivers in the field. This example emphasises at the same time the most important limitation of the new service-- the *HausTeleDienst* was not designed to replace, but to support and augment direct personal contacts.

After a relative short period of time, the personnel at the service centre felt comfortable using the new technology. Even when technical problems occurred during the first months, they could handle the system. This issue was also of less importance than expected for the elderly, as it will be described next.

3.3 Service Use Experience

Issues of acceptability of a video camera in the home were much less important than involved researchers, and especially the service provider organisation, expected. The camera was placed inside a set top box on a regular TV and could be closed and opened by sliding a simple, relatively large shutter back and forth. Because every client was able to handle it without any problems, it immediately gave them security and a feeling of being in power over the technology-- at a glance they could see whether the camera was able to transmit pictures or not. It was a high-quality camera, allowing for an acceptable quality of pictures to be transmitted even with relatively dim lighting in the room.

Much effort was also invested in designing a most simple, easy-to-use remote control unit. It is relatively large in size, about the size of a larger paperback. On the top, it contains 10 large buttons to control the TV; on the bottom, there are 4 large buttons to control the video communications. Both functions are separated by a sliding shutter. Thus, the often severely limited abilities of elderly persons to see and to handle technical devices with little which do not provide sufficient contrast and are not attuned to their declining skills was taken into account. Even very old ladies in their nineties were without any difficulties able to manage the technology.

A more important problem was the fact that at the beginning, the system was not completely reliable. Technical problems led to criticism by some users, stating that technical improvements were necessary. Later, none of the clients had complaints about the technical system, its usability, or its functionality.

In general, the "*HausTeleDienst*" was rated very positively by users. Suggestions for improvements concerned additional personnel and longer service hours, if possible 24 hours a day. The most valuable service component was the active care and information service, although the users did understand the *Haus-Tele-Dienst* services as a general service consisting of different service elements. 10 of the users pointed out that the opportunity to get in contact with someone when *they* want it is most important for them. The second most important advantage of the service is the possibility for immediately getting direct help, if needed.

Almost all of the users emphasised their very personal and close relationships to the staff-- which were not inhibited by the video communications. The new service has had quite an impact on their lives. Five of them believe that the service directly changed their lives. Statements range from "I don't feel lonely anymore" to "I have a more regular daily routines, I've regular meals again" or "I have more joy in my life". Much better than any other research results can these statements describe the real, lasting, positive impact of this video-based social support system on its clients' quality of life.

4. Ethical and Social Aspects in Service Delivery

4.1 The "Big Brother" Syndrome

There is a big fear in society, mainly within younger generations, that there will be no privacy anymore. Any attempt to implement video communications strengthens these feelings: George Orwell's vision that "Big Brother is watching you" becomes reality. Here we are concerned with the ethics of freedom, self-determination, replacement of personal contacts, privacy, etc., versus the ethics of control, dependence, etc.

Our experience has shown that the elderly have far less fear of being observed than researchers expected. None of the participants of the pilot ever used the built-in mechanical shutter to close the camera's lens-- probably because it was so obvious to them that they could manage it whenever they felt like it. Most of them stated that they did not need to have the "picture free-button" to allow the service provider staff to have a look into their flat. Some of them even pointed out that they would like to be observed permanently because "that would give me more security". For most of the younger service provider personnel and the researchers, this has been unthinkable. This example demonstrates that there are different needs and, related to those, different perceptions of the same issue even within one society.

The passing-on of personal data has to be limited and strictly controlled. Nevertheless, there is some need to pass on data: a close cooperation between different outpatient services makes some data-transfer necessary. A responsible use of data, e.g., on chronic diseases and special physical limitations, is mandatory to prevent miss-use. Technical limits and, more importantly, education and training of staff have to assure that there is no unnecessary passing-on of personal data.

4.2 Replacement of Personal Contacts

The main concern against developing and implementing social services based on video telecommunications is probably the fear of replacing direct social communications and relationships with remote connection to an unknown person or, more drastically, to a machine. Such services seem to be helpful and acceptable to most people in a business environment, and sometimes even in a private environment. In the social field mainly, in the field of the elderly and mentally impaired people, this does not seem to be the right way. However, the question one always should keep in mind is: "Do we indeed want to *substitute* personal services with artificial (i.e., telecommunication-based) services?" If this were really the case, ethical criticism would be fully justified.

Rather, however, videophone-based services should be implemented *only in addition* to existing outpatient services. Any service development concept should focus on integration into existing outpatient service networks. Major reorganisation efforts might need to be considered if a more efficient, effective, and client-addressed videotelephone-based social support service is to be implemented. This will lead to additional costs in the beginning of the implementation process; however this will later enable organisations to optimise service delivery.

4.3 Self-Determination

A further key issue is the right of self-determination. Especially in social care, self-determination is a frequent point of discussion. There are countless examples where self-determination is not taken into account, although personnel know that the personal will of the elderly should always be fulfilled. Sometimes there are organisational needs which do not allow the time necessary for persuading an individual to do something, e.g., drink or eat. Sometimes the basic right of self-determination can even mean that the personnel of a facility or of outpatient services have to accept that someone has decided to die. What is to be done if someone just does not want to drink anymore? Is it ethically legitimate to watch someone dying, or would it be more justifiable to force-feed the patient?

As long as service provision can assure self-determination, ethical issues are relatively easy to handle. In our project, this issue did not become important because users were always in the (technical) position to terminate the service (block the camera), or to refuse an incoming call. If this were not the case, but rather for instance the video-phone were used as a monitoring or surveillance instrument-- e.g., for night-time coverage-- then the question is more complicated. In such a case, people would often not be aware of the fact that they were being observed. On the other hand, if one observed the regular practise in night-time care (coverage), one might suggest different ways of service delivery. Is it humane for older people in nursing homes to be awakened by staff just because they are on their regular duty round, or would it be more humane if service provision could be more flexible due to technology which allows personnel to check if a patient is sleeping or not? Among experts, it is unquestioned that uninterrupted sleep is extremely important for the elderly. A humane technology could help do this, but only if the client agrees to this kind of observation.

4.4 Privacy

Another critical point, related to the coverage of the living area, is privacy. This question is ambivalent and can be discussed from different points of view, too. Regarding emergency coverage, it might make sense to cover the whole flat with several moveable cameras, but, respecting privacy, this does not seem to be a desirable aim. In several surveys, some heads of nursing homes brought up this issue by pointing out that most accidents happen in the bathroom or toilet of the flat. They argue that a camera in those rooms would be most helpful for emergency coverage.

Obviously, these rooms especially seem to be the most critical, and at the same time, the most sensitive ones. Does one really want to be observed on the toilet or under the shower? For most of us, this seems to be the ultimate private area of each flat. For some of the elderly, this is obviously different. In interviews, some of them suggested that they would certainly need a camera in this area.

4.5 Budgeting and Social Policy

One major deficit in the situation of the elderly is that there is little money available for social integration, prevention, and rehabilitation for older people living at home. All experts agree that prevention will become more important in the future. Research in gerontology has proved the importance of prevention. Gerontologists are trying to use benefit/costs models to persuade policy makers and economists. If policy-makers accept those long-term effects, there is a possibility that prevention activities will be financially covered in the future. First concepts along these lines can be observed in Germany. The new elderly care insurance system will support technical aids like alarm systems and, hopefully, video telephony services in the future.

Besides this scientific gerontological argument, there is a more pragmatic one: the new generation of the elderly will be able to spend more money and more time on their personal health, i.e., new markets will open. Health classes, special courses for the elderly, etc., are becoming popular. They are already offered by various organisations. This new attitude towards aging will result in new demands, which will necessitate a change in social services policies. New public and individual services need to be offered to fulfill these needs.

5. Outlook

This pilot has proven that video-telephony has a realistic potential to ensure social interaction, medical support, and safety for the elderly and disabled, independently of whether they are living in their homes or in service flats. An integrated service concept can significantly improve the quality of life of the elderly and disabled. It could be shown that the telecommunications component can also support the professional work of personnel in sheltered housing facilities.

patient does not feel "abandoned" to a computer, keeping the therapist accessible and relevant. The Fonetix project represents a study and development of a value-added Internet application that is oriented towards providing a service to people who are hearing impaired. This speech therapy web site is intended for deployment over a traditional Internet or clinical Intranet. The framework includes Web-centric specialised training materials, monitoring software to assist the hearing-impaired person, video and audio conferencing, and illustrates the use of application sharing for a remote diagnostic application. In the past half-decade of development of the WWW, new browser technologies have routinely altered the common view of the Web and on-line communication. Other advances including new protocols, compression techniques and new media formats, as well as helper and plug-in applications to display specialised media formats such as movies and audio files, have facilitated the development of this online consultative environment.

The types of tools being developed here are intended to augment current practices and techniques being used by speech language pathologists. The long term goal of the Fonetix system is to allow speech pathology patients to interact in a meaningful manner with a speech pathologist albeit remotely over the Internet.

2. Methods

Fonetix is a multimedia online software kit developed for the Web for improving speech and hearing perception. Design and writing online documentation is not a one-pass process. It is a continual process of successive refinement [4]. Development of online documentation is iterative, cumulative, and empirical. It is iterative in that several cycles of development are required, cumulative in that we learn and improve through each cycle, and empirical in that improvements are based on testing and experience with working prototypes of the system.

The World Wide Web is the most visual and dynamic part of the Internet, and is accessible with any Web browser (e.g. Netscape Navigator, Microsoft Explorer). The Web refers to a specific kind of Internet interface, complete with text, sound and graphics. The creation of an effective multimedia clinical consultation tool, such as Fonetix, requires the complex blending of technological, methodological and clinical elements. Appropriate design, programming and content are all necessary to create a cohesive on-line speech and hearing therapy site [5]. The current functional model of Fonetix takes advantage of the programming languages and tools for Internet programming. The most basic programming of the web pages have been done using Hypertext Markup Language (HTML), other programming languages such as Java and Javascript were used to increase the interactivity of information transmitted via the WWW. Move advanced languages, such as Perl (Practical Extraction and Report Language) and CGI scripting (Common Gateway Interface) expand static hypertext pages into dynamic ones.

Authoring an online document is a complex process involving multiple activities. With Web technology, we have focused on building reusable information modules (much like *Object Oriented Programming*) (OOP) rather than creating specific linear structures [6]. This process breaks down a complex structure using separate programs for each function. The activities required authoring an online document could be grouped into three phases: data capture, content preparation, and database preparation.

In the data capture phase, individual media elements are created and stored as digital data. Words, pictures, sounds, animation, and video segments are all created or captured electronically and stored in a digital format. In the content preparation phase, the different media elements are integrated into a consistent form. Individual files are imported or referenced from a file or database of topics. In the database preparation phase, the topics are structured and indexed so those users can access individual topics. Links are added to connect topics, keywords are added to let users retrieve topics, and menus are created to permit selecting individual topics.

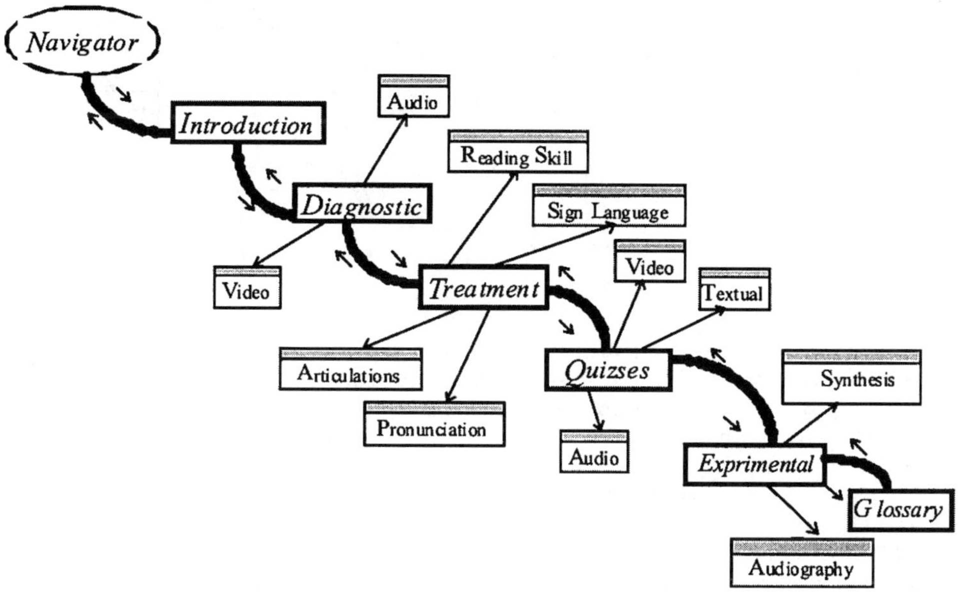

Figure 1. Fonetix navigator sequential cluster

Figure 1 illustrates Fonetix navigation paths, which identify the basic functions and an overview of the Fonetix program. These navigation paths provide a directed and systematic method upon which the Fonetix elements are structures. The methodology for using Fonetix starts with a diagnostic session. Ideally this would use audio and video equipment to record the patient (possibly interactively with a therapist). The results would go to a database and a therapist would analyse them and choose the training plan from the learning section. The Fonetix learning section covers articulation, reading skills, pronunciation, and sign language.

Fonetix includes some quiz or test sessions for practice. These test sessions can be audio or video or textual. Results collected may be sent to the database for problem analysis and provide the therapist with a audio/video patient history to improve the treatment plan.

3. Results

3.1. Diagnostics within Fonetix

Fonetix starts with patient diagnostics. The diagnostics are made in different styles, using combinations of audio and video for problem evaluation. The areas of speech diagnostics are plosives, fricatives, affircatives, aspirates, glides, nasals and blends. The audio and video results can be scored with an error score which therapists can use to determine the patient's problems. Figure 2 illustrates Fonetix diagnostics.

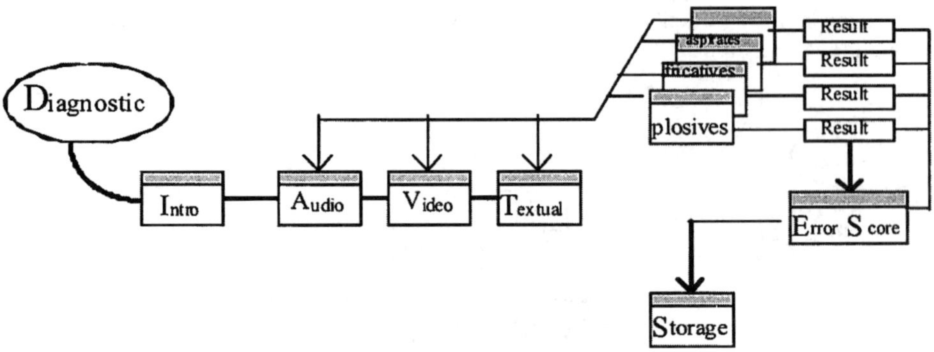

Figure 2. Fonetix diagnostics sequential cluster

For example, Fonetix asks the patient to say and record the words containing affricatives, like: *matches* or *bridges*. The therapist can remotely listen the patient's voice determine whether the pronunciation is correct, has indistinct or simple substitution problem, gross substitution, or omission problems. The therapist is directly involved in the diagnostic section of Fonetix. The analysis however may be off-line using prerecorded audio and video. This process can also be automated. The patient's results can be stored in a database for future reference.

In order to monitor patients over the Internet, Fonetix does web document sharing. This means that any time the patient and therapist are logged on to Fonetix, they are able to see and communicate with each other over the Internet using a video camera, audio equipment, and chat in real-time for textual correspondence within Fonetix. Figure 3 illustrates the use of the Internet as the means of communication between patient and therapist.

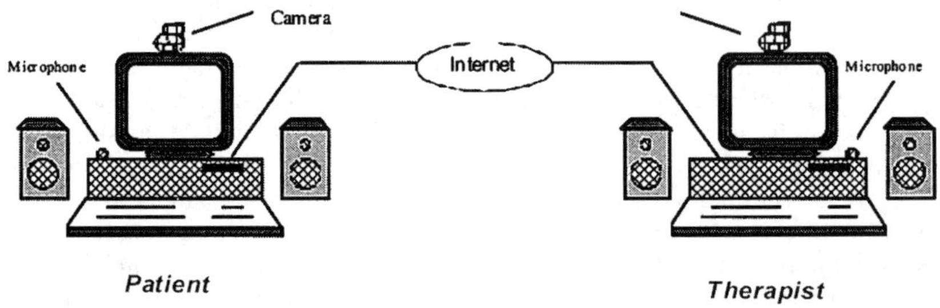

Figure 3. Fonetix Remote Consulting

As mentioned before, Fonetix is an Internet research tool and many of the elements for diagnosis are experimental in nature. With Fonetix we are able to experiment and conduct research on audiography over the Internet. To a large degree we are trying to integrate the patient more directly into his or her therapy. One manner of accomplishing this is by remotely facilitating the patient hearing test. The audiogram is a plot of the faintest sound that can be heard (threshold) at various frequencies. Thresholds are determined with earphones via air conduction (AC) for sound going through the entire auditory system [7]. Fonetix includes this function, which allows the user to record his or her audiogram. The auditory element of Fonetix is still under development, and although we have shown that it is possible to conduct this test remotely, there are still issues of standardisation that must be addressed. It is anticipated that the audiogram function will be used to monitor for departures from a predefined norm, as opposed to being the mechanism to set standards.

Also incorporated into the Fonetix is an implementation of Klatt synthesis program (Klatlk) for synthetic speech waveforms. The Klatlk software reads a file containing synthesis parameters (typically created by a program called gensyn) and writes a synthetic speech waveform file. Gensyn accepts input from a data file, creates as output that is the input file to the Klatlk program. This file can be either visual represented to the user to be used in a feedback manner for speech modification, or forwarded to the clinician for evaluation of a patient's speech patterns.

3.2. Treatment Plan within Fonetix

The basic methods of speech therapy treatment are designed to evoke communicative behaviours. Figure 4 shows the Fonetix treatment plan.

The areas of treatment include articulations, reading skills, pronunciation, and sign language. The articulations include audio, video, and animation examples of the main places of articulation. Reading skills helps patients become familiar with fluency and speed. Pronunciation focuses on isolated words and learning language. The sign language section is included for the severely hearing impaired as well as for persons interested in learning sign language basics.

Various instructions are used in Fonetix to treat articulation disorders. Treatment plans may include combinations of articulations, reading skills for speech fluency, as well as pronunciation treatment for particular types of words and numbers.

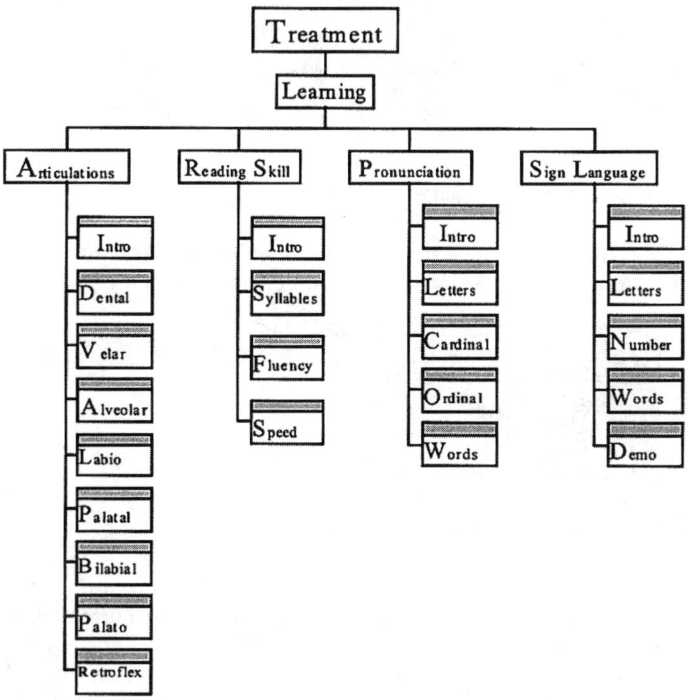

Figure 4. Fonetix treatment hierarchy

In order to form consonants, the airstream through the vocal tract must be obstructed in some way. Consonants can therefore be classified according to the place and manner of this obstruction. The primary articulators that can cause an obstruction in most languages are the lips, the tongue tip and blade, and the back of the tongue.

Articulations are classified into eight sections (Fig. 4). Each articulation section includes an audio, animation, movie and practice component. Figure 5 shows the introduction to dental articulation. Every introduction page illustrates a specific articulation, using sample words with pronunciation and audio. From this page the user may navigate to movie, animation, or practice sessions for that articulation

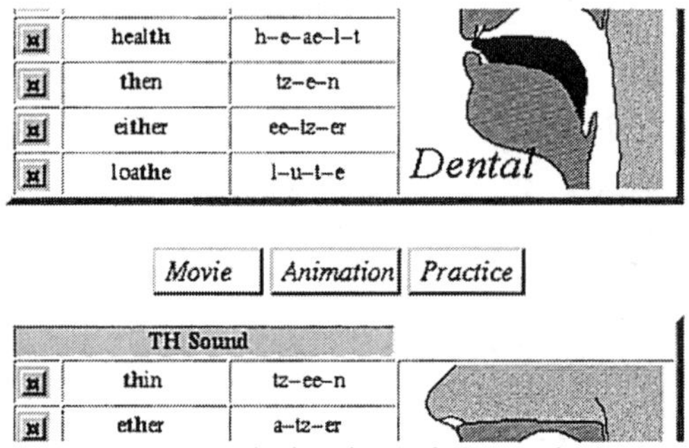

Figure 5. Fonetix dental articulation section

The animation shows the movement of the oral organs, indicating the correct position of the tongue and lips. Figure 6 illustrates frames from the dental articulation animation.

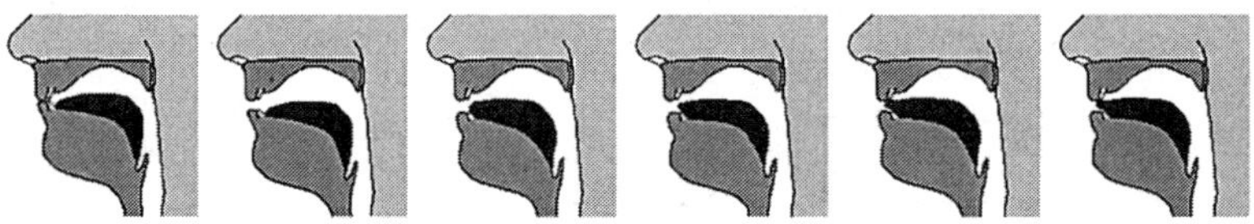

Figure 6. Fonetix dental animation section

The movie section shows the face, lips, and tongue movement of a native speaker during the production of the correct sound. Figure 7 shows some sample movie frames within Fonetix.

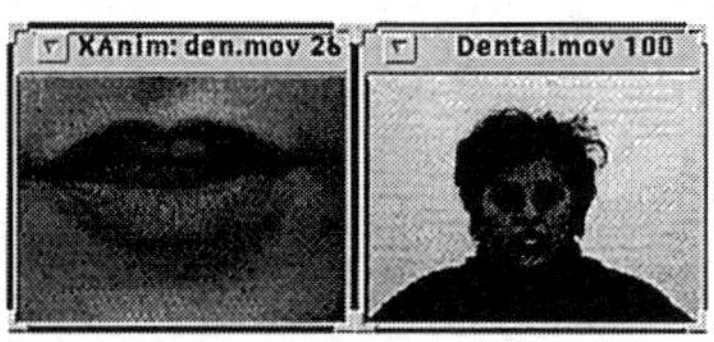

Figure 7. Fonetix dental movie section

Every practice section has sentences, which have the same sound in different words in the sentence. With this practice session a patient can try to produce the sound at the correct way. They also have the ability to step through the sentence, slowing down or speeding up the whole sentence while at the same time saying the words. Figure 8 illustrates the dental practice section. The results of the practice sessions (audio and video) can be recorded and logged for use by the therapist. The therapist may also introduce alternative sentences or isolated words for individualised practice.

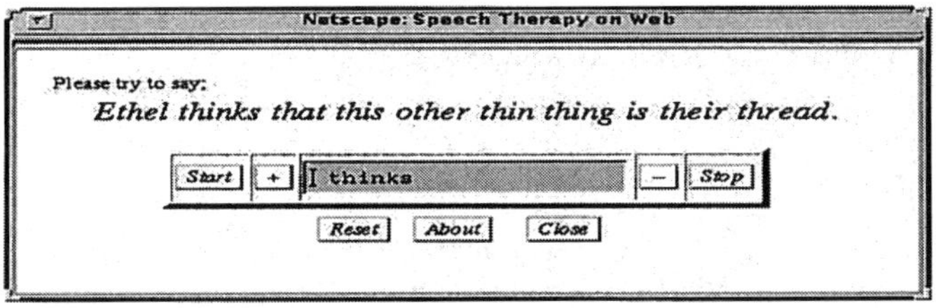

Figure 8. Fonetix dental practice section

Reading skills are useful for treating disorders of fluency. In speech, we control the pitch of an utterance by changing the vibration rate of the vocal cords. The faster they vibrate the higher the pitch. English also distinguishes different phrases, and with different intonation contours. Intonation is the use of pitch in a phonetic phrase.

The intonation system of English is very complex and not completely understood. Fonetix examines a number of typical contours, using English tongue twisters, each sentence of twisters, illustrates different intonation contours. Twisters are useful for learning fluency in speech, controlling the speed of speech, managing airflow, controlling the gentle onset of phonation, and also for reducing the rate of speech through syllable prolongation or to a level where speech is free from stuttering.

3.3. Quizzes within Fonetix

Within Fonetix a therapist is able provide continuous feedback to a patient on his or her performance. Quizzes on different text combinations are useful for treating stuttering and voice disorders. Audio quizzes are useful for hearing evaluation, video quizzes are useful for lip-reading and perception practice. Figure 9 shows the Fonetix quiz cluster.

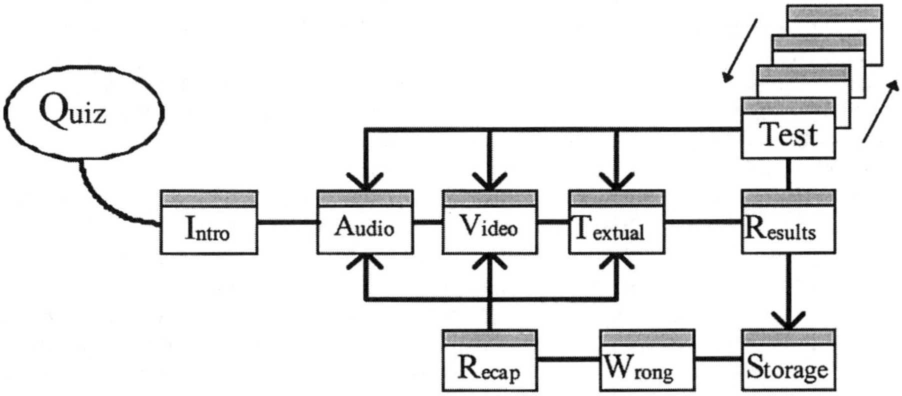

Figure 9. Fonetix quiz sequential cluster

When this information is systematically given to patients, their performance or movement toward a target may be reinforced. The information given back to a person from a system about how the person has been performing is called feedback. Feedback provides reinforcement when it increases the rate of response or some quality of it.

Basically the quiz cluster is able to initially assist in determining a patient's problems, and provide information on the patient's treatment, progress, and recommendations for continuing treatment. Increased use of the Fonetix quiz program in treatment will also facilitate mechanical feedback. Information about the performance levels is feedback and when used systematically, it can increase the rate of responses.

3.4. Summary of Fonetix Design and Implementation

Fonetix is being written to be as a platform independent application, using Java and JavaScript as the development language. This allows for easy access from any browser on the Internet facilitating remote speech language pathology. Extensions currently under development include facilities for improved remote monitoring of progress and remote interaction with a pathologist.

4. Discussion

Although the Internet has been around for over 20 years and has seen unprecedented growth over the past 5 years, there is still uncertainty about how to best utilise this tool within telemedicine and telehealth. At present, it is a massive distributed database housing vast amounts of information accessible from Web based browsers. The real potential of the Internet can only be realised as applications are developed which are truly interactive and effective. At the forefront of interactively are distance learning and remote consultation. Although only in the early stages of development, these applications add value to the Internet. This particular project addresses a specific telehealth application, namely speech therapy for the Web.

Fonetix is one of the first web sites in content development for a value-added Internet application. Even in its experimental state, it provides speech therapy professionals with a model of which aspects of speech therapy that can be developed over the Internet. Fonetix is a functional prototype, in the process of moving from the academic research environment into the practical clinical one. It is only after this transition will we be able to effectively determine the benefits that this types of remote consultation has for both patients and therapists. The attempt to make this transition has unveiled a few challenges that must be addressed.

The first is the necessity for need for *adequate infrastructure*. Community infrastructure must meet the needs of Internet use. There must be a reliable electrical and telephone service. And, of course, both the client and the therapist must both have access to a computer. Although federal programs are dedicated to the 'wiring' of the nation, this does not immediately equate into Internet access in some remote communities. Continued development of the Internet in terms of bandwidth and computing environments will make programs such as Fonetix useful for remote speech therapy, and allow the framework to function in a role of distance training and remote consultation via the Internet

In addition, issues of *technology acceptance* must be addressed. Familiarity with the technology cannot be taken for granted. Fonetix takes full advantage of the multimedia capabilities of the Internet and therefore requires users to be familiar with basic computer usage, as well as being at ease with more advanced audio and video elements. Children seem to adapt with great ease to computer technologies [8]. Since it is anticipated that the initial implementation of Fonetix will be in the school system, the clients will be children. However, the therapist, the paraprofessionals, as well as older patients must also be able to develop the required skills associated with Internet usage in order to expand the usage of the Fonetix application.

Perhaps the greatest facilitator of the successful transition of Fonetix from the research to the clinical environment will be the *willing participation* of the users. The successful development and implementation of any telehealth system requires the active and willing participation of a number of groups-the technology experts, the clinical experts, the patients and policy makers. In Canada, where health services and policies fall under provincial mandates, telehealth applications must include the support of the health departments.

Future research into Fonetix will include more automated analysis of a patient's speech using audio or video [9]. These techniques will exploit clustering methods such as self-organising maps to assist in diagnosis as well as provide guidelines during treatment. Future versions should also include more accurate animation and synchronisation [10]. In addition, the integration of applications such as videoconferences can be used to enhance patient therapist interaction. Other avenues to explore would be the use of Virtual Reality Modelling Language (VRML) to create three-dimensional animation.

The public version of Fonetix can be found at the following URL: **http://www.ee.umanitoba.ca/~morawej/Speech.**

References

[1] P. Jackson, L. Bailey, C. Lee, D. Humenchuk, and L. Dessens. Functional communication for all learners, *Manitoba Special Education Review,* 1998.
[2] L.S. Snyder and D.M. Downery. Developmental differences in the Relationship between Oral Language Deficits and Reading, *Topics in Language Disorders* 17 (1997) 27-40
[3] M. Donahue, D. Cole, and S. Hartas. Links between Language and Emotional/Behavioural Disorders, *Education and Treatment of Children* 17(3) (1994) 244-254.
[4] W. Horton. Design and Writing Online Documentation: hypermedia for self-supporting products, (2nd edition) *John Wiley & Sons, Inc.,* New York, 1994.
[5] B. P. Yuhas, M. H. Goldstein, Jr., and T. J. Sejnowski. Integration of acoustic and visual speech signal using neural networks., *IEEE Commun. Mag.* (1989) 56-71.
[6] D. and J. Wesley. Developing Real-World Internet. *The Coriolis Group Books,* Scottsdale, 1996.
[7] J. T. Jacobson and J. L. Northern. Diagnostic Audiology, *Pro. Ed,* Austin, Texas, 1991.
[8] American Speech Language Hearing Association. Inclusive Practices for Children and Youths with Communication Disorders: Position Statement and Technical Report, *ASHA* (Spring 1996) 35-44
[9] S. Morishima, K. Aizawa, and H. Harashima. An intelligent facial image coding driven by speech and phoneme, *Proc. IEEE ICASSP* (1989) P1795.
[10] E. Caella, F. Lavagetto, and R. Miani. A time-delay neural network for speech to lips movements conversion, *Proc. Int. Conf. Artificial Neural Networks,* 1994.

Address for correspondence

R.D. McLeod
Internet Innovation Centre, Faculty of Engineering,
University of Manitoba,
Winnipeg, Canada, R3T 5V6
http://www.ee.umanitoba.ca/~morawej/Speech.

M. Nerlich and R. Kretschmer (Eds.)
IOS Press, 1999

Evaluation of a Canadian Telepsychiatry Service

Douglas A. URNESS
Ponoka, Alberta, Canada

Abstract: A telepsychiatry pilot project linking five rural general hospitals and Alberta Hospital Ponoka was implemented in June 1996 as a response to both a scarcity of psychiatric resources in the Province of Alberta and the emphasis on community-based care. Psychiatrists located at Alberta Hospital Ponoka provided psychiatric consultations using videoconferencing technology in response to referrals from general practitioners. The project was evaluated through the use of questionnaires administered to consumers, service providers, and psychiatric consultants. Questionnaires were supplemented by interviews, site visits, logs, telephone interviews with consumers, and surveys to general practitioners at the rural sites.

A total of 109 consultations occurred during the pilot stage. Results strongly suggested acceptance and satisfaction with the consultation by consumers, general practitioners and psychiatrists. The patient's perceived benefits included timeliness of service, service within their own community, decreased work time loss for self or family, and positive outcomes as a result of specialist expertise.

Up until September 30, 1998 a total of 535 consultations had been completed, 381 of which were new referrals and 154 of which were follow up referrals. Seventy-two different physicians referred to the service. The practice profile is dramatically different to outpatient psychiatric practice in which approximately 90% of patient contacts are follow-up visits.

1. Introduction

The development of this program took place in the setting of significant structural and funding changes to the healthcare system in the Province of Alberta. Funding had been globally decreased at both the federal and provincial level. Hospital beds were reduced, many physicians moved their practices to other countries or other provinces, thousands of nurses were laid off and healthcare became the number one concern of Canadians. Subsequently a period of re-investment in healthcare occurred but in a more accountable manner. Media sources often quoted the Government as saying "we are not going to just throw dollars at healthcare anymore". The planning doctrine of "medical necessity" as defined by clinicians increasingly yielded to managed care which combined clinical, economic and administrative factors in a rational manner to the planning of healthcare services. Accountability from a clinical, financial, and administrative perspective is increasingly required for new or expanded healthcare services.

A particularly scarce healthcare resource in Alberta has been outpatient psychiatric consultation services. Waiting lists were commonly as long as four months and occasionally longer than a year. Under these circumstances, the development of the telepsychiatry service linked with a careful evaluation project was made possible.

Telepsychiatry is one of the leading applications in the growing field of Clinical Telehealth. Several excellent reviews describe these developments.[1] Telepsychiatry is essentially the provision of psychiatric services through a two-way interactive television. Consultant psychiatrists were located in a studio within a large psychiatric hospital and patients received services in a studio in a small general hospital. The goals of the project included:

- Enhanced ability of general practitioners/consumers to communicate with providers of specialized mental health services;
- Improved access to psychiatrists in a timely fashion.
- Facilitation of quality care within the home community
- Removal of geographic barriers limiting access to specialty mental health consultations.
- Greatly reduced consumer and staff travel time.

The Provincial Mental Health Advisory Board (PMHAB) administered the program. The Board provides province-wide services in dedicated psychiatric hospitals as well as community mental health clinics. General hospitals and public health units are administered through 17 separate Regional Health Authorities (RHA's). The RHA's and the PMHAB report to the provincial Minister of Health. A telepsychiatry partnership agreement between RHA's and the PMHAB detailed each organization's administrative and funding responsibilities. The PMHAB provided equipment, operational training, guidelines, coordination of quality monitoring, technical expertise, and communication planning services. RHA's were responsible for actively participating in the Telepsychiatry Service, funding line installation costs and monthly charges, funding facility renovations, participation in quality monitoring and working collaboratively with the PMHAB. The equipment was made available for purposes beyond telepsychiatry.

2. Material and Methods

Consultation services were provided using high-quality, dual monitor room-style videoconferencing systems. The systems were compliant with ITU Standards, able to operate using a variety of networks and provided a full motion video up to 30 frames per second. Six centrex telephone lines connected the sites. In addition to line installation, videoconference room renovations included installing full spectrum lighting, sound proofing, fabric wallcoverings and window coverings to eliminate natural light.

Consultations were arranged through a relatively traditional process of receiving a request from a General Practitioner's (GP) office followed by a referral letter. Although requests may have originated at a mental health clinic or from the patient's family, a GP's referral was mandatory in order to provide continuity of care within the community. A local telepsychiatry coordinator, usually with a mental health nursing background, served as a facilitator, contact person and as mental healthcare provider. The primary clinical model was to provide initial consultation to the community health care resources with follow-up visits reserved for more difficult cases. Consultation reports were prepared and usually faxed back to the GP's within two days. A variety of psychiatrists provided services.

The initial rollout of telepsychiatry involved the service provision site at Alberta Hospital Ponoka (AHP) and five rural sites. An expansion to a further six sites was approved and rolled out in July 1998. The initial five sites were located in the traditional catchment area for AHP. Four of the six expansion sites lie in northern Alberta, outside the traditional catchment area.

Scheduling of the service is accomplished by allocating blocks of psychiatric consultant time, usually of three or four hour's duration. The number of blocks varied from two to nine a week depending on availability of staff. New consultations were scheduled for 1.5 hours and follow-up consultations for 45 minutes. Consultations were provided to different sites during each block, depending on demand.

The pilot project set out to evaluate the satisfaction of consumers, services providers, and psychiatrists, the appropriateness of the technology, the appropriateness of the program implementation, and the effectiveness and impact of the program. Methodology included obtaining feedback from consumers, service providers, psychiatrists and site coordinators using questionnaires, follow-up telephone interviews and site visits.

3. Results

The pilot project evaluation questionnaires revealed high levels of satisfaction by consumers, service providers and consultants.[2] The only psychiatrist reporting an unsatisfactory experience attributed this to technical problems. Ninety-four percent of patients indicated that they would use the service again and 97% indicated they would recommend it to a friend. See Figure 1 below.

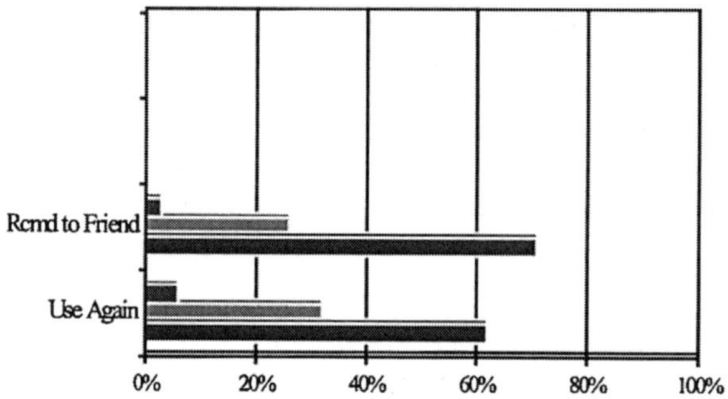

Fig.1: Satisfaction Ratings of Telepsychiatry

Consumers, service providers and consultants felt comfortable in their ability to interact with participants. See Figure 2 below. Psychiatrists commented on a "spotlight" effect giving a sense that the service was something special and one wanted to do a really good job. There also seemed to be less time pressure as a result of the scheduling. There was a very low "no show" rate at approximately 5%. Some psychiatrists commented on a reduced sense of dependency between the psychiatrist and the consumer.

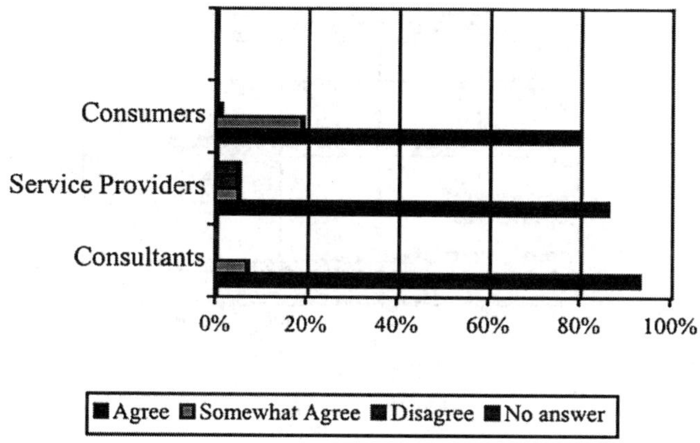

Fig. 2: Agreement with statement: "I was comfortable with my ability to interact with participants"

All surveyed parties largely felt able to present information in the same manner as they would have in person. See Figure 3 below.

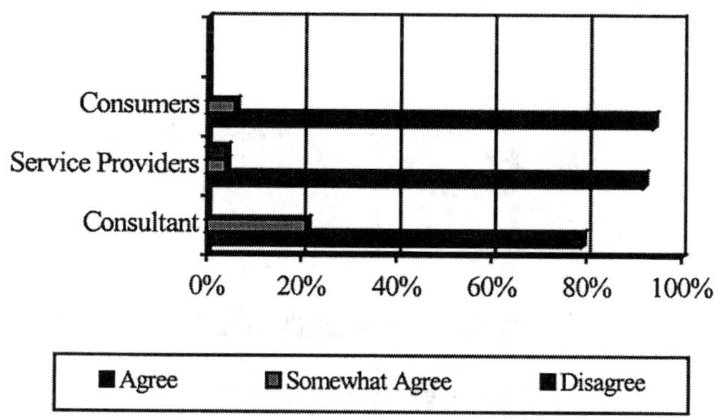

Fig. 3: "The technology was appropriate for the application."

Figure 4 breaks down some technology assessments to various categories. Picture and sound quality were rated least favourably, but the overall assessment was deviated slightly in favour of the higher responses regarding environment and ease of use.

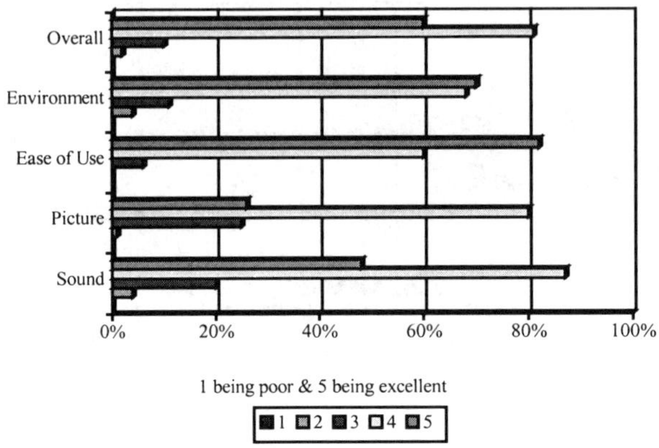

Fig. 4: Technology Assessment – Total Ratings by Question

Eighty percent of consumers agree that they would rather use telepsychiatry than travel. One hundred percent of consumers agree that they would rather use telepsychiatry than wait to see a psychiatrist. Interestingly 42% of consumers indicated they would rather use telepsychiatry than see a psychiatrist in person. See Figure 5 below.

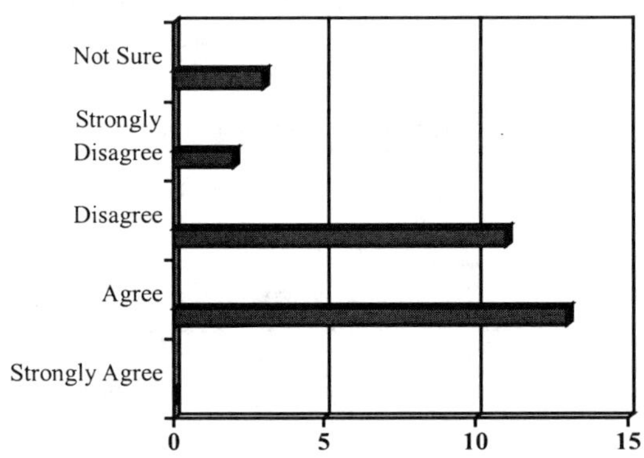

Fig. 5: Consumers' level of agreement with the statement: "I would rather use telepsychiatry than see a psychiatrist in person."

Various speculations may explain these responses. Use of technology is an increasingly acceptable social phenomenon in virtually all aspects of our lives. Many people like the technology and found videoconferencing to be an enjoyable experience. Perhaps the slightly different service delivery model made people feel more respected and cared for.

The threat of boundary violations may be less likely and consumers can easily turn the psychiatrist off with the push of a button.

Other consumer comments from interviews included:

- No family supports so travel difficult – would have to tell someone I needed a ride to the city and why;
- Couldn't wait… would be sicker;
- Expense, parking and driving in the city would make a difference, I probably wouldn't go;
- Would miss a whole day of work to travel.

After approximately two years of operations the service has provided a total of 535 consultations 71% were new referrals and 29% were follow up referrals). Referrals were obtained from 72 different physicians. The practice profile is contrasted to a report on practice profiles in the United States. Psychiatrists in individual practice have 8% patient contacts as new referrals while psychiatrists in group practice have 12 % patient contacts as being new referrals.[3] Only four patients were admitted to Alberta Hospital Ponoka immediately following a consultation. Many patients however, were in local general hospitals at the time of the referral. See Table 1 below.

Patient Profile Male/Female

Age	Median Age	42
	Range	14-91
Gender	Male	28%
	Female	72%
History of Hospitalization	Inpatient in community hospital at time of consult	22%
	Previous history of hospitalization in community or specialized facilities	41%
Population at risk	Referrals -physician indicated suicidal intent or ideation	33%
History of mental illness	Percentage with history of mental illness for over 1 year	55%
Most frequent Diagnosis	Depression	40%
	Schizophrenia	9%
	Panic Disorders	9%
Most common reason for referral	Management of previous diagnosis	64%

Table 1: Patient Profile Male/Female

Recommendations from the pilot project included:

- Telepsychiatry should be planned and implemented as part of a continuum of mental health and other health services;
- Six centrex lines are sufficient for psychiatric consultations;

- Involving physicians, health care provider and community mental health professionals in the planning stages may increase utilization;
- Marketing strategies need to be community based;
- Staged implementation supports local problem solving;
- Implementation plans should include dedicated time of participants
- Consumer data should be integrated with existing data basis
- The project structure includes a method for clinical-administrative decision making

The pilot project and subsequent implementation of an operational telepsychiatry service reaching out from a psychiatric treatment facility to rural communities was seen as successful. Various indicators of this success included:

- Enhanced responsiveness to GP's
- Administrative partnership with RHA's;
- Evaluation as part of service development;
- Integration with local mental health services;
- Improved access to mental health services
- Increased convenience for consumers;
- Increased consumer choice;
- Controlled growth of service;
- User friendly equipment.

The high level of satisfaction by consumers, GP's, and psychiatrists was somewhat surprising given the very personal nature of a psychiatric consultation. This would suggest that barriers to development of telehealth services would not include consumer or physician dissatisfaction with properly functioning technology. Many telehealth pilot projects do not proceed to operational services, more likely due to administrative, funding, and demand variables.

Protocols for evaluating pilot projects and telepsychiatry services will be critical in justifying services and in guiding quality improvement. Our future evaluation plans include further refinement of the database, developing benchmark standards for satisfaction survey results, using qualitative interview follow-ups and quality of life questionnaires. A Donabedian framework of quality assurance as seen as a favourable general model for the clinical evaluation of telehealth services.[4] The specific methodologies and questionnaires require refinement and standardization.

Certain cautions must be applied to telehealth initiatives. Clinicians in general are cautious in adopting new models of service delivery. Enthusiasm by non-clinicians for telehealth projects may be viewed by clinicians as a "technological push" for telehealth projects in the absence of true clinical demand. Careful attention to clinical issues will be critical to the utilization of telehealth.

Individuals familiar with telehealth know that technology will not replace human relationships in the provision of healthcare services. Our experience with telepsychiatry would support the view that telehealth provides an acceptable and in some cases an improved way of facilitating these human relationships.

References

[1] Baer, L.; Elford, R.; Cukor, P., "Telepsychiatry at Forty: What Have We Learned?", Harvard Review of Psychiatry, May/June 1997.

[2] S. Doze; J. Simpson, Telepsychiatry Pilot Project Evaluation, Provincial Mental Health Advisory Board.

[3] Pincus, H., Peterson, B, Suarez, A., Zarin, D. "The Structure of Psychiatrists' Outpatient Practice", Psychiatric Services, June 1998.

[4] Dickey, B.; Hermann R., Eisen, S., "Assessing the Quality of Psychiatric Care: Research Methods and Application in Clinical Practice", Harvard Review of Psychiatry, July/August 1998.

Address for correspondence

Douglas A. Urness
Box 1000
Ponoka, Alberta Canada T4J 1R8
E-mail: PPugh@pmhab.ab.ca

The Impact of Telemedicine on Health Care Management
M. Nerlich and R. Kretschmer (Eds.)
IOS Press, 1999

Functional Characteristics of the Telemedical Network for the Medical Service of the Bundeswehr for Support of Operations Outside Germany and Civil-military Co-operation

C. OTTO[1], M. BOLTE[1], F. LINNEWEBER[1] T. WEBER[2]
[1]*Sanitätsamt der Bundeswehr, Abt. Medizinische Informatik, Bonn, Germany*
[2]*Deutsches Zentrum für Luft- und Raumfahrt e.V., Institut für Luft- und Raumfahrtmedizin, Köln, Germany*

Abstract: The maxim governing the accomplishment of medical tasks by the Medical Service of the Bundeswehr stipulates that the soldiers will, in case of illness, accident or injury, receive medical treatment to the standard they can expect in the Ferderal Republic of Germany.

In this context the introduction of telemedical applications into the Medical Service will improve the quality of the medical care through better and faster access for the medical officer assigned to a unit or a ship for requesting support to expert knowledge from military facilities or the civilian sector.

The telemedical system is based on a high-class commercial PC. This workstation can be extended as needed with medical devices (x-ray film digitizer, dermatoscope, otoscope) and allows linkage to other imaging methods (e.g. videocamera, ultrasound). Currently this system is under evaluation in a multi centre trial.

The participants of this telemedical network communicate via EURO ISDN lines with sufficient bandwidth. If terrestrial lines are not available the communication will be based on satellite capacity.

The application of internet-technology additionally provides access to medical data bases respectively allows civil-military co-operation and the interoperability between medical services of allied armed forces.

This future-orientated telemedical approach with its modular upwards-compatiblity will provide, especially in its mobile version and by using communication standards, the possibility to support necessary civil-military co-operation in the area of disaster relief and missions outside of Germany in the future.

Information technology is currently subject to drastic changes. New technologies for personal computers, server-systems, data-storage, and better, faster and cheaper data-links like ISDN enable us to utilize new forms of health care support like telemedicine.

We define telemedicine as "the investigation, monitoring and management of patients and the education of patients and staff using systems which allow ready access to expert advice and patient information no matter where the patient or the relevant information is located"[1].

Early on, the Medical Service of the Bundeswehr adopted these new technologies to realize a better quality of medical support for German soldiers. Even more challenging demands were introduced by the "out-of-area-operation" in Bosnia/SFOR. In such a situation, the Medical Service of the Bundeswehr is under an obligation to maintain the same standard of medical treatment in case of illness, injury or accident as provided by a civil medical institution in Germany.

Combined missions with allied forces and the need to cooperate with civil hospitals given host-nation-support underline the demand to use common technical standards in telecommunication in order to enable interoperability and thus maximize synergy of services. Examples include videoconferencing with H.320 standard, and transmission and storage of digitalized X-ray-images with DICOM-3 standard. Common technical platforms make use of high-class commercial PCs, ISDN-links with sufficient capacity, and the EURO-transmission protocol. In situations where no terrestrial lines are available, it is required to use adequate satellite links.

The Internet provides access to special medical data-bases and global services with the purpose of acquiring the medical information which is needed to minimize health-risks through better prevention and earlier therapy.

The standards just mentioned are requirements for enabling the exchange of medical information between the requesting physician on the one hand and the expert who is located in a distant military or civil institution on the other hand. Therefore our aim is to ensure a better and faster communication between the medical personnel of our armed forces within Germany, as well as those out-of-area and on-board of ships.

This communication can be constructed through either "online forms" or "offline forms". An example of the online form is the dialogue between the requesting physician and the expert. The offline form could be performed by file-transfer, e.g., with the transmission of digitalized X-ray-films or email messages with embedded still-images, scanned ECG-/EEG-strips, clinical laboratory reports, etc. A combination of both forms is also possible.

To evaluate the benefit of telemedicine for the Medical Service we started a study in 1997 with the German Aerospace Centre, Institute of Aerospace Medicine. Having analyzed user requirements, the study group committed itself to the functional specification for a standard telemedical workstation.

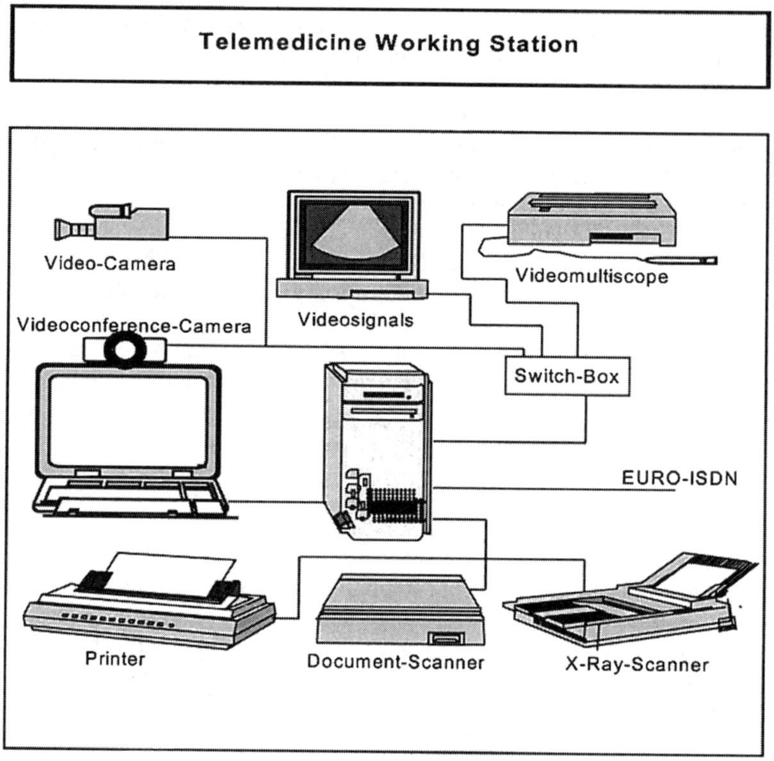

Figure1: Telemedicine Working Station

This computer system is composed of „commercial off-the-shelf" products. If required, it can be extended with medical devices, e.g., X-ray film digitizers, document-scanners, plain survey cameras, dermatoscopes, and otoscopes. Communication is performed *via* ISDN-lines with the additional option of using the TCP/IP protocol.

The telemedical workstation in the stand-alone version is an interim solution on the way to an integrated medical information and communication platform. It can be seen as a first step towards the implementation of the Electronic Patient Record, as it provides a solution for the storage and data-processing problems of multimedia patient data which result from the use of digital medical devices.

The following figure demonstrates the geographical extension of the telemedical systems in the Medical Service of the Bundeswehr.

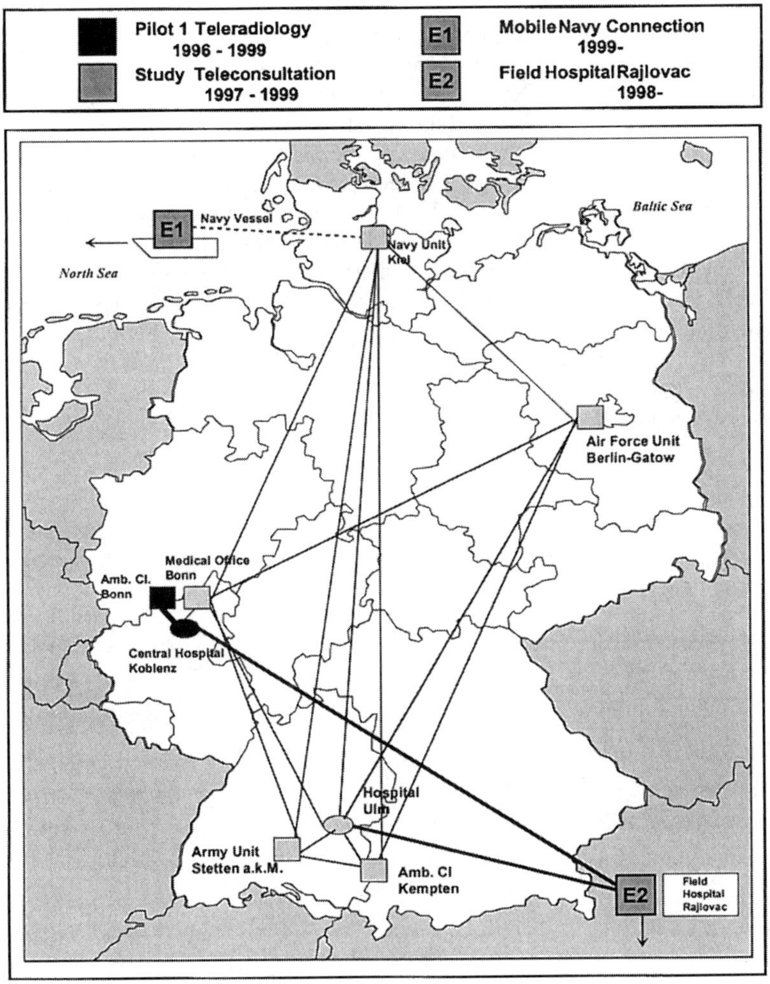

Figure 2: Extension of Telemedical Projects

The central concept of this discussion is being tested in a pilot project with the Bundeswehr Hospital in Ulm, one Army, one Air Force, one Navy Medical Center, and an Outpatient Clinic of the Central Services of the Medical Service have been assigned to this expert facility. Currently this system is under evaluation in a multi-user study in cooperation with the German Aerospace Centre. Upon completion of this study in 1999, we will extend telemedical support to the Medical Service of the German Armed Forces.

As previously considered, we want to establish all kinds of civil-military cooperation which are demanded and necessary to improve medical treatment on both sides. One option could be requesting contact with civil medical institutions, e.g, in order to transfer a digitized bloodpicture to the Institute for Tropical Diseases in Hamburg with the suspicious diagnosis of a Malaria disease. The Medical Service of the Bundeswehr is able-- in special cases and if wished-- to support medical treatment of civilians and to cooperate with civilian Non Governmental Organizations (NGO) during humanitarian missions based on common agreements with the United Nations and the OSCE.

These sorts of situational realities encourage cooperation not only within military and civil organizations and structures, but also between different allied forces, NGOs, host-nation-facilities and government organizations. Therefore, we take advantage of modern telemedical technologies in order to share knowledge, divide financial burden, and profit from better and faster cooperation-- especially where such cooperation has already existed.

Prerequisite for the further propogation of civil-military cooperation is the willingness to work together and to focus on what is required in the near future. Therefore the existence of common telematic standards should also be regarded and underlined especially during forums like this G-8-Symposium, during telematic-meetings of the European Union, and in the national and regional frame.

Address for correspondence

C. Otto
Sanitätsamt der Bundeswehr
Abt. Medizinische Informatik
Platanenweg 29
D-53225 Bonn, Germany

---

[1] *Nyno B J., Telektronik 89:4-11, 1993*

Webliography

Suggested Telemedicine Websites

We wish to provide a set of links that would each act as portals to a significant number of resources. Given the volatility and often ephemeral nature of Web information it is impossible to provide a comprehensive list of relevant sites, especially in a static print volume. Instead, we have tried to identify rich, well-tended, up-to-date (as of early 1999) starting points for finding whatever may be available in the near future. Additionally, we have included a few single-project sites that were substantial and active, primarily to offer examples of on-going real-world telemedicine efforts. Again, many others exist and will be arriving in the near future, hopefully accessible from links such as these.

We have not included many interesting corporate and descriptive product sites in order to avoid the appearance of any commercial endorsement. The exceptions to this rule of thumb were some commercial sites (e.g. a couple of journals) with dedicated sets of publicly-accessible resources, especially links to other sites. We encourage readers to use the links below as suggested starting points to launch into their own explorations - our goal has been to make this process as fruitful and easy to begin as possible. Many other commercial sites are extremely valuable and worth your attention as well.

Address for correspondence

David E. Moxley
University of Missouri - Columbia
Health Management & Informatics
324 Clark Hall
Columbia, Missouri, USA
E-mail: MoxleyD@health.missouri.edu

Category	URL	Title	Organization
Telemedicine	**http://208.129.211.51/**	Telemedicine Information Exchange	Telemedicine Research Center
Comments	*major support from the National Library of Medicine*		
Telemedicine	**http://telemedicine.partners.org/**	Partners Telemedicine	Partners HealthCare System
Comments	*Harvard Medical School, Mass. General Hospital, etc. consortium*		
Telemedicine	**http://www.atmeda.org/**	American Telemedicine Association Website	American Telemedicine Association
Telemedicine	**http://www.atsp.org/**	Association of Telemedicin Service Providers	Association of Telemedicin Service Providers
Telemedicine	**http://www.dis.port.ac.uk/ndtm/**	UK National Database of Telemedicine: A database of Telemedicine and Telecare projects in the UK	Department of Health; Healthcare Computing Research Group, University of Portsmouth
Comments	*information collected during separate surveys of Telemedicine and Telecare activity in the United Kingdom, commissioned by the UK Department of Health.*		
Telemedicine	**http://www.ehto.org/**	European Health Telematics Observatory	European Health Telematics Observatory
Telemedicine	**http://www.gets.cadrus.fr/**	European Telemedicine Center	
Telemedicine	**http://www.hostnet.org**	Healthcare Open Systems and Trials (HOST)	Healthcare Open Systems and Trials (HOST)
Comments	*non-profit consortium*		
Telemedicine	**http://www.lib.uiowa.edu/hardin/md/telemed.html**	Hardin Meta-Directory - Telemedicine	University of Iowa
Comments	*quality links*		
Telemedicine	**http://www.nlm.nih.gov/research/telemedinit.html**	NLM National Telemedicine Initiative	US National Library of Medicine
Telemedicine	**http://www.nlm.nih.gov/research/telfront.html**	National Library of Medicine's NGI and Telemedicine Projects	US National Library of Medicine
Comments	*describes current NLM telemedicine contracts, grants, etc.*		
Telemedicine	**http://www.telemed.med.ecu.edu/**	East Carolina University School of Medicine Telemedicine Program	East Carolina University School of Medicine
Telemedicine	**http://www.telemed.virginia.edu/**	University of Virginia Office of Telemedicine	University of Virginia Office of Telemedicine
Comments	*Incorporates Commonwealth of Virginia Telemedicine Network and other projects*		

Category	URL	Title	Organization
Telemedicine	**http://www.tmgateway.org/**	The Federal Telemedicine Gateway	multiple US government agencies, including Defense, Ag, and NASA
Comments	*The Federal Telemedicine Gateway contains: (1) The Joint Working Group on Telemedicine (JWGT) Inventory, which includes information on active, federally funded telemedicine projects that provide direct patient care; (2) Links to other federally funded telemedicine projects that do not provide patient care; and (3) Links to other telemedicine resources, activities, and databases.*		
Telemedicine	**http://www.va.gov/telemed/**	US Veterans Administration Telemedicine	US Veterans Administration
Telemedicine	**http://www.vtmednet.org.:80/telemedicine/**	Telemedicine Program at Fletcher Allen Health Care	Fletcher Allen Health Care, University of Vermont
Comments	*thorough program description and outside links*		
Telemedicine	**http://www2.kumc.edu/telemedicine/index.asp**	Kansas University Medical Center Telemedicine Program	Kansas University Medical Center
Comments	*Not many resources, but describes many ongoing projects in KS*		
Telemedicine	**http://www.telemedtoday.com/**	Telemedicine Today Magazine	Telemedicine Today Magazine
Telemedicine – commercial	**http://www.itwm-trier.fhg.de/**		Institut für TelematikTrier
Comments	*German telemedicine consulting/outsourcing company*		
Ambulatory Adult Primary Care	**http://www.nmh.org/netreach/netreach.html**		
Comments	*clinical pathways, educational materials, "virtual patient cases", links, etc.*		
Family Practice	**http://www.virtualpresence.org/**	Virtual Presence Telemedicine Program	Women & Infants Hospital, Providence, Rhode Island
Comments	*southern New England's first telemedicine network*		
Imaging	**http://icsl.ee.washington.edu/**	Image Computing Systems Laboratory	University of Washington, Department of Electrical Engineering
Comments	*Project descriptions and links*		
Informatics Online Journal	**http://maddog.fammed.wisc.edu/hmid/hmid.html**	Health and Medical Informatics Digest	University of Wisconsin - Madison
Comments	*contains many links with each issue*		
Legal	**http://www.arentfox.com/telemedicine.html**	Telemedicine and the Law	Arent Fox (Washington DC law firm)
Comments	*commercial sponsor, but covers much US legislation, federal and state, and case law*		

Category	URL	Title	Organization
Legal	**http://www.ctl.org/**	Center for Telemedicine Law	Center for Telemedicine Law
Military	**http://www.matmo.org/**	DoD Telemedicine	US Department of Defense
Comments	*This is the premier site for DoD Telemedicine in the Pacific Region.*		
Nephrology	**http://www.imac.georgetown.edu/telemed/phoenix/phoenix.htm**	Project Phoenix	Georgetown University Medical Center
Comments	*joint effort between the Imaging Science and Information Systems (ISIS) Center, Department of Radiology, the Clinical Economics Research Unit (CERU) and the Division of Nephrology in the Department of Medicine at Georgetown University Medical, Center, Washington, DC.*		
Ophthalmology	**http://www.jdigital.com/**	Justice Digital Solutions	Justice Digital Solutions
Comments	*US commercial firm, but with significant free links and resources*		
Pathology	**http://europath.imag.fr/**	EUROpean Pathology Assisted by Telematics for Health	
Pathology	**http://www.jr2.ox.ac.uk/ndp/telepathology.htm**	Telepathology City	University of Oxford, Department of Pathology and Bacteriology
Comments	*take a peak, it's lively*		
Radiology	**http://www.mgh.org/education/telemed.html**	Upper Peninsula Telehealth Network	Marquette General Hospital
Comments	*extensive rural Michigan Teleradiology Network*		
	http://hiru.mcmaster.ca/cochrane/default.htm	The Cochrane Collaboration	The Cochrane Collaboration
Comments	*The Cochrane Collaboration is an international organisation that aims to help people make well-informed decisions about healthcare by preparing, maintaining and promoting the accessibility of systematic reviews of the effects of healthcare interventions*		
	http://hiru.mcmaster.ca/nce/default.htm	HEALNet Health Evidence Application and Linkage Network	HEALNet/RELAIS
Comments	*links a wealth of Canadian programs and initiatives*		
	http://www.ncl.ac.uk/~nphcare/PHCSG/Journal/index.htm	The Journal of Informatics in Primary Care	Primary Health Care Specialist Group and the British Computer Society
	http://www.telemedmag.com/	Telehealth Magazine	Miller Freeman, Inc
Comments	*commercial magazine with considerable links and resources*		
Telemedicine	**http://www.psychiatry.uq.edu.au/qtn/index.htm**	Queensland Telemedicine Network	Queensland Telemedicine Network
Comments	*catalogs many Australian projects, including mental health services, Paediatric Care, Radiology, Cardiology, Dermatology, Intensive Care, Ophthalmology, Pathology, Renal Medicine, Flying Doctor Service, Rural Support*		

Author Index